A Tradition of Soup

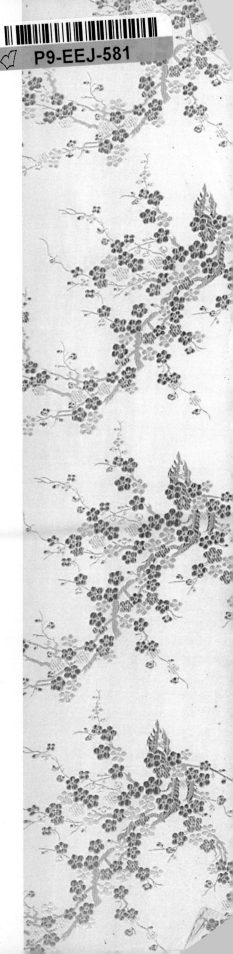

A Tradition of Soup

Flavors from China's Pearl River Delta

Teresa M. Chen

Foreword by
Martin Yan

North Atlantic Books
Berkeley, California

Published by
North Atlantic Books
P.O. Box 12327
Berkeley, California 94712

Cover photo by Teresa M. Chen
Cover design © Ayelet Maida, A/M Studios
Book design by Susan Quasha
Printed in the United States of America

Delta boundary map on page 15 used by permission from *The Record of San Joaquin*.

A Tradition of Soup: Flavors from China's Pearl River Delta is sponsored by the Society for the Study of Native Arts and Sciences, a nonprofit educational corporation whose goals are to develop an educational and cross-cultural perspective linking various scientific, social, and artistic fields; to nurture a holistic view of arts, sciences, humanities, and healing; and to publish and distribute literature on the relationship of mind, body, and nature.

North Atlantic Books' publications are available through most bookstores. For further information, call 800-733-3000 or visit our website at www.northatlanticbooks.com.

MEDICAL DISCLAIMER: The following information is intended for general information purposes only. Individuals should always see their health care provider before administering any suggestions made in this book. Any application of the material set forth in the following pages is at the reader's discretion and is his or her sole responsibility.

Library of Congress Cataloging-in-Publication Data

Chen, Teresa M.
 A tradition of soup : flavors from China's Pearl River Delta / Teresa M. Chen ; foreword by Martin Yan.
    p. cm.
 Includes bibliographical references and index.
 Summary: "Integrates traditional Chinese medicine with the culture and cuisine of China, with a focus on soups. Offers many healthy and healing recipes"—Provided by publisher.
 ISBN 978-1-55643-765-6 (alk. paper)
 1. Soups—China—Pearl River Delta. 2. Cookery, Chinese. 3. Medicine, Chinese. I. Title.
 TX757.C465 2009
 641.5951—dc22

                                        2008033001

1 2 3 4 5 6 7 8 9 UNITED 15 14 13 12 11 10 09

This book is dedicated to the fond memory of Ah-Bu,
who taught and nurtured me in more ways than cooking.

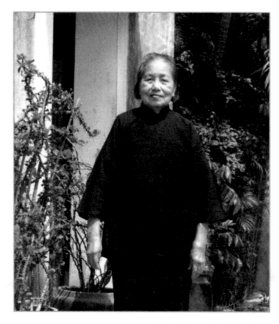

Sui Wong (1903–1991)
My Ah-Bu

Acknowledgments

Scores of people contributed ideas, recipes, and technical support to make this book a reality.

Recipe Providers: I solicited recipes only from people over the age of seventy, and affiliated with Jene Wah, Inc. in Stockton, California. Those who provided recipes also granted interviews. They also generously supplied the ingredients for the soups and tested the recipes in Jene Wah's kitchen. They are (in alphabetical order by last name): Lai King Chan 陳林麗瓊, Lin Chan 陳蓮, Yuen Chin Lee 錢茵姆, Bevin and Judy Hong 湯伯垣、湯趙碧霞 (Judy is an exception to the age requirement), Bob and Meeyoke Hong 湯伯榮、湯黃美玉, Sun Kwong 鄺黃銀新, Wai Tak Lau 劉惠德, Yin Kan Lau 劉雷賢近, Wong Lai Kuen Lee 李黃麗娟, Sun Ma 馬黃新月, Wai Kuen Szeto 司徒惠娟, Wai Ying Lee Tam 譚李惠英, Shu Shing Tan 譚淑笙, Thelma Yim 嚴梁杏嫦, and Kim and Henry Yip 葉天仕、葉黃金珠.

Culinary Advisors: Among my friends in Stockton are many professional chefs. I asked them for advice but not for recipes because they are too young. Among them are Mr. and Mrs. Lai Wong 黃雅禮 of Golden Palace Restaurant, Jack Ju of New Yen Ching Restaurant, and Ivy Leung, former owner of Wok Inn Restaurant. Amy Kong, wife of Ken Kong, the chef of Jene Wah, Inc. shared her expertise in making sweet dessert soups. Mr. and Mrs. Kai Pang 彭啓, former owners of Wing Wah Deli & Market, clarified for me, once and for all, the beef cut called *ngaauh naahm.* Henry Yip 葉天仕, a soup recipe contributor, is also the former owner of Gan Chy Chinese Restaurant and one of the founders of Jene Wah, Inc.

Interviewers: Eileen Phillips, Jene Wah's former program analyst from the San Joaquin County Department of Aging, suggested that we interview all of the seniors who provided me with soup recipes. From the point of view of oral history and cultural anthropology, this was a great idea. Besides Eileen and myself, Diane Barth and Beth Luna conducted the interviews.

Photographers: Calixtro Romias, a photographer working at *The Record of San Joaquin,* volunteered to take pictures during the interviews. Fritz Chin 陳純良, founder of Fritz Chin Photography, not only helped with every test-cooking session that took place at Jene Wah's kitchen, but also taught me how to take pictures of soups and ingredients, such as chicken feet and fish heads.

Ben Clark shared his photo of a sea turtle that he took when diving in Hawaii. Janet Fong shared her pictures from a sea turtle farm in Grand Cayman Island, Panama. Stephanie Jan provided me with a picture of the fruiting spike of a rice plant. Donna S. Yee contributed a picture of the rice paddies in Southern China, taken during her last trip there in 2005. Fritz and Lisa Chin's trip in 2005 gave me excellent pictures of an old-fashioned Chinese kitchen and a pot of soup slowly cooking in the courtyard. Charles Hwang took pictures at the Martyrs' Mausoleum in Guangzhou to show the historical connection between the two deltas and the two continents. Mary Wei shared her picture of Tibetan hot pot and Julie Low shared her picture of hot pots made with cloisonné, both taken during their respective trips to China in 2007.

Closer to home, Kathy Crump provided me with beautiful pictures taken on her estate along the Five Mile Creek. Mr. and Mrs. Kwei-yu Chu 朱貴昱、謝明暐 of

Modesto, California, shared pictures of lotus blooming in their Lotus Gardens. Tony Wong did the white-balancing act and produced great pictures of my pantry while his wife Tana Lee took the best-ever picture of my dendrobium nobile in bloom. The staff of Gluskin's Cameras Audio Video have always been attentive in processing my pictures, both film and digital.

I was able to take pictures of the Pearl River Delta in the summer of 2006, thanks to my sister Bernie's arrangement and the hospitality of Mr. and Mrs. S. Sun 孫逢亮先生夫人, their son Vincent 孫向榮, and their friend Mr. Ji-fa Zhu 朱集發 of Panyu District in Guangzhou. Those pictures are priceless.

Photoshop Wizards: Adler Chan and Andrew Kazakes helped me Photoshop pictures of the many ingredients used in the soups. Andrew's attention to detail elevated my photography from being amateurish to semi-professional and publishable.

Map-Maker: My daughter Yvonne worked on the maps of California and of the Pearl River Delta and its tributaries.

Illustrators: Shirley Fong did most of the line drawings for this book. Adam Doi helped with the fluid design of *yin-yang* in constant motion. They express well what lies beyond the reach of photography.

Buyers and Suppliers: Some ingredients required trips to San Francisco. Ivy Fung and Josephine Li have kindly gone on buying trips for me in the City. When I was hunting for special ingredients, many friends either went to get them for me or gave me some from their own pantries or gardens. These generous people include Yuk Chau (long-life noodles), Tip Kwan Hui (black moss), Ivy Leung (*sehk-chyuh* ginseng), Wai Tak Lau (hasmar), Jack Ju (abalone and sea cucumber), Walter and Laura Sun (purple laver), Susan Wang (mock meat and fermented sweet rice), Lin Chan (dried bitter melon and duck gizzard), Wai Kuen Szeto (home-grown dried bok choy), Sui Lun Wong (home-grown winter melon), and Janice Chan (home-grown fuzzy melon). Mr. and Mrs. Lai Wong brought me dried osmanthus flowers from China, while my sister Bernie Lai sent me knotted dendrobiums from Hong Kong. Once again, I have to acknowledge all the recipe providers who also supplied ingredients for their soups. They are both kind and generous.

Tureen- and Pot-Lenders: I was told that professional food photographers use a different soup bowl for each soup they photograph, so I started borrowing soup bowls from my friends as well as shopping for new ones. George and Shu Fang Wang, Kathy Ho, Janet Fong, Josephine Li, Shirley Fong, and Thelma Yim all kindly let me use and photograph their heirloom pieces and tureens from their china sets. Marj Fries' fine collection of ceramic bowls, some of them her own creations, added beauty and charm to many of the photographs. Esther Chan also gave me two lidded from-stove-to-table ceramic pots at Christmas of 2005. Julie Low loaned me her chimneyed Hot Pot while Dr. George Wang 汪理 let me photograph his Yunnan clay pot, also with a chimney for steaming soup. Dr. Susan Wang let me try her steamer, which is deep enough for my lidded porcelain urn.

Translator: Many people suggested that the book should also be available in Chinese, at least the part about the people and their stories. Since I was already up to my elbows in soup, Josephine Li recruited her husband Desmond to help me translate the text into Chinese. I appreciate the fluidity of his style and his great sense of humor. The Chinese version will be published separately at a later date.

Typist: I am blessed with an assistant who can type in both Chinese and English. Connie Lui also helped me organize my digital photo files and Google for information. Without her, many good ideas might still be just ideas, not committed to words and images. I appreciate her efficiency.

Manager: Through every step of the development of this book, Josephine Li was there. From scheduling and shopping to measuring and recording, she took care of details. I appreciate her patience and dependability.

Critics: Dr. Jean Johnson critiqued an early manuscript. My harshest critic by far is my daughter Suzanne, a journalist. She questioned both the form and substance of the book with the eyes of an editor. She helped me focus on the task at hand. Consequently I have restructured and rewritten several drafts. I appreciate her professionalism.

Supporters: Numerous people gave me support, but my biggest supporter is my husband and my boss, Dr. Yi-Po Anthony Wu, medical director of Pacific Complementary Medicine Center (PCMC). I appreciate his input, feedback, and infinite patience.

Members of my AAUW Creative Writing Group have been cheering me on through the metamorphosis of the book. I especially wish to thank Mildred Tucker and Lois Clark for their encouragement. Ivy Fung and Rebecca Gin have provided valuable resources about Cantonese cooking. They have helped raise my standards.

Promoters: Before the book was even finished, Sue Mow and Winnie Wong volunteered to go on road shows with me. So did Diane Barth and Eileen Phillips. I appreciate their enthusiasm.

Introducers: As a first-time author, I sorely needed introduction. First, Esther Yip Chan, former director of Jene Wah, Inc., wrote a foreword for me. Sadly, Esther's untimely death in 2006 prevented her from seeing the completion of this cookbook project, which she helped to start. Then Doreen Leung—author, columnist, gourmet food judge, and healthy-cooking authority in Hong Kong—also agreed to write a foreword to introduce this bowl of soup steeped in the Chinese tradition of health and healing. Finally, Martin Yan, host of the evergreen *Yan Can Cook* television show and author of numerous books on Chinese cooking, has extended his role as Ambassador of Chinese Culinary Art to take me under his wing. I am grateful for their confidence in my work.

Proofreaders: Paul Fairbrook, Jean Johnson, John Morearty, Eileen Phillips, and Laura Sun helped proofread the English text while Karen Wong, a foodie from a family of restaurateurs and chefs, helped with the laborious job of proofreading the recipes.

Editors and Designers: Robin Donovan would not allow me to take anything for granted, and her baby beat this book to the finish line. Picking up where Robin left off, Adrienne Armstrong completed the manuscript. Art director Paula Morrison orchestrated the layout while Susan Quasha provided the artistic design and Ayelet Maida created the elegant cover. Emily Boyd kept the book project on course and stabilized me whenever I felt overwhelmed. I am grateful to the competent team at North Atlantic Books.

Publisher: Richard Grossinger of North Atlantic Books, with his cross-cultural perspective and natural, holistic view of healing, is undoubtedly the publisher most suited for this book.

Contents

Foreword by Martin Yan

In the West, soup is often thought of as a first course, the beginning of a meal. Back in the Pearl River Delta of Guangdong, where I grew up, soups are also first courses, yet they are a lot more than "just the beginning" of a meal. Ask any Cantonese about his favorite soup and watch his eyes light up. Mine is a duck soup, made from a rich broth flavored by roast duck carcass. Or is it a simple vegetable broth with watercress, silken tofu, red dates, and dried shrimp? I was lucky that my mother was a great home cook and a true soup whiz. Like so many Cantonese families, we enjoyed our soup not only as a first course but also throughout the entire meal. And her soups were so remarkable that often they were the highlight of the meal.

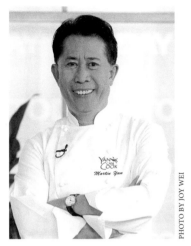

Martin Yan

With all my television and business projects, I am constantly on the go. Much of my life revolves around hopping on and off airplanes and adjusting to different time zones and diets. Even when I am home, I keep a busy schedule, one that often does not allow for the luxury of a relaxed meal. Whenever I feel worn down and haggard, I remember my mother's words of wisdom at the dinner table: "Drink your soup!"

Soup is my way to get back to basics. Others may prefer vitamin pills or scientifically balanced dietary supplements. For me, it's a well prepared, nourishing bowl of soup. In Western culture, the magical "chicken soup" is often hailed as a cure-all. In China, we believe both in the preventive and the curative power of our soups. But it's not a case of pure faith. We add medicinal herbs and roots to our daily thirst-quenching soups to make them into elixirs at our dinner tables. For centuries, Chinese doctors have used soup as a way of administering natural medicinal herbs that would cure or ward off diseases.

When Teresa first discussed this book project with me, I was overjoyed. Over the years I have tried to stress in my cookbooks the importance of soups and the prominent place that they deserve in our diet. I am therefore delighted to see that finally someone who is well versed in the subject has put forth the tremendous effort for a complete book on Chinese soups. The great care that Teresa has put into detailing every aspect of our soup culture, down to preparation and storage instructions for the essential ingredients, is a true testament to both her boundless enthusiasm for this subject and her professionalism as an academic.

For soup enthusiasts like me, this book is simply invaluable. I would further recommend *A Tradition of Soup* to all health-conscious (and who isn't these days?) people who are engaged in active lifestyles. Take it from my mom: "Drink your soup!"

—MARTIN YAN, bestselling author and host of *Yan Can Cook*

Foreword by Doreen Leung

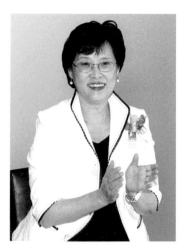

Doreen Leung

When I was approached by Dr. Teresa M. Chen to write a foreword to her book on healthy Chinese soups, I gladly agreed. It is not only that I hold Teresa in high esteem as a person, but also because of the meaningful content and interesting coverage of the book.

China has enjoyed at least five thousand years of history. The Chinese are very sophisticated in using food as medicine for maintaining health and increasing vitality. In particular, the people in the Pearl River Delta region of Southern China have cooked up a rich culinary culture, notably with their slow-cooking soups. Ingredients are selected and combined according to season, climate, physical constitution, and health needs. There are soups to moisten dryness in the system, to lubricate skin, to improve complexion, and to strengthen the body. Passed down through generations, Grandma's soups are reputed for their many wonderful health benefits.

On top of that, a bowl of soup can also convey the tender loving care of a mother for her children or a wife for her husband. Traditionally a pot of soup draws the family together around the dining table with a power similar to that of the Thanksgiving turkey. Better still, while the turkey wields its magic only once a year, Chinese soups can be served weekly or even daily. Soup magic is easily accessible.

During her twenty-some years as a volunteer at Jene Wah, Inc., Dr. Chen has made friends with many Po-Pos (Grandmas) and Gung-Gungs (Grandpas) at the Chinese senior center in Stockton, California. Impressed with their energy and looks in spite of their age, Teresa set out to learn their secret. She found it in the slow-cooking soups they make from unwritten recipes passed down in their families. Discovering further that all of these people had interesting stories to tell about their immigration to the United States, Teresa decided to record their stories as well as their recipes, which will distinguish this work as a bridge between the East and the West in three significant areas: cuisine, health, and socio-cultural history.

Embracing the project with great enthusiasm, Teresa and her friends interviewed the Jene Wah people, took notes, took pictures, and tested the soup recipes. Though these soups are healthy and delicious, I still feel sorry for Dr. Anthony Wu, Teresa's "better half," who had to drink his fill of all the soups she tested in her own kitchen, occasionally two or three soups in one day during re-takes. Fanatic about details, Teresa consulted many people and thoroughly researched the literature, making sure that the information was as accurate as possible.

Coming from the healthcare field, Teresa did not know what I have known all along, that it is always easier to write a book than to get one published. Indeed, Teresa had agonized over it for a while. It is great that she found a publisher on her first try, and the type of publisher she had hoped for, with a similar philosophical orientation and non-profit inclination. The world is made better and more beautiful by people who exhibit such selfless dedication.

I sincerely wish the best, health, and happiness for Dr. Chen and the readers of this book.

—DOREEN LEUNG, *Hong Kong Economic Times* columnist
Hong Kong, China
December 8, 2007

Foreword by Esther Yip Chan

Care for our own elders and extend that care to all elderly;
Love our own children and extend that love to all the children.

—Confucius

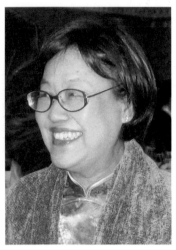

Esther Chan

Confucius' teaching is the foundation of Jene Wah, Inc.'s community service, faithfully upheld by its founders and successors, directors, and staff. Having served Jene Wah, Inc. for over twenty years, I have witnessed Jene Wah's growth and development into a one-stop, multi-service agency for the Chinese elderly. The center has become instrumental in overcoming language and cultural barriers for first generation immigrants, young and old alike, and helping them make a smooth transition into their new country and town of Stockton, California, which they now call home.

The directors of Jene Wah, Inc. are unpaid volunteers. They contribute generously of their expertise and guidance, time and labor, and make up for shortfalls in funding with donations. Dr. Teresa M. Chen served on Jene Wah's Board of Directors from 1984 to1996. During her tenure, Dr. Chen wrote many grant proposals for Jene Wah, Inc. She also initiated the publication of Jene Wah's newsletter and a bilingual Chinese telephone directory, chairing the Editorial Committee and raising funds to finance the printing. The Yellow Pages advertisement sponsored by local businesses made it possible for us to distribute the Chinese Directory free of charge. The biannual directory serves as a handy guide as well as a valuable record for the Stockton Chinese community.

"Nutrition Lunch" has always been part of Jene Wah's program. Initially, the lunches were provided by the Senior Service Agency. Noticing a lot of waste because the Chinese seniors did not like Western-style food or could not tolerate the lactose in the milk, Dr. Chen came up with the idea to propose a Chinese-style Nutrition Lunch Program to the San Joaquin County Department of Aging. The preparation work was at once educational and inspiring. It was in 1992 and 1993, when Teresa was President of the Board, that she arranged for the entire Jene Wah Board to visit On Lok and Self-Help for the Elderly in San Francisco. We learned from the nutritionists there, and gathered sample menus and recipes. We studied costs and surveyed food preferences. Teresa was able to get the support of Mr. Paul Fairbrook of the University of the Pacific who agreed to lend his expertise in food service and chair Jene Wah's newly formed Nutrition Committee. Then Teresa wrote the proposal with technical assistance from Mr. Joseph Chelli. And that was only the beginning. Now, thanks in large part to Dr. Chen, Jene Wah seniors enjoy their daily Chinese-style Nutrition Lunch prepared in Jene Wah's own commercial grade kitchen.

Teresa's interest in good food and good nutrition, however, does not begin nor end with Jene Wah's success story. She came from a family of food connoisseurs and was raised by a gourmet cook. Professionally, as a health educator at the Pacific Complementary Medicine Center, Dr. Chen promotes traditional Chinese food therapy and exercise. Teresa is a volunteer health educator for Jene Wah and teaches breathing and *Liutong* exercise to the seniors. Because of her connection with Jene Wah and her rapport with the seniors there, Teresa is the ideal person to collect their slow-cooking soup recipes and write about them. I highly recommend that you take the time to savor the flavors of the Pearl River Delta introduced in this book.

—ESTHER YIP CHAN, executive director, Jene Wah, Inc. (1985–2006)

Stockton, California

May 1, 2006

Preface

This cookbook is written to promote Chinese food and culture, and to promote health. It pays tribute to my kindred Cantonese people from the Pearl River Delta and to our soup tradition that explicitly links food to health and healing.

Professionally, I am a health educator at Pacific Complementary Medicine Center, which was founded by my husband Dr. Yi-Po Anthony Wu and me, in Stockton, California. Our medical practice is dedicated to combining the best of Eastern and Western medicine for comprehensive and holistic health care. The goal is to help our patients attain optimum health in mind, body, and spirit. Through the practices of acupuncture, herb and food therapy, relaxation techniques, health exercises (including *taijichuan,* yoga, *qigong,* breathing exercises, and self-massage), and healthy eating in our Western clinical setting, we strongly emphasize what is now fashionably called "lifestyle." As a member of the team, I learn on the job and practice what we preach.

Personally, I like to cook and I appreciate good food. I also like to write. Of course, it takes much more to write a cookbook. In my case, it took a long journey home.

It all started with a lecture I attended in 1981 when Dr. K.C. Chang, Peabody Professor of Anthropology at Harvard University, talked about his book *Food in Chinese Culture.* Dr. Chang and his constellation of contributors, while acknowledging the health benefits of food and herbs, did not offer any recipes. I decided then and there that one day I would compile recipes to enable readers to put these concepts to use.

Years went by and the desire to write a cookbook was relegated to the back burner. Fortunately, that is the best way to make a great pot of soup.

As I continued to learn and grow, I had the good fortune of serving on the Board of Directors of Jene Wah, Inc., a multi-service senior citizen center, where I got to know many of the seniors personally. I found much inspiration in the active lives they led, the indomitable spirit they demonstrated, and in the traditional soups they made to keep themselves and their families healthy. The dormant seed from 1981 finally germinated in the fertile soil of the San Joaquin Delta. Instead of writing just another cookbook on Chinese food, I decided to zero in on Chinese soups, and, specifically, on healthy soups from the Pearl River Delta, where most Chinese-Americans come from.

Though all Chinese regional cuisines include soups, Cantonese cuisine is unrivaled in its repertoire of health-promoting soups. My search for recipes that would demonstrate a close link between food and health in Chinese culture has come full circle, bringing me back to my ancestral home in the Pearl River Delta, in the form of healthy and delicious soups, not so much from book research as from my contact with Chinese seniors in Stockton.

I started to collect soup recipes in 2003 from twelve people, all seventy years of age or older, at Jene Wah, Inc. (Judy Hong was the only exception because she stood in for her mother-in-law Mrs. Yuk Hung Hong). I recorded and test-cooked each of their recipes in Jene Wah's kitchen, with the help of the contributors themselves. Then I decided to also record the life stories of the recipe providers. This was certainly a worthwhile project as it provided me a means to give the soup tradition a human face. Traversing two continents across the Pacific Ocean and connecting the Pearl River Delta and the San Joaquin Delta with their past and present, these common folks from Southern China wrote Chinese-American history with sweat and tears, and with hard work and silent endurance. Their stories can be found in this book's appendix.

I must say that people from the Pearl River Delta have always been the standard bearers of the Chinese soup tradition. They continued to make traditional soups in their new home in America, not just once in a while, but weekly and daily for general health maintenance. They also made every effort to transport and transplant traditional Chinese ingredients across the ocean. I feel duty bound to introduce all of these soup ingredients to the English-speaking world. What I cannot do with taste and smell, I have tried my best to present in words and illustrations in the section of the book devoted to ingredients.

When I proposed the project of compiling soup recipes, it was greeted with much enthusiasm and support at Jene Wah and in the community. So many people came forth to offer their resources that I had to prepare an unusually long list of acknowledgments. Each of these people has ownership in the soup culture. They have all contributed to this pot of Stone Soup that I make.

While I have had wonderful soup-making and photography teachers, I have also been blessed with colleagues who guided me to a better understanding of Traditional Chinese Medicine (TCM), especially where food and nutrition are concerned. Consistent with the principle and practice of TCM, food therapy aims to correct imbalance and harmonize opposing and interacting forces. Food as medicine is both preventive and therapeutic. We eat to stay healthy—to nurture and to defend ourselves. We eat in accordance with the seasons, the weather, the environment, and with our own physical and mental conditions in mind. Even with the inclusion of some medicinal soups, this entire cookbook is wellness- and health-oriented, not disease-oriented.

To see a doctor when you are sick is like forging weapons in battle or digging a well when you are thirsty. So said the ancient sages. The mission of doctors is not so much to make the symptoms go away as to help patients maintain optimal health and attain longevity. To get there, we all have to learn to eat right, to relax and rest well, and to exercise regularly.

At Pacific Complementary Medicine Center (PCMC), our goal is to guide our patients beyond pills, scalpel, and even acupuncture needles to a real appreciation of healthy lifestyle. For almost a quarter of a century, we have conducted free seminars, led *tai chi, qigong,* and yoga classes, held cooking demonstrations, and offered regular group and individual sessions in nutrition counseling. As a result, PCMC can boast the most enlightened patient population in California's central valley. Hopefully, our patients are also healthier, happier, and will live longer.

In our Western society, especially where food is in abundance, people do not eat well. For many Americans, fast food is the norm. It seems that people abhor cooking, especially those who live alone. My experience is that women with hot flashes, more often than not, would rather take *danggui* pills three times a day than take the time to make themselves a pot of delicious Danggui and Chicken Soup. Their symptoms do go away with the pill, but do they know what they are missing? To me, the former is medication while the latter is nurturing. Do we really prefer to eat like astronauts in space?

I invite you all to pause on your fast track to smell the roses, and, aah … the aroma of soup cooking on the stove. Entertain your taste buds with the myriad flavors nature has to offer and nourish your family and yourself with ancient wisdom in the modern kitchen.

People often assume that healthy food is, by nature, uninteresting food. These healthy soups will certainly prove otherwise. Fortified with health-promoting intentions and good nutrition, they will entice you with their colors, aromas, and flavors. And in case that isn't enough, I have made an additional effort to simplify procedures for busy cooks. The end product should be simply delicious and healthy. Maybe you'll treat yourself to a soup tonight?

A Note on Language Designations

Throughout the text, with the highest concentration in Part Three—Ingredients, Chinese terms are given in Mandarin and/or Cantonese pronunciation. Whenever possible, common English names are given. Unless it is already in prevalent use, a Latin botanical or zoological name is given as a last resort for clear identification.

In the Ingredients section, Chinese characters accompany Mandarin *pinyin* and Cantonese Romanization. I have chosen to use the so-called complicated form 繁體 instead of the simplified form 簡體 because most overseas Chinese newspapers and magazines are printed in the former font. This may be somewhat inconvenient for those who know only the simplified form, but the *pinyin* 拼音 pronunciation is included as a guide. A Chinese storekeeper will probably recognize both forms of writing. Besides, with the picture guide and Cantonese pronunciation, it is highly unlikely that you would be given the wrong food or herb item.

Pinyin Notation

The phonetic spelling of Mandarin Chinese, Guanhua 官話, also called Guoyu 國語 or Putonghua 普通話, was designed by a national committee of linguists and educators. Two parallel systems were proposed—one using Romanization like the English alphabet, while the other, following the style of Japanese phonetic spelling, came up with its own unique set of symbols. In the 1930s the Nationalist government adopted the latter version and that system is still in use in Taiwan. The Romanized pinyin system was officially adopted by the People's Republic of China after 1949 and major universities in the United States began converting to pinyin in the 1960s, replacing the Wade-Giles or Yale University system in textbooks and dictionaries.

Cantonese Romanization

My Cantonese spelling is based on an old dictionary published by Yale University Press. Subsequent textbooks, such as the one by Elizabeth Boyles for the United States Department of State, also followed the Yale system. Standard Cantonese, also known as Gwongjau Wa 廣州話 or Saangsehng Wa 省城話, is used widely in the Pearl River Delta, Hong Kong, Macao, and up the Western River, Sai Gong (or Xi Jiang 西江).

A pronunciation guide for both the *pinyin* notation and Cantonese Romanization can be found in this book's appendix.

Weights and Measures

When it comes to traditional Chinese herbs, an entirely different apothecary weight system is involved. The units are jin 斤, liang 兩, qian 錢, and fen 分 in *pinyin*. 10 fen = 1 qian, and 10 qian = 1 liang, it takes 16 liang to make one jin (approximately 1.33 lbs). Confusion sets in as we translate liang loosely into "ounce," incorrectly making jin the equivalent of "pound." Because American merchants trade in pounds and ounces, Chinese herbal formulas (or recipes) often cause confusion. Here I have included a conversion table for your reference. Also included is the metric equivalent used in China, Japan, and most European countries. For measuring medicinal herbs, it is useful to have a small scale that measures weight under 1 liang or 38 grams, as liang and qian are the most frequently used units in Chinese herbal formulas.

Weight Conversion

Metric System	U.S.	Traditional Chinese
608 g	21.28 oz	1 jin
500 g	17.6 oz	
250 g	8.8 oz	
200 g	7.0 oz	
150 g	5.25 oz	
100 g	3.5 oz	
50 g	1.75 oz	
38 g	1.33 oz	1 liang
20 g	0.70 oz	
10 g	0.35 oz	
3.8 g	0.13 oz	1 qian
1 g	0.035 oz	
0.38 g	0.013 oz	1 fen

Measure Conversion (1)

Cups	Fluid Ounces	Tablespoons	Teaspoons	Milliliters
1C	8 oz	16 Tbsp	48 tsp	237 ml
¾ C	6 oz	12 Tbsp	36 tsp	177 ml
⅔ C	5 oz	10 Tbsp	32 tsp	158 ml
½ C	4 oz	8 Tbsp	24 tsp	118 ml
⅓ C	3 oz	6 Tbsp	18 tsp	79 ml
¼ C	2 oz	4 Tbsp	12 tsp	59 ml
⅛ C	1 oz	2 Tbsp	6 tsp	30 ml
1/16 C	½ oz	1 Tbsp	3 tsp	15 ml
1/48 C	⅙ oz	⅓ Tbsp	1 tsp	5 ml

Numbers are rounded and approximated.

Measure Conversion (2)

Gallon	Quart	Pint	Cup	Liter	Milliliter
1	4	8	16	3.785	3785
¼	1	2	4	0.946	946
⅛	½	1	2	0.473	473
1/16	¼	½	1	0.236	236

To simplify the conversion, we roughly equate 1 quart to 1 liter and 1 cup to ¼ liter.

It is not easy to translate Chinese weights and measures into the American measurement system. American cooks often use volume instead of weight with dried beans, grains, nuts, seeds, and flour and meal. As each matter has its own unique density (by Archimedes Law), there can be no uniform conversion between volume and weight. For example, 4 ounces of almonds can be referred to as one cup of almonds, but one cup of mung beans weighs approximately 8 ounces whereas 4 ounces of black sesame seeds equal about ¾ cup by volume.

Also, the Chinese use bowls instead of cups for measure. Please refer to page 51 for equivalents of Po-Po's bowl measurement.

PART ONE

Overview

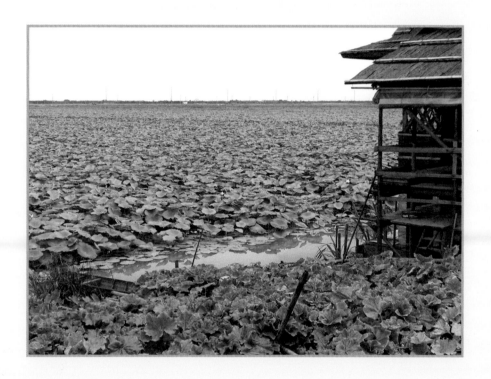

1
The Chinese Healing Tradition

Traditional Chinese Medicine (TCM)

Traditional Chinese Medicine is a system with solid theoretical foundation and clinical application that is based on Chinese philosophy, empirical observation, and logical thinking. Its practical aspects include diagnosis and treatment on the one hand and prevention, recovery, and health maintenance on the other. Efficacy of TCM treatments is improved and fortified by thousands of case studies, faithfully recorded by generations of Chinese doctors.

The Chinese people gave credit to their legendary sage king, the Yellow Emperor, for laying the foundation of Traditional Chinese Medicine more than five thousand years ago. *The Yellow Emperor's Inner Classic (Nei Jing)* 內經, written during the period of the Warring States (403–221 BCE), is thought to be the earliest medical text in the Chinese language. Another legendary sage king, Shen Nong, whose *Shen Nong's Herbal (Ben Cao* 本草*)* appeared at the end of this period, at the transition into unified Qin and Han Dynasties, was credited with the discovery of the healing properties of herbs. Over the millennia, the Chinese continued to pass down their medical knowledge relatively uninterrupted. It is from these classic texts that the basic TCM tenets of *Yin-Yang* and the Five Elements were born.

The Yin-Yang Theory is the foundation of Chinese philosophy and TCM. Etymologically, the two words *yin* and *yang* were originally used to designate the shady side and the sunny side of a hill, but they have come to represent the two sides of any object or phenomenon under the sun. More than just opposites or polarities, yin-yang embodies the unity of opposites and the law of change. Yin and yang, while in opposition, are not mutually exclusive. There is the seed of yang in yin, and there is the seed of yin in yang. The two are interrelated and interdependent, representing dynamic and cyclical processes, such as the change of the seasons and the cycles of day and night. The universe is always in flux and we human beings are always in the midst of change. Life, and hence health, is dependent on the interplay and balance of yin and yang.

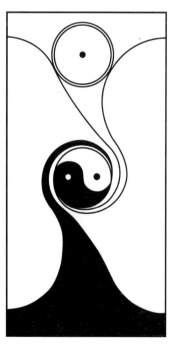

Yin-Yang Transformation

In TCM, internal organs are considered yin while their corresponding functions are yang. Yang functions burn up yin substances, while yang functional energy is expended to generate yin nutritional substances. The mutual dependency between yin and yang is such that only with ample yin can the human body function well, and only when the yang functions are in good order, can the substances be properly replenished. In TCM terms, there are four typical cases of disease-causing imbalance: excess of yin, excess of yang, deficiency of yin, and deficiency of yang.

Taoist philosophy further classifies things in terms of the Five Elements—Wood, Fire, Earth, Metal, and Water—along with corresponding seasons, climates, tastes, colors, emotions, viscera, and bowels to further define the five phases and the cyclic nature of life and health. The intricate web of interrelations and interactions among the five elements and their correlates underlies the Chinese way of thinking and dictates how generations of Chinese doctors discern disease patterns and formulate treatment with medicine and food.

Five Elements and Their Correspondences

ELEMENTS	Wood	Fire	Earth	Metal	Water
SEASONS	spring	summer	late summer	autumn	winter
CLIMATE	wind	heat	humidity	dryness	cold
DIRECTIONS	east	south	center	west	north
COLORS	green	red	yellow	white	black
TASTES	sour	bitter	sweet	sharp	salty
VISCERA	liver	heart	spleen	lungs	kidneys
BOWELS	gall bladder	small intestine	stomach	large intestine	bladder
PORTALS	eyes	tongue	mouth	nose	ears
EMOTIONS	anger	joy	sympathy	sadness	fear
PLANT PART	leaf	flower	grain	fruit	root

This chart serves as a guide for traditional Chinese food therapists when they design diets for the sick as well as for health maintenance. To strengthen spleen and stomach, whole grains are the natural choice. To counter dampness or edema, grains like pearl barley and foxnuts and legumes like aduki beans and hyacinth beans are recommended. The correlations are by no means random, nor are they that simplistic. Many factors come into play to affect our health and I greatly respect a Chinese doctor's ability to restore balance in this intricate web.

The five elements interact with one another in a cyclic way. While the season of spring replaces winter, it brings forth summer, which in turn brings forth autumn. The sequence is represented in the theory as the Generating and Subjugating Cycles. The way the generating and subjugating arrows go, each element is linked to the other four, forming a network of interrelations. When something goes wrong, everything else is also taken into account. It is never the simplistic "one symptom, one drug" approach. The synergy of several herbs is employed to balance the various elements.

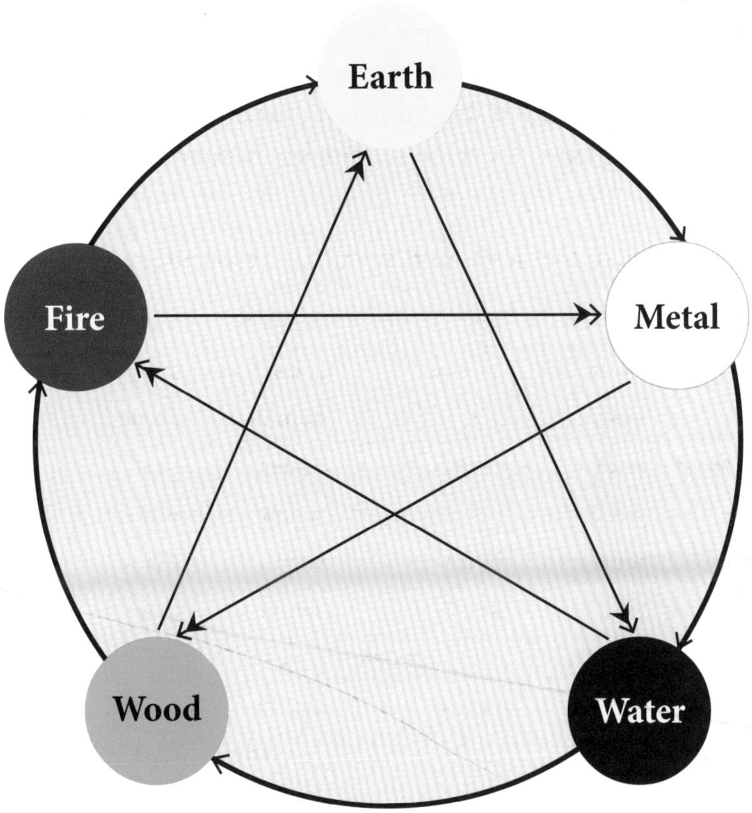

The Five Elements
Generating or Supporting (→), Subjugating or Restraining (↠)

In order to strengthen the lungs (the metal element), TCM teaches that one should first strengthen spleen and stomach (the earth element) and minimize the influence of the fire element. Translated to taste, one should seek out naturally sweet and neutral food to support the lungs. At the same time, if there is a lung ailment, one should treat the heart as well.

In TCM, viscera and bowels refer to both the organs and their functions, which constitute the meridian/channel network within the body. Whenever the name of an internal organ such as kidney, liver, lung, or large intestine is mentioned in TCM, we have to interpret it as the label of the meridian that runs through that particular organ. One can say that the meridians are the highways and byways whereas the organs are major stops along the way.

There are also meridians without specific organ names. Examples are the Triple Burners (*san jiao* 三焦) and the two connected meridians of Conception (*ren* 任) and Governing (*du* 督). These meridians are best defined by their functions even though they too are associated with various internal organs. In the case of the Triple Burners, as we shall see in the next section, the Middle Burner (*zhong jiao* 中焦) features prominently in the digestive function and is associated with the stomach and the spleen (including the pancreas), as well as the heart, the lungs, the liver, the kidneys, and the intestines.

Another important concept in TCM is life's endowment of *Jing* (essence), *Qi* (vitality), and *Shen* (spirit). In short, according to TCM, to squander away our endowment of essence, vitality, and spirit through an unhealthy lifestyle leads to premature aging, sickness, and early death. On the other hand, if we conserve and cultivate our life's endowment, we can all enjoy healthy, long lives. We replenish our endowment through the food we eat, the water we drink, and the air we breathe, as well as through our feelings and thoughts.

The goal of traditional Chinese nutrition is twofold: to heal and to prevent disease. Food, as well as medicine, restores health by bringing our systems into balance and thereby correcting the conditions of disease. More importantly, good nutrition helps prevent illness, thus protecting our bodies from unnecessary wear and tear. Eating right keeps our systems balanced and in optimal health, nurturing and prolonging life.

The Digestive Process as Viewed in TCM

The classic *Treatise on Spleen and Stomach* (*Pi Wei Lun* 脾胃論), written by Li Dong-Yuan in the thirteenth century CE, had a profound influence on the development of TCM with its theory that the spleen and stomach are the source of life-sustaining nourishment (ying qi 營氣) and are central to warding off disease (wei qi 衛氣). Nutrition in TCM terms is more than what we eat. It involves the proper functioning of the digestive mechanism.

TCM likens the process of digestion to that of distillation in what is known as the "triple burner" system. Food is chewed and mixed with saliva in the mouth where it is reduced to a mash before swallowing. The spleen and stomach form the middle or central burner of the system. The spleen supplies the heat or fire, while the stomach serves as the pot or vat in which the mash

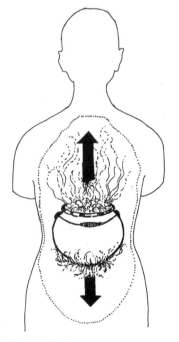

The Middle Burner

is further broken down with 100-degree heat, transforming the mash with the pure essence rising to the top, just like in distillation, and the dregs being left behind. The pure and clear essence rises to the heart and lungs and becomes blood and qi, which are circulated throughout the body to support life. The impure and turbid dregs are sent downward, to be excreted.

According to this view of digestion as a process of transformation by heat, it follows that cold food and drinks lower the temperature of the "soup" in the cauldron, hence impeding the breaking down of food in the middle burner and, therefore, impairing digestion. The more a food is like a 100-degree soup, the easier it is for the body to digest and absorb its nutrients. In other words, the stomach and spleen need to expend less energy to process hot, cooked foods, leading to a greater net gain for the body.

When cold negates heat, leading to the failure of the stomach and spleen to adequately transport and transform foods, a sludge accumulates. The stomach must work harder to try to burn off this sludge and becomes like a car stuck in overdrive, chronically overheated. This, in turn, causes the stomach to register hunger, which leads to overeating and a vicious cycle is created. Overeating begets stagnant food, which begets stomach heat, which reinforces overeating. Further, persistent stomach heat may eventually waste stomach yin, or fluids, causing chronic thirst and preference for cold drinks and chilled foods.

Poor food transformation leads to many chronic conditions like malnutrition, obesity, edema, anemia, and diabetes, to name just a few. To strengthen the spleen and stomach, then, is our first line of defense against metabolic problems. To promote good digestion is to promote health of the entire body.

Healthy Eating

Within TCM, diet and nutrition are integral to health maintenance and life preservation. To use the yin-yang analogy, food and medicine are two sides of the same coin, the former for wellness and the latter, sickness. We use food for health and medicine for healing. As yin and yang share the same source, so do food and medicine; hence the understanding that "Food and medicine share the same origin" 藥食同源.

Longevity is a universal human desire. The search for a life-prolonging elixir has been a medical quest since antiquity. A deeper understanding of TCM, and the Taoist philosophy behind it, reveals that the elixir of life is within us, cultivated by us through activities, rest, and diet in tune with the natural rhythm.

Consistent with TCM's characterization of all objects and phenomena in terms of yin-yang, the Chinese describe food using yin-yang attributes— hot/cold, warming/cooling, dry/moist, ascending/descending, and floating/ sinking—using a taxonomy that applies equally to medicinal herbs, as well as to physiology and pathology. By classifying foods in this way, Chinese doctors and lay people can easily determine what to eat on the basis of symptom observation.

For optimal health, we are urged to eat local and seasonal foods: tender greens in the spring, cooling melons and squashes in the summer, nuts and pumpkin in the fall, and root vegetables and preserved food in the winter. Rarely does a TCM doctor recommend eating meat except when it is necessary to correct a deficiency or vacuity. Eating a diet that consists of mostly grains and vegetables, with perhaps a little fish now and then, reduces the risk of cardiovascular disease, high cholesterol, diabetes mellitus, and cancer.

Because the ideal temperature for digestion in the middle burner is approximately 100 degrees, traditional Chinese doctors seldom recommend cold or raw food, much less dousing the fire with ice-cold drinks, which dampen the fire under the cauldron, leading to undue taxation of the spleen. Hot, warm or room temperature water, tea, broth and soup are recommended for hydration so as not to shock your system. Because we view the stomach as a cauldron containing a 100-degree soup, it is not difficult to see that soup-making is a perfect form of pre-digestion, breaking down the food and preparing it for ingestion, thus conserving spleen and stomach energy and nourishing the body for health and longevity.

2
The Soup Tradition

Lean Times and Fat Times

There is a Western parable about soup in lean times. Two hungry travelers started with stones in water and ended up with a pot of soup big enough to feed the entire village. Almost everything the villagers had went in—a piece of soup bone, a few potatoes, a cabbage, an onion or two, and a few beets. Before they knew it, the aroma of borscht filled the air.

During the Depression, soup enabled the Chinese families in Locke, California, to eat well off the land. A boy might catch a pigeon roosting in the barn or get a fish head from the fishmonger. His mother would make it into a soup, adding seasonal vegetables and herbs grown on their little plot of land. It was made heavenly with rice.

The Chinese soup tradition started back in the old country, where people knew many lean times. With humble ingredients, the Cantonese prepared a flavorful soup stock, to which practically anything on hand could be added. The most commonly used ingredients for the stock were pork neck bone and chicken rib bones, saved from the butcher after being carved of meat. For vegetarian soup, the base was usually made from soybean sprouts or white turnips. Napa cabbage also made a tasty stock. They all had a natural sweetness.

Wealthy households and restaurants expanded the possibilities by using a whole chicken, a whole fish, or a whole hunk of pork to make stock. After cooking for hours on end, with medicinal herbs and complementary ingredients, the broth would be strained and served hot. Fancy restaurants, in order to prove the authenticity of the broth, dished out the dregs in a bowl and brought them to the table. Etiquette forbade diners from reaching for the chicken feet, spareribs, or duck gizzards in the bowl. Besides, the dregs were considered fibrous and tasteless because all the flavor had been boiled out of them.

Beef was hardly used in the villages because the peasants revered the water buffalo as a valuable farming companion. Beef was introduced to the Chinese diet by returned sojourners from the United States or Australia, who acquired a taste for it and flaunted it as a status symbol. In China, the cattle breed for meat is the yellow cattle (*huángniú* 黃牛) or *wòhng ngàuh* in Cantonese.

Chinese home cooks are frugal. Scraps and trim go into the soup pot. Nothing is wasted. Chicken bones, pork bones, fish bones, and ham bones will all do. For vegetarians, flavor is coaxed from tough vegetable leaves and mushroom stems.

Old hens and ducks, whose egg-bearing days are over, are used in slow-cooking soups, yielding remarkably tasty broths. Making soup stock with the breasts of young chickens or expensive cuts of meat, such as beef or pork tenderloin, is not only more costly but also wasteful, because boiling would render these tender meats chalky and bland, hence unfit for eating, once the fatty particles and flavor have been extracted.

Chinese markets feature a wide offering of scraps and trim for soup. These include pork neck bone, chicken chest bone and back bone (after the breast meat has been carved away), chicken feet, giblets, ham hocks, pork snout, old stewing chickens, fish heads, fish tails, and bones of big fish like halibut or sturgeon (after fillets are cut away). When Cantonese people get a good-sized grouper, they prepare their favorite dish, called *yāt-yú-léuhng-hek* 一魚兩吃, meaning "one fish, two ways to eat." The fillet may be steamed, poached, baked, or stir-fried while the head, fins, tail, and backbone go into the soup pot with tofu and mustard greens (see recipe on page 190).

Leftovers such as the carcass of a roast duck or a roast turkey, trimmings from a lobster or shrimp shells can all be turned into soup stock. Leftover rice serves as the foundation of rice soup or porridge. This frugal way of cooking is both economically and ecologically sound. And the bones are rich in calcium and other minerals. It is therefore advisable to use scraps not only in lean times, but at all times. Results of these recycling efforts are actually considered gourmet, not compromises. Try my recipes and you'll understand.

The Pearl River Delta is a fertile area compared to the rest of China; it is the least prone to famine. Most of the time it is blessed with an abundance of rice, fruits, and vegetables, as well as a great variety of foods proffered by the river. This has made Guangzhou (also known as Canton, a name given by Westerners) the most renowned city for gourmet eating. In areas around Guangzhou, soups have evolved from ordinary fare to a culinary art involving exotic ingredients. While original recipes like winter melon soup, cabbage soup, fish head soup, and turnip soup are relegated to the home kitchen, restaurants catering to city folks and rich people developed soups with pricey ingredients such as shark's fin, sea cucumber, hasmar, abalone, and snake meat. In the last hundred years at least, shark's fin soup has become a status symbol at wedding banquets.

Soups for Health, Healing, and Longevity

As detailed in the previous chapter, the Chinese have long recognized that "medicine and food share the same origin," with food holding the honored position of "superior medicine" that is both nurturing and preventive. According to traditional Chinese medical theory, our prenatal life force (qi) comes from our genes, while our postnatal life force is sustained and balanced by the nutrition we get from the food we eat and the air we breathe. Indeed, of all folk traditions, Chinese medicine has probably developed and preserved the most complete medical system involving the use of herbs and other natural ingredients, both as food to nurture and as medicine to heal. The cook, then, holds the key to our health and for generations, cooking in the traditional Chinese home kitchen has been seasoned with wisdom and care. According to the Chinese way of cooking, food should be chosen in harmony with the season and consistent with diners' physical conditions and activities. This is especially true of old-fashioned Cantonese cooking and menu planning. In general, warming (yang) foods are served in winter and cooling (yin) foods in summer. Within a given recipe, a yin ingredient, such as mustard greens, is often balanced with ginger, a yang ingredient.

Traditional Chinese nutrition is very specific about the correlation between food and the human body. To select proper food for disease prevention and life nurturing, one pays attention to such energetic properties as the Four Temperatures (*si qi* 四氣), Five Flavors (*wu wei* 五味), Direction or Tendency (*qu xiang* 趨向), and Meridian Entered (*gui jing* 歸經). These properties are consistent with those applied to Chinese herbs, and they are more than food labels; they are relational terms. Proper choice of food requires knowing these properties in relation to the condition of the human being.

Wellness means harmony within this network, while disease is viewed as the manifestation of imbalance within the system. TCM aims to restore balance and harmony through various forms of treatment including acupuncture, acupressure, herbal remedies, and food therapy. By tapping the energetic properties of food, the six disease-causing "evils"—heat, wind, dampness, cold, dryness, and fire—can be dispelled and any imbalance between yin and yang can be corrected.

Food is an integral part of Chinese medicine for health maintenance and restoration. This is especially true of soups, which can be looked upon as a palatable form of herbal tea. There are therapeutic soups for all reasons, as Bevin Hong, Jr. said of his grandmother: "She had a soup for putting on weight, a soup for losing weight, and a soup to get rid of zits" (please see the Hong story on page 359). The tradition is passed on from mothers to daughters and from mothers-in-law to daughters-in-law. The Cantonese have developed the making of healing soups into a high art form, capturing both their efficacy as medicine and their delicacy as food.

Special healthy and healing soups are regularly prepared to maintain or restore balance in the system. There are yin tonic soups and yang tonic soups. There are also soups to tonify qi and blood. In general, yang tonic soups restore vitality in older people and those recovering from illness. Yin tonic soups, on the other hand, counter-balance excess heat and dryness in the system, conditions often attributed to yin deficiency.

Revival of the Soup Tradition

Early Chinese immigrants to California prepared *louhfo tong,* or slow-cooking soups, on portable camp stoves and on the pit stoves at the back of their shops or laundries. The louhfo tong would be started in the morning to be served at dinner, by which time the nutrients would be well dissolved in the soup. The aroma would transport one down memory lane to the smell of soup wafting down narrow alleys at dusk, welcoming the men and children home at the end of the day. The community of lonely Chinese men longing for home conserved the healing soup tradition, and the tradition conserved them. These healing soups are still being prepared by grandmothers (and grandfathers) for their families and by a few choice restaurants in Stockton, California.

Back in China, for nearly a hundred years since the overthrowing of the imperial dynasty, educated Chinese women aspired to be men's equal by "walking out of the kitchen" to become doctors, nurses, teachers, writers, and other professionals. My mother's generation despised kitchen work and prided themselves on sparing their daughters from kitchen chores. As a result, my generation was brought up not knowing how to cook. But for domestic helpers, I would not have known about slow-cooking soups at all.

After coming to the United States, we quickly adopted the American way of life. We began to eat out more, and to eat more fast foods. We shied away from spending hours in the kitchen, even though somehow we learned to cook on our own. We looked for quick recipes and shortcuts. What use did we have for slow-cooking soup?

In general, soup is not the forte of American cuisine, as witnessed by the small number of cookbooks devoted to soups. Restaurant soup offerings are limited, and soup is rarely a priority on special occasion menus. The younger generation prefers milk, juice, soda, or water with their meals. Who needs soup in the U.S.?

I embarked on the project of collecting *louhfo tong* recipes fearing that this style of soup cooking was fast becoming a lost art. While I was disappointed with the lack of information on Chinese soups in the English-language cooking literature, I was pleasantly surprised when I searched the literature in Chinese. On a recent trip to a bookstore in Shenzhen across the border from Hong Kong, I discovered a whole section of cookbooks dealing exclusively with Guangdong slow-cooking soups. Demand for healthy soup cookbooks is not limited to the Guangdong area, as witnessed by the fact that Cantonese medicinal soup recipes are also published in Beijing, Shanghai, and Taipei, as well as in Guangzhou (Canton) and Hong Kong. There is no doubt that the soup tradition is experiencing a renaissance, especially soups with health merits. Its sphere of influence has expanded from provincial to national, and possibly global, spurred by a renewed interest in natural healing and traditional medicine.

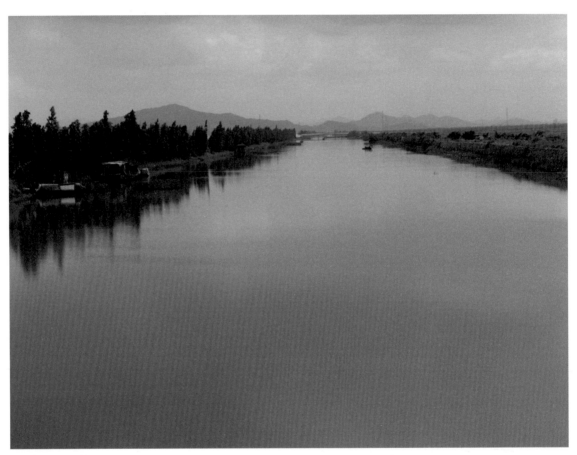

Pearl River Delta

3
The Cantonese People

A Tale of Two Deltas

Sacramento-San Joaquin Delta

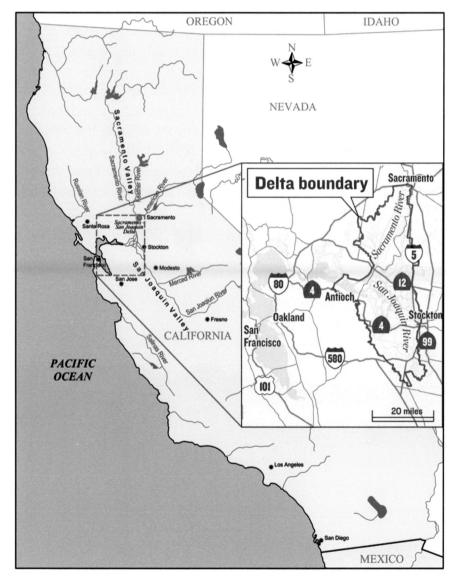

Map of California Showing Sacramento-San Joaquin Delta

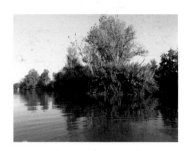

Scene of San Joaquin Delta, Cormorants in a Tree

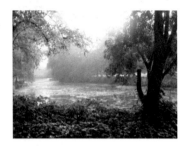

Scene of Five Mile Creek, San Joaquin Delta

Feeding into Shasta Lake are headwaters issuing from Mt. Shasta in the north and from the Warner Mountains in the northeastern corner of California. From Shasta Lake, the Sacramento River travels southward for 382 miles (615 kilometers) through the Sacramento Valley, meeting the Feather River and American River shortly before it enters the delta. There it is joined by the San Joaquin River which also originates from the western slopes of the Sierra Nevada, albeit hundreds of miles to the south. San Joaquin River turns northward near Fresno and winds 330 miles (530 kilometers) through the San Joaquin Valley toward the Sacramento-San Joaquin Delta. Together the Sacramento Valley and the San Joaquin Valley constitute the Central Valley of California.

The fertile sedimentary soil, the ample supply of water from melted snow, and the dry summer heat provided the valley with great agricultural potential. After the Gold Rush, efforts were directed toward fulfilling this potential. Asian laborers were imported to cultivate the land. Marshes were drained and levees built. Thousands of acres of arable land were reclaimed. Pears, peaches, plums, cherries, melons, grapes, tomatoes, almonds, walnuts, oranges, lemons, as well as a long list of Asian introductions including kumquats, loquats, persimmons, pomegranates, and pomelos were planted, leading to the valley's distinguished title of "Fruit Basket of America."

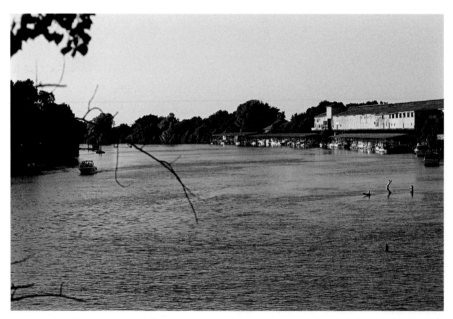

Boat House, San Joaquin Delta

Before they reach Suisun Bay, San Pablo Bay, and then San Francisco Bay—all estuaries into the Pacific Ocean—the Sacramento and San Joaquin rivers deposit sediments to form a delta made up of numerous islands and "a thousand miles of inland waterways"—an uncanny maze of sloughs, old rivers, cuts, canals, and channels. The sedimentary soil in the area, known as peat dirt, is especially hospitable to the green spears of asparagus, winning Stockton the title of "The Asparagus Capital of the World."

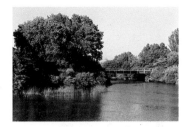

Scene of San Joaquin Delta

From the Gold Rush days into the mid-twentieth century, before highways were built, transportation of fresh produce and livestock was done on the waterways. Chinese "coolies" were hired to load the boats. Some Chinese entrepreneurs became grocery brokers or buyers, while others worked as street peddlers carrying their goods in two baskets at the ends of a long pole across their shoulders. The Chinese built levees and farmed the land. They leased land from white owners and grafted different kinds of pears and cherries. Some specialized in Chinese vegetables like bok choy, long beans, snow peas, winter melon, and bitter melon to supply the Chinese in California. Grocery stores sprang up in every Chinatown or Chinese settlement. Some featured meat and poultry departments, as well as produce. Shipments from China of preserved foods, like salted duck eggs and *laap cheong* (pork sausage), traveled up the river after crossing the ocean. Locally, the network of growers, buyers, and sellers developed into a chain of Chinese markets after WWII, the Centro Mart of the Central Valley.

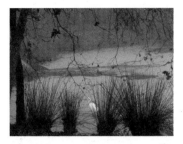

Tulle Fog, San Joaquin Delta

Pearl River Delta

A map of the Pearl River and its tributaries resembles that of California rotated 90 degrees counter-clockwise. Instead of a north-south orientation, the rivers going into the Pearl River Delta sport an east-west orientation. The terrains, however, are similar—rivers coming from the mountains, creating fertile valleys and deltas before draining into estuaries that lead into the sea.

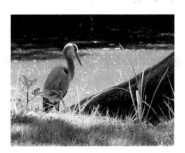

Blue Heron, Five Mile Creek

Three rivers—the West River, the North River, and the East River—flow into the Pearl River, which itself is relatively short and consists of many islands and miles of inland waterways.

The Pearl River Delta is a fertile area. Compared to the rest of China, it is the least prone to famine. Hundreds of islands bathe in high tide and sustain a wide variety of fish, shellfish, reptiles, waterfowl, and amphibians. On land, semi-tropical fruits—including lychees, longans, pineapples, bananas, papayas, guava, and star fruits—grow in lush groves. During peaceful years, rice paddies and mulberry groves—mulberry leaves being the main staple of silkworms—feed and clothe the people of Southern China, with excess left over for export. This made Guangzhou (Canton) China's most renowned city for gourmet eating.

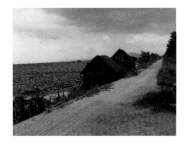

A Farm House by the Pearl River Bank

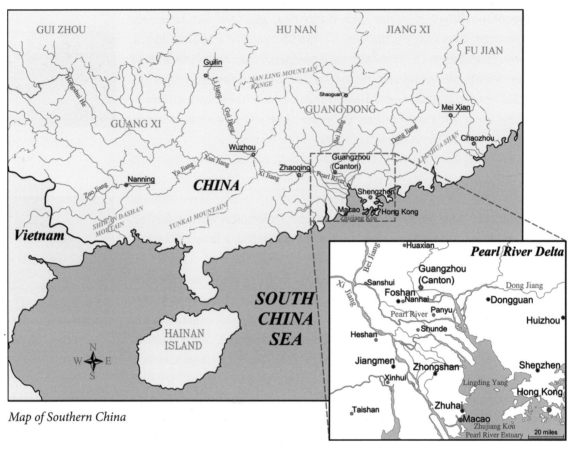

Map of Southern China

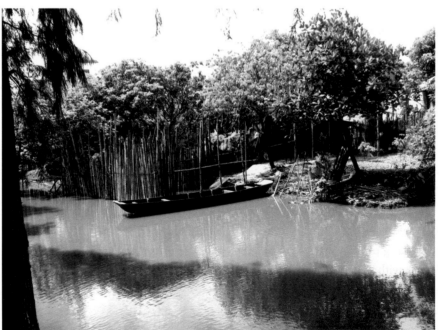

A Residence by the Pearl River Bank

Because of the climate, the delta yields two crops of rice each year. However, rocky land away from the riverbanks is less productive. Only sweet potatoes and taro roots can be grown there. Such was the general condition of the region known as Seiyup, the four counties covering Toishan (Taishan), Hoiping (Kaiping), Yunping (Enping), and Sunwui (Xinhui). Poorer soil and the lack of water for irrigation made the Seiyup people more adventurous. The men ventured out to the Port of Canton and sought work. Eventually, these same men ventured across the Pacific to seek their fortune in gold.

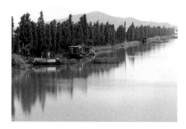

Pearl River Delta

Historical Link Between the Two Deltas

Hong Xiuquan who led the Taiping Rebellion (1850–1864) and Dr. Sun Yat-Sen (also known as Sun Zhongshan), who led the revolution that overthrew the imperial dynasty in 1911, both hailed from the Pearl River Delta.

Hong was a Hakka peasant from Hua Xian 花縣, on the northern end of the Delta. Hong was a Christian convert, and his Taiping rule promoted monogamy and banned foot binding. Women fought alongside men in the Taiping Army. In 1853, 500,000 Taiping soldiers stormed and captured Nanjing, making it the capital of the Heavenly Kingdom of Taiping. They even tried to push toward Beijing.

Dr. Sun was from Xiangshan 香山, later renamed Zhongshan in his honor. Sun and his revolutionary party made many attempts to overthrow the Manchu rule of the Qing Dynasty. An armed revolution took place on March 29, 1910, when seventy-two young intellectuals from the Guangzhou area were killed, only months before the successful October 10 revolution of the same year led to the founding of the Republic.

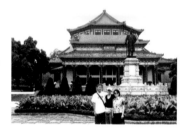

Dr. Sun Yat-sen's Memorial, Teresa Chen and Children

Sun's connection to the Sacramento-San Joaquin Delta marks an important chapter in Chinese revolution. Sun came twice to the United States to raise funds for his cause. Because there was a price on his head in San Francisco posted by the Qing consulate, and because many Xiangshan people were working in orchards and farms along the rivers, it was only natural for Sun to take to the elusive Delta. From Suisun to Isleton, and from Locke to Sacramento, there are many places reputed with the claim that "Dr. Sun slept here."

A mausoleum was built in Guangzhou for the seventy-two martyrs. A pyramid of seventy-two stacked boulders was made; but, instead of the names of the young men who died, on each stone was engraved the name of an overseas locale with organized Nationalist Party supporters who donated toward the memorial park. On a recent visit to the mausoleum in 2002, my children and I were thrilled to discover Sacramento, Stockton, Fresno, Modesto, and Suisun named on separate stones.

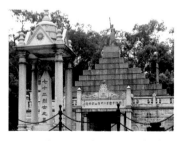

Mausoleum and Memorial of 72 Martyrs in Guangzhou

Feminism: Pearl River Style

Amahs (au pairs) from Shuntak distinguished themselves with their skills preparing dishes like stuffed dace fish and crab shells, making them very desirable as domestic helpers for the urban gentry. These culinary skills also allowed some Shuntak women to liberate themselves from subservience to marriage and become independent contractors. They joined a Sisterhood that provided them with support and job referrals. They worked in silk factories in Shuntak or hired themselves out as domestic helpers in the city. Had it not been for a series of political upheavals, many more Sisters could have retired comfortably in so-called "Vegetarian Halls," homes for women who had sworn to Buddha and the Goddess of Mercy that they would never marry. (An account of the Sisterhood from 1930s to the 1950s can be found in Gail Tsukiyama's two novels: *Women of the Silk* and *The Language of Threads*.)

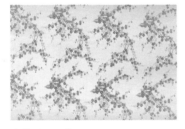

Silk Brocade

My own Ah-Bu was from the Shuntak Sisterhood. She was already working for my family when the Japanese invaded Guangzhou. She lost all her relatives, including her only brother during an air raid. When my family fled to Hong Kong in 1949, she came along and we became her adopted family. My siblings and I were fortunate to be brought up with her attentive care and superb cooking. At Jene Wah, Inc. there was a lady affectionately nicknamed "Sau Po-Po," meaning "Skinny Granny," who was also from the Sisterhood. She was here because her "adopted" kids refused to leave her behind when they emigrated from Hong Kong. She was no blood relation, but somehow they managed to match-make her to a widower from Stockton and she married at the age of sixty-five and moved to the United States.

Ah-Bu and Sau Po-Po's stories signaled the demise of the Sisterhood, and it has since ceased to exist, though feminism will never die. Everywhere one turns, one finds stories of hardworking, resilient, resourceful, and enduring women. In the spirit of Fa Mulan—popularized by Maxine Hong Kingston in *The Woman Warrior* and by the Disney movie *Mulan*—and the woman-warriors of the Taiping Rebellion, which broke out in the West River region of the Pearl River, Chinese women show their strength in their daily dealings with life. They don't necessarily have to do battle in the front, nor claim men as their archenemy.

The Golden Mountain

History and Her Story

News of gold in California reached Southern China just as the port of Guang-zhou was suffering an economic setback as a result of the Opium War. Arriving in San Francisco, the Chinese came inland, up the river on steamboats to work in the gold mines. When they were denied mining rights, they worked the land or became cooks and laundrymen to serve the white miners. With the Chinese Exclusion Act, they were further forbidden to own property or become citizens. For nearly an entire century after gold was discovered at Sutter Creek, the Chinese came to California as sojourners, with the understanding that they had to temporarily leave their families behind and eventually return to China themselves, alive or dead.

As fate had it, during the 1906 San Francisco Earthquake, all immigration records were burned. The few Chinese merchants, who were exempt from the Chinese Exclusion Act and were naturalized citizens, took advantage of the opportunity to claim sons when they registered themselves anew. Since all of the original records were destroyed, some even came forward and claimed that they were native-born. As offspring of U.S. citizens could be admitted to the U.S. even if they were born in China, each claim could be sold for a handsome price ($100 for each year of age, the minimum age being 12 years). The U.S. government was quick to catch on. These "paper sons" were later the victims of atrocities at Angel Island, the immigration station where all prospective immigrants from Asia were detained and interrogated from 1910 to 1940. The "paper sons" who managed to sneak through kept a low profile and had double identities. Maxine Hong Kingston wrote about both these "paper sons" and Angel Island in her book *China Men,* while *Island,* an anthology of documents, oral histories, and writings edited by Him Mark Lai, Genny Lim, and Judy Yung provides a more academic exploration of these events.

Hardly anyone claimed his daughters. Until the Chinese Exclusion Act was finally repealed, the Chinese community was largely a bachelor community in inner-city enclaves or ghettos. Except for the lucky few who were able to find and marry young women who were daughters of Chinese ministers or merchants, most bachelors had to save up enough money to return to China to get married. In most cases, the wives stayed behind to take care of aging in-laws and to raise families. The men would send money home and cross the ocean every so often to beget more children and to bring the older boys over to Golden Mountain, as San Francisco, or California in general, was called.

These Chinese men worked hard in the U.S. at menial jobs and endured discrimination, but the U.S. dollar went a long way in China. In the hilly and arid areas especially, families with Golden Mountain connections were considered well off. Poor families were eager to find their daughters Golden Mountain husbands, regardless of age differences as great as forty years. An arranged marriage to a Golden Mountain man meant a handsome monetary gift up front to the woman's family and a steady monthly income for the wife; the latter often referred to as a "long-term meal ticket." For many of these women, however, their status was little better than that of a domestic servant, serving the master's family. Women were rarely sent for, and daughters born in China were not even registered (please see Sun Ma's story on page 361).

After the repeal of the Chinese Exclusion Act in 1943, Chinese men with citizenship could put their names on a long waiting list to bring their women and children over. As the quota for Chinese admission was a meager 105 per year, the wait could have been as long as a lifetime.

After WWII, Civil War between the Nationalists and the Communists escalated in China. When it culminated in the founding of the People's Republic and Chiang Kai-Shek's retreat to Taiwan in 1949, families with Nationalist and/or overseas connections were forced to flee China to avoid prosecution. With drought and famine plaguing Southern China, thousands tried to cross the border every day. Hong Kong became a way station, its population swelling from about a million to more than three million in one decade. The Refugee Act, designed to admit some educated elite to the United States, did little to speed up the reunion of families split between China and America.

It wasn't until 1963, when President John F. Kennedy raised the Chinese immigration quota to equal those of European countries, that the congestion in Hong Kong was somewhat eased. Many women who married in the 1930s were finally able to join their husbands thirty years later. They brought with them the war experience, the communist experience, and the refugee experience. The once-young bride arrived on American soil an older woman. By then the children were grown up. She might even be a grandmother. She hardly knew her husband, much less the American environment. Her world shrank to the confines of Chinatown and the Chinese immigrant community, which was male-oriented due to decades of gender imbalance. Women became mere appendages to the men who brought them here, joining their husbands in their lines of business—laundry, restaurant, grocery store, etc.

Most women also became caretakers, babysitting grandchildren and taking care of their aging husbands who, in the majority of cases, were many years the women's senior. They relied on their husbands to take care of them until, finally, many of them were widowed. Widowed Chinese women living alone did not, as a rule, cook nor care well for themselves. They became socially isolated. The help they needed was beyond reach because of the language and cultural barriers.

As early as the 1970s, there were quite a few of these helpless elderly women in every Chinese-American community. Spurred by the Civil Rights Movement in the 1960s, many community service agencies sprouted up in cities across the United States. Most noteworthy of these agencies are Self Help for the Elderly and On Lok in San Francisco.

Jene Wah, Inc. in Stockton, California

The hardship of Stockton's elderly Chinese widows caught the attention of Ray Wong Quen, a New York Life insurance agent and volunteer court interpreter blessed with a vision and a lion's heart. In 1975, Ray Wong Quen, along with Samuel Chan and Henry Yip, chartered Jene Wah, Inc. as a non-profit service agency dedicated to helping Chinese elderly and new immigrants transition into their lives in the United States.

Jene Wah was so named because it was conceived to "improve the lot of the Chinese" elderly and newcomers. It became one of the first agencies funded in 1979 by the newly established Department of Aging in San Joaquin County. Starting with translation and interpretation, Jene Wah's service expanded to include assistance in filling out forms and filing tax returns, language and job training, Green Card renewal, doctor's office visits, and hospital admission, as well as daily lunch, recreational activities, and health exercises. Not only was Jene Wah able to bring the Chinese elderly out of their isolation, it was also instrumental in introducing the Chinese to mainstream ways of life and establishing their own ethnic identity. They began to participate in the annual Senior Awareness Day of San Joaquin County and the Spring Festival sponsored by the Chinese Cultural Society of Stockton, to attend health and dental fairs, and to go on field trips to Martinez and Reno. Volunteers began teaching English and citizenship classes and providing nutrition, insurance, health, and voter education. Since its beginnings in the 1970s, Jene Wah has evolved into a one-stop service agency and a home away from home for Chinese seniors. The programs are meant to empower them to live independently, free from insecurity and fear.

One may credit Jene Wah's success to the founders' vision, the directors' dedication, and the staff's diligence, but it is always the clients who carry the agency. Here is a true story, a Stockton-Chinese chicken soup for the soul.

In April 1995, Jene Wah's Board President Rowena Chen arranged a purchase of a building on East Church Street in Stockton. For the past few years, the agency's future had been uncertain due to a nonrenewable lease contract. Before the move could be consummated, however, $200,000 had to be raised to cover the purchase and repairs to the property. The Board of Directors, under Rowena's untiring leadership, decided to go forward—it was our only choice. A fundraising committee was formed, and grant proposals were written. Little did we know that the seniors had a plan of their own.

Jene Wah's seniors took a field trip of sorts, walking to the new site en masse. They were pleased with what they saw. Early the next morning, they surprised staff members Lucia Miao and Esther Chan by forming a long line outside of the office, cash in hand. They had talked among themselves after the site visit and agreed to contribute $100 each toward the building fund. Lucia, who arrived first, was dumbfounded. Esther, who arrived minutes later, broke down in tears. Months of agonizing over the future of the agency had been rewarded with a generous show of support from Jene Wah's own clients. Their spontaneous giving warmed everyone's heart and healed the wounds of struggle. In the ensuing weeks, donations came in the mail from out of town, with notes indicating that it was their mothers' wish for Mother's Day. This outpour of support made it possible for Jene Wah to raise $20,000 in the first month, and to retire its loan within two years.

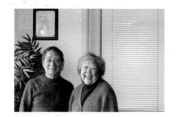

Mr. and Mrs. B.P. Lee

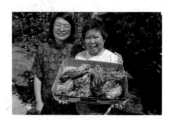

Teresa and Wai Kuen Szeto

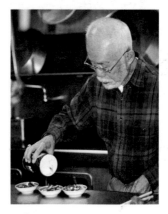

Bob Hong

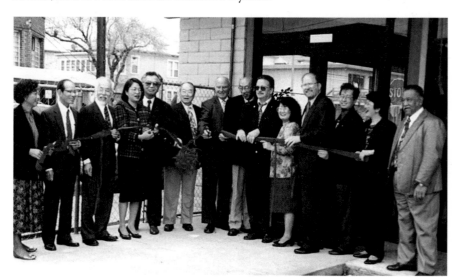

Jene Wah's Ribbon Cutting Ceremony at Grand Opening, 1996

Our elderly may be physically frail, but they demonstrate an indomitable spirit. It is exactly this spirit that carried them across the Pacific, and through numerous adversities encountered in the old country as well as in the new one. Instead of little old ladies and passive recipients of goodwill, I see them in a new light as armor-clad woman-warriors, fighting demons of land and sea.

Jene Wah Cookbook Chefs*

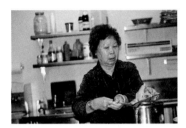

Wai Kuen Szeto

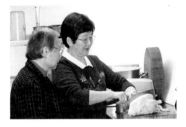

Y.K. Lau and Fee Lau

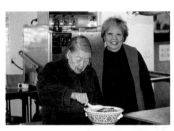

Lau Wai Tak and Lai Kuen Lee

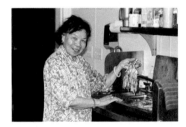

Lin Chan

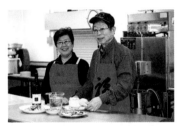

Judy and Bevin Hong

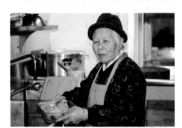

Yuen Chin Lee

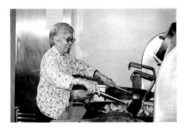

Sun Kwong

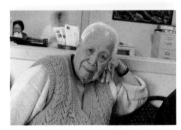

Lai King Chan

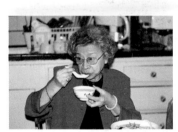

Thelma Yim

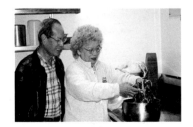

Mr. and Mrs. Henry Yip

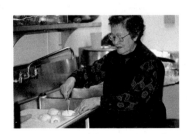

Tam Lee Wai Ying

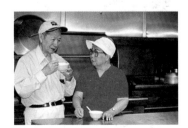

Mr. and Mrs. Ying Ming Ma

*(see Profiles of Contributors on pages 357–365)

PART TWO

Soup Basics

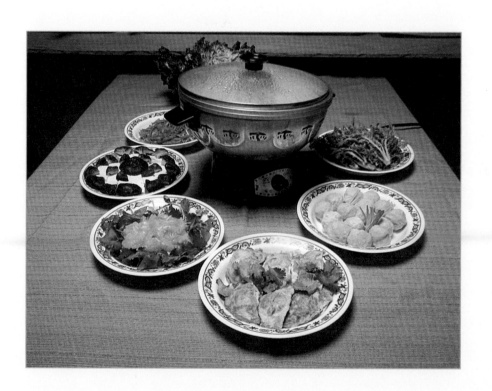

4
Cantonese Soups

Types of Soup

Cantonese soups can be classified in terms of "what" and "how." The "what" involves "what it is like" and "what goes into it." There are four major categories:

Tong: broth, soup, and stew.
Gang: thickened soup or bisque.
Juk: rice soup or porridge.
Tohngseui: sweet soup.

When noodles or dumplings are added to a soup, it becomes a noodle soup or dumpling soup. When medicinal herbs are added, it becomes a medicinal soup.

湯 Tong: Broth, Soup, and Stew

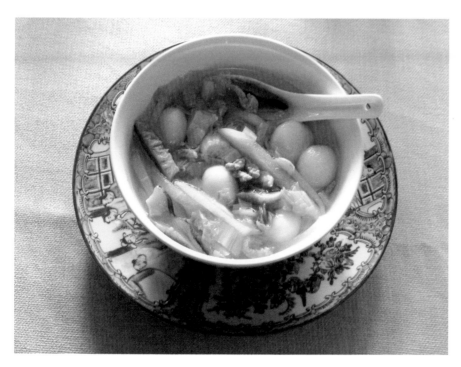

Tong: Winter Solstice Savory Dumpling Soup (see recipe on pages 203–204)

What the Chinese call soup may include what Westerners call broth, soup, and stew. In the West, it is a common understanding that a broth contains only clear liquid. Both a stew and a soup are served with its cooked ingredients. With Chinese slow-cooking soups, the line between a stew and a soup is often muddled because starchy roots, grains, and legumes will thicken the soup after hours of cooking.

Most people strain a soup and discard the medicinal herbs and soup bones. Only the broth is offered to people recovering from serious illnesses or on a liquid diet. The broth may also be mixed with rice to make a porridge for the sick.

羹 Gang: Thickened Soup or Bisque

Cantonese like to thicken a clear soup with starch (such as cornstarch, lotus root starch, arrowroot starch, water chestnut starch, or potato starch) and call it gang (pronounced "gung"). The thickening provides a glossy finish and often, with seasoning and garnish, enhances expensive but bland ingredients, such as fish maw or shark's fin, to give the soup a richer presentation.

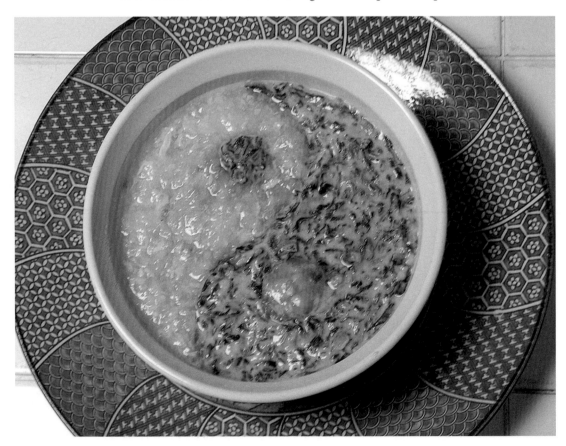

Gang: Tai Chi Bisque (see recipe on pages 251–253)

粥 Juk: Rice Soup or Porridge

Rice soups, with or without added ingredients, are always called juk (pronounced "joke") in Cantonese, to distinguish them from other soups. Besides rice, other grains, seeds, or beans may be added. I have included simple instructions for preparing the juk base below, in order to allow the reader to be creative in converting a soup recipe into a juk recipe. The reverse is not necessarily true. Some of the juk recipes included in this book are unique and do not have a soup counterpart. When using fish in juk, Cantonese people prefer using only thinly sliced fish fillets so as to avoid the danger of choking on fish bones.

糖水 Tohngseui: Sweet Soup

A soup or juk may be sweetened and served as a dessert or snack between meals. Made with grains, beans, nuts, and fruit, these soups are generally referred to as tohngseui, literally "sweetened liquid," in Cantonese. A pureed sweet soup is further specified as wu 糊 (e.g., hahptouh-wu, "walnut paste")

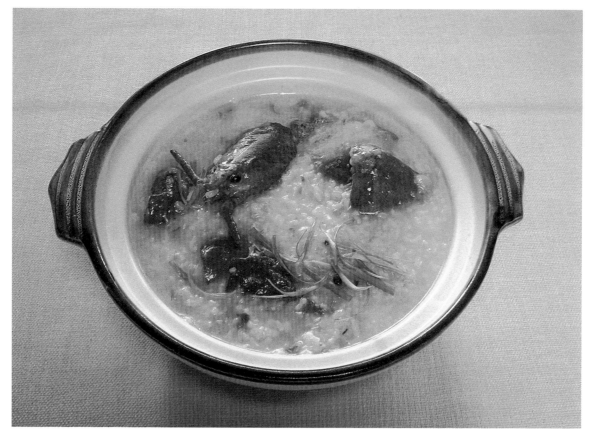

Juk: Lobster Trim Porridge (see recipe on page 311)

while a sweet soup with clear liquid is often called a tea, chah 茶 (e.g., hohng-jou-chah, "red date tea" and the Wedding Tea; see recipe on page 197).

上湯 Seuhng Tong: Top Stock

A top stock is made of soup bones (pork bone, beef bone, duck or turkey carcasses, neck bone, and/or ham hock), giblets, or shrimp or lobster shells when available. The ingredients are boiled for hours. After fat and scum are skimmed off, the liquid is separated from the solids by using big strainers. The resultant broth is the "top stock," which is kept handy in a big pot in a corner of the kitchen. Water is added to the strained solids and boiled again. The liquid obtained the second time around is called the "second stock," also kept handy in a big pot in the kitchen corner for making noodle or wonton soups.

Chinese restaurant chefs always keep big pots of stock on hand for use in soups or sauces. However, traditional Chinese home cooks normally start a pot of soup from scratch, adding ingredients at different stages of cooking or

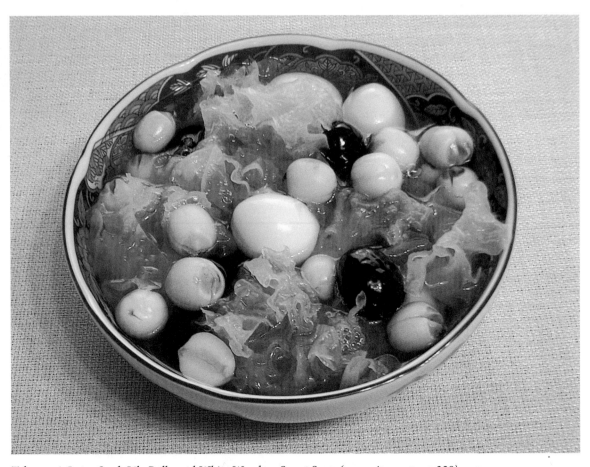

Tohngseui: Lotus Seed, Lily Bulb, and White Woodear Sweet Soup (see recipe on page 329)

all at once after some initial preparation. A broth is obtained after the boiling process by straining out the solids. Hard-to-swallow herbs should be placed in a mesh bag, which can be removed before serving the soup. Bony fish like dace should also be cooked in a mesh bag in order to ensure that all bones are removed before serving.

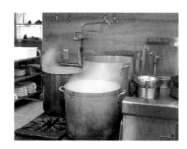

Huge Stockpots in a Restaurant

The Way of Fire

To classify Cantonese soups in terms of "how," that is, the processes by which the soups are prepared, we have four major categories:

Bou: boiling.
Gwan: quick boiling.
Dahn: double-boiling.
Louhfo: slow-cooking.

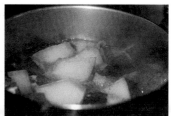

Winter Melon Boiling

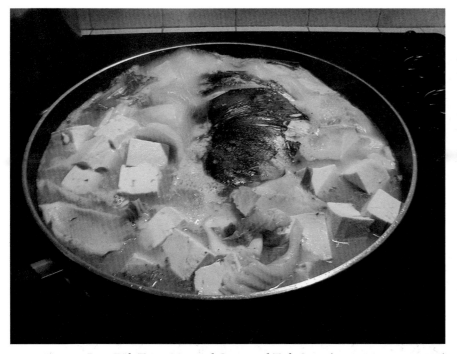

Bou: Fish Trim, Mustard Geen, and Tofu Soup (see recipe on page 190)

The most important factors in the process are temperature and time, called *fohauh* 火候, roughly translated as "the way of fire" here.

Bou 煲 refers to the method of boiling for more than 30 minutes, which is the most common. Gwan refers to the method of quick-boiling for fewer than 30 minutes. The Hot Pot combines the bou and gwan methods with an even shorter cooking method called *luhk* in Cantonese, which means steeping raw food in hot liquid without requiring it to boil before the food is consumed. Thinly sliced raw fish fillet is often treated this way in a bowl of piping-hot rice soup, a process we call *luhk juk*.

For gwan 滾 or quick-boil soups, as well as for noodle and wonton soups, either second stock or plain water may be used. Often the only necessary additions are condiments like soy sauce and sesame oil. Exotic and expensive ingredients, on the other hand, always call for the use of top stock. I have included only one basic top stock recipe, made with soup bones and giblets *(see recipe on pages 44–45)*. Top stocks are always made in advance.

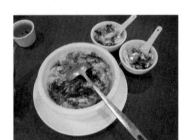

Purple Laver and Tofu Soup (see recipe on page 142)

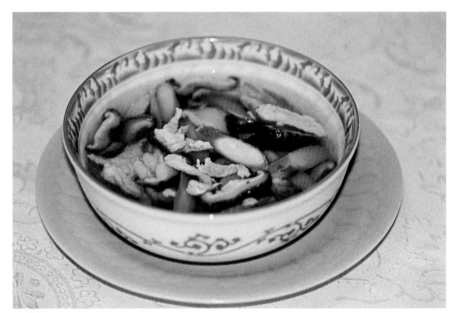

Gwan: Asparagus, Shiitake Mushroom, and Sliced Chicken Soup (see recipe on page 227)

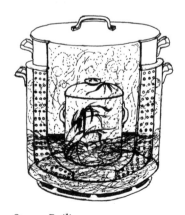

Steam-Boiling

Most soups are cooked in a pot sitting directly on the fire, but some medicinal soups, in individual or smaller portions, are cooked in a covered porcelain container sitting atop a pot of boiling water, by the heat of the steam. This steam-boiling or double-boiling method is generally referred to as dahn 燉 (pronounced "done") in Cantonese. Only a small amount of hot water (not quite enough to cover the solid ingredients) is put in the lidded steaming container called *dahnjung*. The juice or liquid in the food is sweated out in the steaming process. Instead of a dahnjung, people from Yunnan designed a clay pot with a chimney for steaming called *qiguo* 汽鍋 in Mandarin Chinese. The *dahn* 燉, or double-boiling method, which is hailed for producing the purest essence and flavor of the ingredients, never requires a separate soup base or top stock.

Alternatively, ingredients may be placed in a covered container inside a steamer. Depending on the recipe, hot water is sometimes used to submerge the raw ingredients inside the inner container, which is usually a decorated porcelain jar or ceramic bowl featuring a matching lid. The outer pot can be simply a bigger lidded pot or wok equipped with a rack to elevate the inner container. The fancy porcelain inner container is the dahnjung, meaning exactly 'the inner vessel for steam-boiling.'

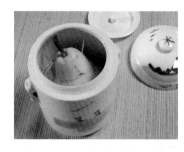

Pear in Urn for Double-Boiling

It is a hassle and a hazard to replenish boiling water in a steaming pot. Be sure to start with enough water to last the entire duration of the steam-boiling process, which may be as long as 3 hours. An electric rice cooker, with its double layers, can be used for a similar purpose. Not only is hot steam rendered unnecessary by its design, but the rice cooker also has the distinct advantage of a built-in timer, so one does not need to hang around the kitchen for hours just to make sure that the water in the outer pot has not dried up.

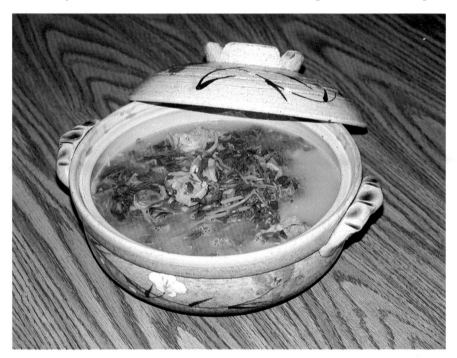

Louhfo: Watercress Soup (see recipe on page 127)

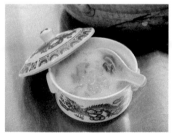

Hasmar Soup or Bisque

A slow-cooking process that lasts more than 3 hours may also be referred to as dahn, but is more appropriately referred to by the Cantonese as *louhfo* 老火 or "aging by fire." As more and more people abandon the tedious double-boiling method, and turn to electric slow cookers, the term dahn has shifted to mean the making of all slow-cooking soups. You will encounter this nomenclature of soups in Chinese cookbooks and menus.

In the old days in the old country, straw or sawdust was used as fuel and it took time for the fire to get really hot. A pot of soup would sit on a portable stove for hours against one brick wall in an open courtyard. As the soup cooked, its aroma would drift down the alley in the village, welcoming home the hungry men and children in the late afternoon, one whiff revealing whether a turnip soup or a watercress soup awaited them, or whether it was cooked with pork or chicken. There is something at once magical and nostalgic in the flavor and aroma of a slow-cooking soup.

In the modern kitchen, fueled by natural gas or electricity, cooking time can be greatly reduced since water boils much faster over high heat, though the simmering time required remains the same for the ingredients to release their nutrients and flavors.

Different ingredients must be added to the soup at different times. For instance, beans take much longer to cook than fruit. When making a slow-cooking soup, for example, I would always add goji berries toward the last 30 minutes of cooking, while dried beans must first be soaked overnight and then slow-cooked in a thermal cooker for several hours before mixing in with other ingredients toward the final stage of cooking.

The success of a great soup also depends on the amount of water in relation to the amount of ingredients and the size of the pot. Too much water and the soup will taste like hogwash. Even after hours of cooking, the flavor will not be released. Too little water, on the other hand, runs the risk of the soup drying up, thus sticking to the bottom or burning. A similar problem may arise if the pot is too small for the ingredients. With grainy and starchy ingredients, checking the water level at least once during the 3-hour cooking span, on medium heat, is crucial to make sure there is still enough liquid in the pot.

When Chinese cooks are making soup, they normally look at the food in the pot instead of at the kitchen clock. The amount of time required is a dependent variable of so many things including the quality of your pot, the power of your stove, and the size of your ingredients that the time indicated in the recipes is not to be taken as absolute. Within bounds, soup-making, unlike baking, is rather flexible and forgiving. Maybe this is the difference between the arts and science, and between the right brain and left brain of cooking.

5
Techniques

Reconstitution of Dried Ingredients

Many ingredients used in traditional soups require rehydration. Soaking time varies for each dried ingredient, from less than half an hour for dried Mandarin orange peels to overnight for some dried beans. Below are tips on preparing some of the dried ingredients. Consult the recipes for specific soaking times and for additional tips in the ingredients section.

Preservatives, such as salt, lime, ashes, and sulfite, are sometimes attached to dried ingredients and must be removed, by rinsing or soaking in water, before the ingredients can be used for cooking.

Most of the time we reconstitute with cold water, which is best for soaking dried ingredients with higher carbohydrate content and lower protein content, such as dried Chinese cabbage and seaweed. Small shellfish, such as dried shrimp and mussels, are also rehydrated in cold water. Rehydrating in hot water, on the other hand, achieves faster and better results for some ingredients, such as black mushrooms, which yield a stronger aroma when steeped in hot water. The size of the ingredients also matters. For instance, the bigger and thicker black mushrooms always take a longer time to reconstitute. In the recipes, I tend to enter the minimal time required to get an ingredient ready for the soup pot. Please remember, in most cases, additional soaking time will not hurt. As people are always in a hurry, I also adapted to using warm water to hasten rehydration.

Some dried ingredients with high protein content, such as dried abalone, fish maw, dried bean curd sticks, shark's fin, conch meat, sea cucumber, and deer tendons, remain tough and rubbery even after steeping in hot water. These ingredients should be added to a large pot of boiling water and allowed to steep, covered, overnight with the heat turned off. For abalone, conch meat, fish maw, shark's fin, or deer tendon, this process must be repeated three times. It may even take four rounds of covered steeping in boiling water to rehydrate large sea cucumbers that have turned rock hard. The extra water change and soaking is necessary to get rid of the taste and smell of lime or alkaline. Alternatively, some may resort to boiling the tough ingredients for hours on end to soften them, but since most shellfish will emit a strong smell, the water must be changed repeatedly. This process is more laborious and consumes more energy than covered steeping.

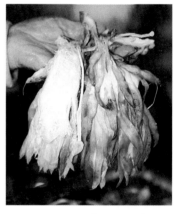

Reconstituted Cereus Flowers

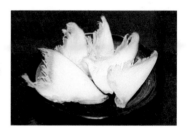

Dried Shark's Fin

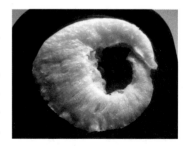

Reconstituted Shark's Fin

Other methods for rehydration are sometimes used for certain ingredients. For instance, dried scallops may be steamed after first being soaked in hot water for 10 minutes. Steaming allows you to retain the flavorful soaking liquid as well as the shape of the scallops. For a tough, rubbery ingredient like dried octopus, baking soda may be added to the soaking water to facilitate tenderizing.

Dried seafood, including abalone, fish maw, sea cucumber, octopus, squid, shark's fin, and scallop harden like leather, because of the combination of gelatin and protein they contain. As a matter of fact, fish air bladder is the source of isinglass, a strong commercial glue. It is quite a challenge to reconstitute them and reclaim them as food.

The traditional way of rehydration by heat and water is rather tedious. It is a job that requires tremendous patience. Repeated soakings every 12 hours in a covered pot of hot water (with the heat turned off) are called for. Depending on the grade and size of the ingredient, the process may take three to four days. Add another round of rinsing and soaking for sea cucumber to get rid of its briny and chalky taste. Ginger and green onion are often added in the last round to enhance the flavor.

For home chefs, I would suggest using smaller-size ingredients. The finger-size sea cucumbers recommended by Jack Ju of New Yen Ching in Stockton take only one round of soaking, while the 5-inch shark's fins my mother used require only two rounds. Fortunately, rehydrated sea cucumbers and shark's fins, in larger sizes, are available frozen in specialty stores and even some Asian supermarkets. However, I have yet to find dried abalone and dried octopus already reconstituted for our convenience. Use canned abalones instead of dried ones.

It is a common practice in the Pearl River Delta area to "refresh" dried squid with a mild alkaline solution of potassium carbonate and sodium bicarbonate. Bottled and available in most Asian grocery stores, this solution, called *gán séui* 梘水 in Cantonese, is used to macerate the leatherlike substance and restore softness. Amazingly, the squid thus reconstituted regains the texture of fresh squids. Along the same line, baking soda and boric acid have been suggested.

As I shy away from the use of chemicals, which also remove the natural flavor, I opt to take the long road with octopus and squid—not only to soak but also to boil. If they are still tough and rubbery after all that work, so be it. At least I would have retained and captured their flavor in the soup.

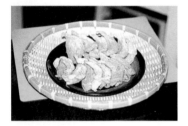

Dried Swallow's Nest

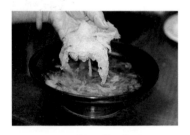

Reconstituted Swallow's Nest

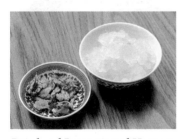

Dried and Reconstituted Hasmar

Cutting and Trimming

Vegetables

Leafy vegetables are usually added last to soups. For preparation, wash thoroughly and remove yellow leaves before cutting. Use scissors to cut watercress into 3-inch pieces. For Chinese cabbage or mustard greens, remove the base and separate the stems, wash thoroughly to remove sand and dirt, then slice into 2-inch pieces.

Root vegetables like carrots, potatoes, turnips, burdock, taro, bamboo shoots, lotus roots, and arrowroot are usually cut into large pieces for soup. They are most commonly peeled and cut crosswise into thick (½-inch to 1-inch) slices. If you think the round root sections are too big, cut in half lengthwise to produce half-moon-shaped pieces. You may even quarter arrowroot discs if they are very large. Cucumbers and bitter melons are first halved lengthwise then, after removing the seeds and pulp, cut crosswise into thick slices that arch like rainbows. The lotus root is especially suited for cross-cut disc-like treatment because of its attractive pattern of holes.

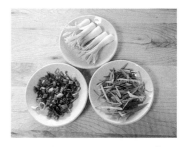

Green Onions Cut Three Different Ways

Long cylindrical roots like carrots and daikon lend themselves to an angled cutting method known as "roll-cutting." Use a vegetable peeler to remove the skin, slice off the base, then make a diagonal cut, rotate the cylinder about 120 degrees and make another diagonal cut. Roll again and cut again. The tip of a bamboo shoot may look better cut in wedges, but its chunky body fares better with roll-cutting.

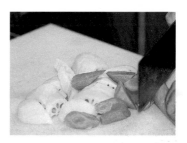

Roll-cutting Carrots

Winter melons are best cubed after scrubbing the white powder from the outside, halving them, and removing their seeds and pulp. Some people prefer to cut off the thick rind while others prefer to leave the skin on for added flavor. The cubes are made by first cutting a cross-section about 2 inches thick and then making cuts at 2-inch intervals all the way around. Kabocha pumpkins can also be cut into cubes with the thick green skin on.

Dicing refers to cutting into ¼- to ½-inch cubes. Dicing is a delicate way to prepare winter melon and fuzzy melon for soups. Start by peeling the melon and cutting it into ½-inch slices, then cut the slices into ½-inch strips (to julienne) and finally cutting the strips into ½-inch cubes. Bamboo shoots and carrots may also be cut into smaller dice this way.

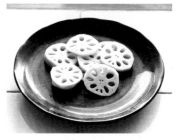

Cross-section of Lotus Root

Chinese broccoli stems and asparagus can be sliced at a slant or cut crosswise into coin-size disks for aesthetic effects.

Fresh vegetables and fruit are rarely thinly sliced for slow-cooking soups, as doing so would cause them to disintegrate in the cooking process. Generally,

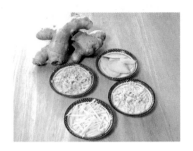

Fresh Ginger Cut Four Different Ways

fresh vegetables and fruits, such as chayote and papaya, are cut into large wedges after the seeds, pulp, and skin are removed.

Fresh ginger is used both for seasoning and as a condiment. Scrape off the skin before cutting. Ginger can be sliced, shredded, or minced. Standard slices are two to three millimeters (about ⅛ of an inch) thick. Ginger slices are always added to the hot water for the *feiseui* or parboiling process. They are also added when pan-frying fish in preparation for soup. In both cases, the ginger slices are discarded early on. Cut ginger crosswise into wide slices to allow for easy removal. Stack up the slices and you can cut the ginger into strips. If finer shreds are desired, start with thinner slices, half the thickness of the standard slices above, then stack them up to make fine cuts. Gathering the strips or shreds together, you can chop or mince the ginger. If fresh ginger is called for, do not substitute with ginger powder.

Some *louhfo* (slow-cooking) soups with chicken and exotic ingredients like abalone and shark's fin call for a chunk of ginger about the size of a walnut to be there throughout the cooking process but removed at the end. Most people do not even scrape off the skin. Just wash the ginger and smash it with the side of a cleaver or crush it with the handle of a knife.

Most dried root vegetables such as wild yam and foxglove root (rehmannia) are purchased pre-sliced and ready to use, needing only to be rinsed. Dried cabbage and cereus blossoms are sold whole, but since they are used like herbs for flavoring and are usually removed before serving the soup, cutting is unnecessary. For those who like to eat them, it is best to cut them into manageable lengths, about 2 inches long.

Poultry

Chicken and duck require special trimming. Because of the thick layer of fat under the skin, it is advisable to remove the skin even before parboiling. Small game birds like partridge and squab do not need to have their skin removed.

Old chicken and duck can be stewed whole while younger ones may be chopped into large chunks.

Before cooking chicken feet, cut off the toenails with a pair of scissors.

For quickly boiled soups, thinly slice chicken breast meat and lightly marinate before cooking in hot broth. If minced chicken is called for, also use white meat and lightly marinate.

Meat

Fresh pork loin should be thinly sliced or shredded for use in quick-boiling soups. For noodle soups, sliced or shredded pork should be marinated and stir-fried.

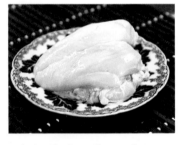

Whole Chicken, Skin and Fat Removed

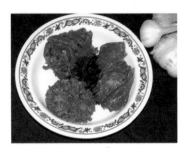

Beef Cut Three Different Ways

Large pieces of meat like pork spareribs, beef shanks, and outer flank should be parboiled before being cut as it will render them easier to cut neatly.

Ground beef, pork, or turkey for making wontons or meatballs should be lightly marinated with seasoning and cornstarch to give the meat cohesion and a smooth texture.

Marinade for Meat and Poultry

Quickly boiled soups are lighter than slowly cooked soups. For flavor, the cook either relies on the use of soup stock or on marinating the thinly sliced ingredients. The following is a basic marinade you can use for 12 ounces of meat or poultry.

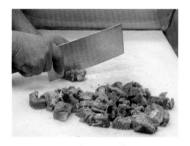

Cutting Parboiled Beef Outside Flank

> 2 teaspoons soy sauce
> 1–1½ teaspoons cooking wine
> ¼–½ teaspoon sugar
> ¼–½ teaspoon salt
> ⅛–¼ teaspoon ground white pepper
> 1½–2 teaspoons cornstarch
> 1 tablespoon of vegetable oil, to be stirred in last

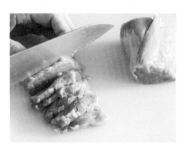

Slicing Pork Loin

I tend to season light. Instead of 2 teaspoons of soy sauce, I would cut it down to 1 teaspoon but add 1 teaspoon of water so there is enough moisture to spread the cornstarch. Depending on personal preference, the following may be also added to the marinade.

> ⅛–¼ teaspoon garlic powder
> ⅛–¼ teaspoon ginger powder
> 1 egg white, beaten

Shrimp (and Prawn)

After the shrimp are shelled and deveined, you may use the small ones whole, and the large ones coarsely cut in sections, halved vertically, or butterfly-cut along the center back line.

Combine 1 tablespoon of salt (to 1 pound shrimp) with 3 cups of ice-cold water and soak the shrimp for 1 hour. Drain. The shrimp is now ready for soups.

If you want to marinate shrimp for stir-fry dishes, for every 12 ounces of shelled and deveined shrimp, mix 1½ teaspoons of salt and 1½ teaspoons of cornstarch with 1 beaten egg white, then stir in the cleaned and pat-dried shrimp, and refrigerate uncovered for 2 hours.

Fish

When cleaning a whole fish, be sure to remove the gills, guts, scales, and black lining inside the belly. Rinse well and pat dry.

To fillet a fish, use a sharp knife to cut as close to the bone as possible from tail to head, then cut as close to the skin as possible in the same direction.

You may ask the fishmonger to clean and fillet fish for you at a fish market.

Preliminary Cooking

飛水 Feiseui—Parboiling Meat or Poultry

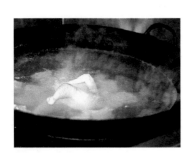

Feiseui—Parboiling Chicken

Meat and poultry, no matter how fresh, will yield an unpleasant smell and some foamy coagulation when they are boiled. Chinese soup-makers insist on a step called *feiseui*, literally translated as "flying [through] water," before these ingredients are acceptable for adding to the soup pot. It is standard procedure to put the raw meat, bone, or poultry (preferably skinned and with fat trimmed) into a pot of boiling water, often with a few slices of fresh ginger, and boil it for 5 to 10 minutes until a foamy coagulation rises to the top. The water will then be discarded and the parboiled meat or poultry thoroughly rinsed with cold water and drained.

Tendons

Beef tendons and chicken feet take much longer to cook to the desired tenderness. After feiseui, bring them to a boil again in a fresh pot of cold water with some fresh ginger slices in the inner pot of a thermal cooker. Place the inner pot inside the thermal cooker, cover, and let slow-cook overnight. Dried deer tendon takes a long time to reconstitute.

Preparing Fish for Soup

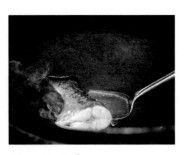

Browning Fish

People of the Pearl River Delta have more access to seafood than people who live inland. With the high tide, fish and crustaceans are channeled into shallow ponds through small gateways on the levees. As the tide recedes, fish, crab, and shrimp are gathered with nets. The fish gathered in this manner are usually small, around 1 foot long, because the grids of the gates are kept small so as not to endanger the levee system. Fishermen must go out on boats to obtain larger fish, but the small fish are preferred for making soup as they fit into a soup pot more easily. The heads, collarbones, or tail sections of larger fish, however, can also be used for soup.

Some fish, such as dace and silver carp, have small, sharp bones, which must be carefully removed. After proper preparation, including scaling and cleaning, the fish is usually placed in a bag made of cheesecloth or gauze. While only the broth is served to the family, the frugal cook often opens the bag to pick the meat off the bones, to eat on the side. Less bony fish, such as grass carp, bass, and catfish, can be cooked without a bag after the skin has been browned on both sides to keep it from falling apart during the boiling process. Cautious cooks, especially those with young children, still strain the soup before serving.

Most carp and catfish have a muddy taste, which can be eliminated by cleaning thoroughly, removing the black lining inside the belly, and poaching the fish with ginger in a pot of boiling water. Discard that first pot of water before proceeding to make soup.

Making Soup Stocks

From Soup Bones

Chinese cooks use scraps and bones—most commonly pork neck bones, chicken rib bones, and perhaps chicken feet and necks—to make soup stock. These soup bones, trimmed of meat, are available at Chinese butcher shops. Roast turkey and duck carcasses, as well as ham bones, are welcome soup ingredients when they are available. Since most soup bones fall apart after hours of cooking and are usually strained out of the stock, there is no need to cut or chop them into smaller pieces, but be sure to remove the fat and skin and rinse them thoroughly before using.

With Meat

In this country of abundance, people use whole chunks of meat to make soup stock, but doing so can render the meat tough and flavorless. To salvage the situation, remove the meat after less than an hour of boiling, chill, and thinly slice. This meat can then be arranged on a platter and served as a side dish with condiments like oyster sauce. This is done routinely with beef shank and pork loin. It is a practical and delicious way to utilize the meat's protein.

With Poultry

To make a soup stock with poultry, one may use it whole or cut into pieces. To minimize the amount of fat in the soup, start by removing the skin, then do the preliminary step called feiseui described above. The parboiling will remove additional fat. If you intend to serve the chicken later as a separate dish to complement the soup, you do not need to remove the skin first. Simply cut up the chicken and arrange on a bed of lettuce along with chopped ginger, sliced green onions, and soy sauce, oyster sauce, or even chile sauce for dipping. Be sure to skim off all visible fat in the soup after you remove the chicken and once again before the soup is served.

Vegetarian Soup Stock

Stems of bok choy and napa cabbage, green and white icicle turnips (daikon), soybean sprouts, and carrots are all favorites for starting a pot of vegetable soup. Stems and soaking liquid of the aromatic black mushroom (or shiitake) add to the flavor, while the cap may be used separately. Dried straw mushrooms are also recommended. Put everything in a stockpot and boil for at least 1½ hours.

Top Stock 上湯

An All-Purpose Soup Stock

Personally, I am not in a habit of making a lot of soup stock and storing it up for future use. While soup stock made from soup bones and/or meat does well with refrigeration, fish and vegetable soups lose their freshness overnight. Hence, I offer only one recipe for making a generic soup stock, to be used with quick-boiling or gwan soups, wonton and noodle soups, and with gourmet rice soups.

> **2 pounds chicken breast bone**
> **2 pounds pork neck bone**
> **1 ham shank bone (optional)**
> **10–20 black mushroom stems (optional)**
> **1–2 cups shrimp shells (from peeling ½–1 pound of shrimp) (optional)**
> **1 pound chicken gizzards**
> **1 pound chicken feet, toenails clipped off (optional)**
> **4 ounces fresh ginger, peeled and cut into thick slices**

Rinse all ingredients.

Bring 5 quarts water to a boil in a large soup pot. Add half of the ginger and all of the bones, chicken gizzards, and chicken feet (if using) to the boiling water. Boil until fat and scum rise to the top (about 10 minutes). Drain and rinse the solids after discarding the liquid.

Fill a large stockpot with 5 quarts of water and add the parboiled solids, shrimp shells and mushroom (if using), and the remaining ginger. Bring to a boil, boil for 10 more minutes, and then reduce the heat to medium-high. Continue to boil, with lid elevated by a pair of chopsticks, for 3 hours or more.

Strain the stock. Skim off any obvious fat. Cool stock, then pour into lidded containers or double-zipped storage bags to go into the freezer, stacked upright. Be sure to label and date each storage bag. The stock will keep for a month in the freezer, but it is best to use it sooner.

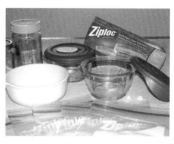

Containers for Storing Soup Stock

This should result in 2 quarts of top stock.

Restaurants may boil the strained solids once more to make a thinner stock for noodle and dumpling soups. This is called the second stock (*yitong* 二湯).

If you want an extremely rich stock, slow-cook extra meat and/or poultry with the soup instead of taking them out early to make a side dish. The stock thus obtained is referred to as the supreme stock (*díng seuhng tòng* 頂上湯). It is the soup stock preferred by the majority of my Jene Wah chefs. It is most flavorful.

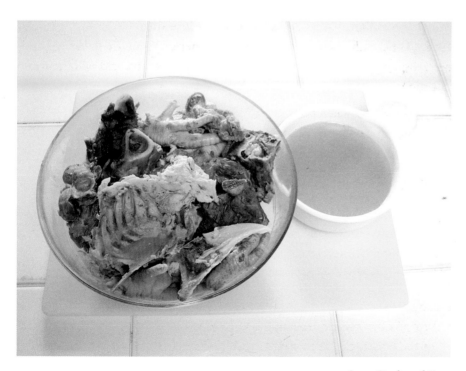

Soup Stock and Dreg

6
Equipment

Soup Pots and China Service

Clay Pots

Both slow-cooking soups and herbal remedies were traditionally prepared in clay pots. A medicinal pot sports a slanted spout for pouring, while a soup pot is shaped like a watermelon standing on its end. Both have a single handle. This type of porous cookware cracks easily if subjected to cold water while hot, or to heat when bone dry. Wires are wrapped around clay pots to prevent cracking. Submerging the bottom half of a clay pot in rice water (the water used to rinse rice before cooking) prior to putting it on the stove is an old-school method said to prevent cracking. Personally I have never experienced breakage during use, but I can testify to the brittleness of clay pots because a new red clay qiguo that I hand-carried on an airplane cracked in half en route from Hong Kong to San Francisco, probably due to luggage shifting in the overhead compartment.

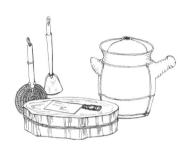

Equipment in a Chinese Kitchen

Soup Pots and Stockpots

The sizes of soup pots range from 2 quarts to 10 quarts. My favorite is a 4-quart stainless steel soup pot. It is the ideal size to make a soup for four. A soup pot should be no more than sixty percent full with liquid and solid ingredients.

The smallest stockpot holds 8 quarts. I use my 8-quart stockpot only when I am dealing with big soup bones or turkey carcass. In general, I find the stockpot too heavy to handle, though it is meant to sit on the fire for many hours.

Soups tend to boil over if they contain starchy ingredients like grains, beans, and potatoes, so it is helpful to raise the lid by setting a pair of bamboo chopsticks across the rim of the pot to allow steam to escape. This will result in the liquid boiling down faster, so to be safe, check the soup 1 hour into simmering to see if more hot water needs to be added.

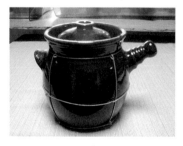

Traditional Soup Pot

Wok

A wok is so versatile that it may be used as a steamer for individual servings of dahn (double-boiled) soup, or just for making gwan (quick-boil) soups. I also prefer to make fish soup in a wok. After browning the fish on both sides with ginger, it is much easier to simply add water and other ingredients into the wok to complete the soup than to transfer the fish into a soup pot.

Hot Pot

The hot pot is used for tabletop cooking, thus it is both decorative and functional. All over China, hot pots made of shiny copper or with showy cloisonné exteriors and filled with steaming hot soup are presented to diners year-round in air-conditioned restaurants that serve Mongolian, Tibetan, Sichuan, Beijing, vegetarian, or maham (the Islamic equivalent of kosher) meat hot pots to tourists and locals alike. Instead of charcoal, the modern-day individual-sized hot pot is fueled by propane.

In the United States, electric hot pots made in Taiwan have dominated the market. Aluminum pots have been replaced by stainless steel, and see-through glass lids generate more anticipation and excitement at the table. The fake chimney at the center of the hot pot has disappeared altogether to allow for more cooking space.

Pressure Cooker

A pressure cooker may be used to shorten the cooking time for tough meats and tendons, or for cooking beans. Care should be taken that the pot is only half full and that beans are never cooked to the point that they burst open, as the skin will then clog the escape hole for the hot steam. It would be a waste to slow-cook an expensive cut of meat because in the end it would be tough and tasteless after yielding up its fat particles. Therefore, stewing beef is an ideal candidate for pressure-cooking. Chinese chefs invariably use cheaper cuts like beef brisket and shank, pork spareribs and neck bones, and old chicken, duck, and domesticated pigeon to make slow-cooking soups. To pressure-cook stewing meat and stewing chicken first will dramatically cut down the time it takes to make those ingredients tender. Follow the instructions on your pressure cooker manual.

Crockpot

Making soup in a crockpot requires some initial preparation. After feiseui, simply follow the instructions in the crockpot's manual. Cover the pot with a

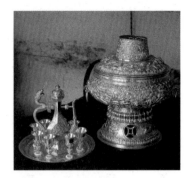

Tibetan Hot Pot

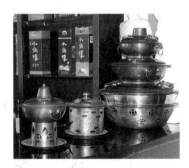

Bronze Hot Pots

lid, then set the cooking temperature and the timer and leave the kitchen. The crockpot is especially good for making porridge. With sufficient water, the ingredients will not stick to the bottom.

Electric Rice Cooker

An electric rice cooker is also good for making slow-cooking soups. Like the crockpot, it has the advantage of a built-in timer. The rice cooker serves as an outer pot for making dahn (double-boiling and slow-cooking) soups. The cook does not need to be present when the soup is cooking. Most rice cookers made in China and Japan also feature a setting for making juk (rice porridge). The brands are Sanyo, National, and Zojirushi.

Thermal Cooker

A green alternative is the thermal cooker. A thermal cooker is essentially a thermos with an inner pot in which the soup ingredients are first heated on the stove. Also known as "vacuum flask cooking," this method traps the heat in the inner pot, allowing the soup to continue cooking without a continuous outside heat source, saving gas or electricity.

A removable inner pot, with handle and lid, fits inside the outer thermos or vacuum flask, which is also made of stainless steel. To cook, the prepared ingredients are put in the inner pot along with the desired amount of liquid and heated to cooking temperature, boiling for at least 10 minutes, with the lid on. The pot is then removed from the heat and placed inside the thermos or vacuum flask. The vacuum flask not only minimizes heat loss, it also continues the cooking process with the retained heat, at a steady temperature somewhat below the boiling point. The thermal cooker works like a slow cooker, but does not require electricity. And it does not need supervision, either.

Slow cooking in the thermal cooker is especially good if you want your ingredients to hold their shape instead of turning to mush. For instance, I like to cook aduki beans or black beans in the thermal cooker first before adding them, hours later, to the cooking liquid in the big soup pot during the last 15 minutes of simmering. This way the soup will not stick to the bottom of the pot and the beans will be soft yet still hold their original shape. For those who prefer a starchy or creamy soup, take the inner pot out of the thermos and simmer on direct fire for 30 minutes before serving. The already softened beans or root vegetables will begin to fall apart, offering a thicker constituency.

I have owned a thermal cooker since the early 1990s when it was first introduced to the U.S. market. It was manufactured in Japan by Nippon

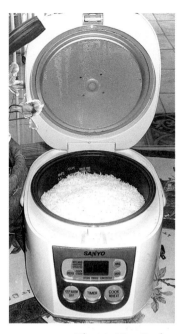

Electric Rice Cooker

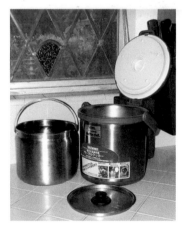

A Thermal Cooker Showing the Inner Pot

Sanso Corporation under the trademark THERMOS®, makers of vacuum flasks of various designs. The model I have is called Thermos Shuttle Chef, with the inner pot coming in 3.0-, 4.5-, 6.0-, and 8.0-litre capacities. Thermos Shuttle Chef is especially suited for making louhfo (slow-cooking) soups and stews. After 6 hours, the residual temperature of the food inside the thermos is around 158˚F (or 70˚C), a perfect simmer.

Tureens and Serving Bowls

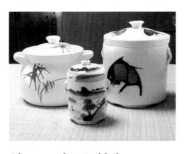

Blue-on-white Lidded Containers for Steaming

Considering the term chinaware etymologically came from "China," one should not be surprised to find a rich array of ceramic ware for making and serving Chinese soups.

Chinaware, prized in Europe and America, is made of fine porcelain with customized designs. Most notable is the blue-on-white Canton design as found in George Washington's collection on Mt. Vernon. It has been imitated by the Dutch and the Japanese, and duplicated by Wedgwood of England. Western sets do not, as a rule, include Chinese-style soup bowls or soup spoons. Instead, European-style tureens and shallow soup bowls come with these sets.

In the old days, very few Chinese could afford fine porcelain. Bowls used by the common people were earthenware with hand-painted designs. These cruder bowls have never been popular objects for export. Those that survived in the United States were probably carried here by immigrant families and handed down through a couple generations. According to some younger Chinese-Americans, these old pieces were not appreciated and most likely sold at garage sales. It is heartwarming, however, to see Martin Yan and Grace Young use some of these dishes in their cookbooks and for Ellen Blonder and Annabel Low to recreate the patterns and designs in their illustrations for *Every Grain of Rice*.

Artifacts recently excavated in Stockton (2000 CE) show that "Food preparation and consumption items used at the laundry were predominantly Chinese porcelain (69.6 percent), followed by white improved earthenware (14.8 percent). The Chinese porcelain sets include six cups, six tiny cups, four small dishes, three large bowls, sixteen medium bowls, twenty-six small bowls, one small plate, one medium plate, and twelve porcelain spoons. Five teapots were also found. Patterns include Four Flowers, Longevity, Bamboo, Double Happiness, Shuang Hsi, and celadon glaze." (See Annita Waghorn's research report.) The bachelor men who kept house in the laundry probably acquired their hodge-podge of porcelain ware in San Francisco's Chinatown.

The researchers at Sonoma State University estimated the date of deposition to be between 1894 to circa 1937, based on records from the Sing Lee Laundry then operating at 123 East Channel Street in Stockton, California.

Beginning in 1937, the Sino-Japanese War, then WWII, and then the Civil War between the Chinese Nationalists and Communists, threw China into great turmoil. Trade embargoes on Communist China from 1949 to 1979 meant a complete halt to the direct import of Chinese porcelain into the United States. Chinese-style dinnerware was primarily imported from Taiwan and, to a small extent, brought here by immigrants from Hong Kong. Meanwhile, the quality of Chinese porcelain suffered during the Cultural Revolution from 1965 to 1976, and took almost twenty years to be revived. With U.S.-China trade flourishing again, good-quality chinaware from many famous kilns in China once again became available in the U.S. market.

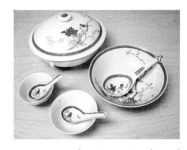

Fine Porcelain Soup Bowls and Tureen

Echoing the era of hand-painted bowls is the blue-on-white fish design that shows up on big soup bowls and *dahnjung* (steaming urns), as well as on condiment dishes, rice bowls, and porcelain spoons. Its staying power is probably due to popular demand of Western buyers.

Where soup tureens and soup pots are concerned, recent innovations leading to dishwasher-safe, from-stove-to-table, lidded, and hand-painted ceramic pots have provided us with really convenient vessels for making soups and stews—and they double as attractive serving bowls.

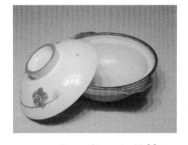

From-Stove-to-Tabletop Ceramic Pot

In this book, I refer to bowl sizes as small, medium, and large. In general, a small bowl is about 4 inches in diameter (with a capacity of ¾ cup), a medium bowl is about 6 inches in diameter (with a capacity of 1½ cups), and a large bowl measures 8 inches in diameter (with a capacity of 3 cups).

Individual soup and rice bowls are small. When food is served it is not good etiquette to fill it to the brim. As a result, each "bowl" of broth is about half a cup in liquid measure.

Utensils and Gadgets

Blenders and Strainers

The closest a Chinese soup comes to being a pureed soup is by simmering finely chopped vegetables until they are very soft and then finishing the soup off with a thickener. I have only once had winter melon pureed through a blender and I can't say I like the texture. The Chinese delight in detecting flavorful morsels in their creamy soups, no matter how soft or tiny, and pureeing takes away that pleasure. Canned cream of corn is a favorite starter for quite

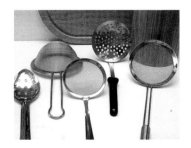

Strainers

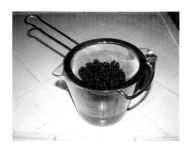

Straining Schisandra Liquid

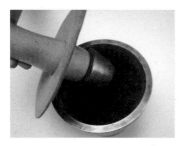

Mortar and Pestle

a few Chinese soup recipes, probably because one may still detect the bits of corn. Even so, minced chicken and "egg flower" are often added to enhance the mouthfeel of a thickened soup.

The only occasion on which I would use a blender for making a Chinese soup is when I am making a sweet soup with nuts or seeds. For some strange reason that I cannot explain, the Chinese readily accept the smooth mouthfeel of a sweet soup while they tend to reject it in savory soups. Blanched peanuts, walnuts, almonds, or toasted sesame seeds are processed in the blender with water until they become fine grains. A small amount of white rice, to be used as a thickener, is also powdered in the same manner. Strain out coarse pieces, mix the powder into hot water, and then simmer until thickened to desired texture. Sweeten and serve. If you do not have an electric blender, you may grind the nuts or seeds by hand in a mortar or grinding bowl with a pestle. A grinding bowl with coarse grooves on the inside does well with a few ounces of nuts at a time. You may want to work the paste through a strainer and repeat the grinding until you get the desired consistency.

When adding medicinal herbs to soups, the herbs should be boiled separately and strained with a generic kitchen strainer, saving the liquid to add to other food such as meat or poultry. Sometimes I run the liquid through a strainer with fine mesh a second time to get rid of any fine grit or debris from the herbs.

Instead of running a pot of fish soup through a strainer to get rid of fine bones, the Cantonese chef puts the fish, after it is slightly browned with oil and ginger, in a mesh bag. The fish falls apart inside the bag and yields its flavor into the soup. These fine mesh bags for boiling fish are available, in various sizes, in Chinese grocery stores.

Chopsticks, Ladles, Knives, and Other Utensils

Making Chinese soups requires surprisingly few pieces of equipment besides those already mentioned above.

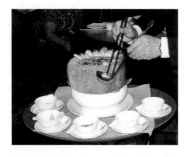

Winter Melon Soup Being Served with Chopsticks and Ladle

Chopsticks are very versatile tools in the Chinese kitchen. I use them to beat eggs, to mix cornstarch with water, to stir-fry, to stir a soup, for ventilating (by raising the lid of a soup pot so that steam can escape), and for scaffolding (building a platform at the bottom of a wok to elevate a steaming dish or urn just like a rack above boiling water). Upon serving, the chopsticks can again be used to remove bones or other unwanted ingredients and to arrange the food for presentation. As the Chinese pick up the individual soup bowl and lift it to the mouth, one can actually consume the soup with a pair of chopsticks instead of a spoon.

A ladle picks up the liquid in a soup. A ladle can be used in conjunction with a pair of chopsticks to pick up soup noodles or ingredients and transfer them into individual serving bowls. One can count and distribute equal amounts of wontons or meatballs or any other ingredients in the soup with a ladle.

A ladle is not made for stirring. Use a wooden spoon or a pair of long cooking chopsticks for that purpose.

A Chinese-American kitchen has an inventory of cleavers and knives, chopping boards, colanders, spatulas, and other kitchen tools that most American families would have. Since these tools are not specific to making soup, I shall not go into details here.

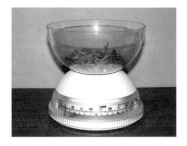

Herb/Food Scale

Measuring Cups and Measuring Spoons

While po-po (grandmas) can get away with not using exact measurements, I feel compelled to be more precise in a recipe than just saying "a pinch of this" and "a handful of that." For the English-speaking readership, I have tried my best to follow the U.S. standard of weights and measures in this book's recipes.

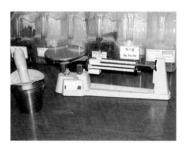

Scale for Herbs in Herb Dispensary

When it comes to traditional Chinese herbs, an entirely different measuring system is involved. The units are *jin* 斤, *liang* 兩, *qian* 錢, and *fen* 分 in Pinyin. While 10 *fen* = 1 *qian,* and 10 *qian* = 1 *liang*, it takes 16 *liang* to make one *jin* (approximately 2 lbs). Confusion sets in as we translate *liang* loosely into "ounce," thus making *jin* the equivalent of "pound." As American merchants trade in pounds and ounces, each time a Chinese herbal formula (or recipe) is presented, we cannot know for sure. When this happens, I always refer to the metric system. As dried Chinese herbs are rather light, sometimes it is easier to measure by volume or pieces, instead of by fractions of an ounce. (Please refer to the conversion tables under Weights and Measures on pages xx-xxi.)

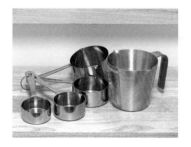

Measuring Cups

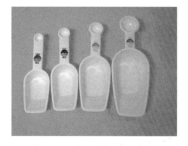

Measuring Spoons

PART THREE
Ingredients

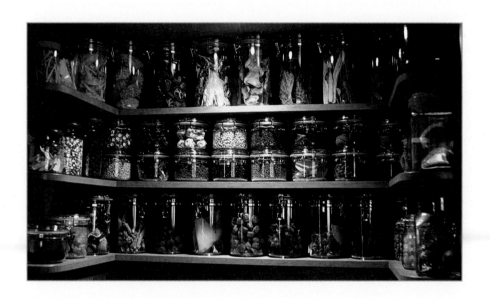

7
Animal Sources

The traditional Chinese diet consists of a high percentage of complex carbohydrates and low percentage of animal protein. Country folks get their protein from legumes, bean products, nuts, and seeds. Though most households raise a few chickens, they are more for the eggs than meat. People on the Pearl River Delta get their protein by working with rising tides that send small fish and shrimp through the gates on the levee into small ponds.

Though this cookbook is written for omnivores, the amount of meat used in each recipe should be indicative of the Chinese dietary practice of leaning more toward vegetables and grains. This does not mean that the Chinese diet is deprived of the proteins that provide the building blocks of body tissues.

Every ingredient listed in this section is accompanied by its Mandarin and Cantonese Romanized spellings. Please refer to the pronunciation guide in the appendix for the correct articulation of these terms in two of the most prevalent Chinese dialects.

Meat 肉類

Beef (niú ròu; ngàuh yuhk) 牛肉

Beef is rich in protein and iron. In Chinese cuisine, beef is most commonly prepared by braising, stir-frying, or boiling in soups.

Beef is high in saturated fat, so the amount of beef taken should be watched carefully and lean cuts like shank and round steak should be used whenever possible.

In the Cantonese diet, beef appears mostly in stews and soups. Since these dishes are cooked slowly for long periods of time, expensive cuts like porterhouse and prime rib would be a waste. As a result, Chinese cooks tend to use cuts of beef that are priced in the "low to moderate" categories by American standards. These lower-priced cuts like shank, rib, brisket, or outside flank, and oxtail offer better flavor and better eating, while more expensive cuts only become tough and flavorless in soup.

Outside Brisket and Outside Flank (níu năn; ngàuh náahm) 牛腩

For years I thought of this delicious fatty cut of beef as the brisket, but Cantonese butchers use this term to describe the belly instead of the chest. Grace

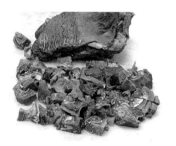

Beef Outside Flank

Yang has identified the belly part as the outside flank, a ½-inch layer of muscle plate outside of the flank steak. Further research reveals that the Cantonese term náahm 腩 covers both the outside brisket and the outside flank, in fact, the entire underside of the cow.

Toward the front, by the first eight ribs, is the brisket, which Cantonese butchers call *ngàuh náahm tàuh* 牛腩頭 (literally, the head or frontal end of *ngàuh náahm*). This is the biggest and thickest piece, lined with a thick layer of fat that needs to be trimmed before cooking. In the United States, the brisket is the part commonly used to make corned beef and cube steak. The meat is marbled with fat and yields the richest beef flavor in stews.

Beneath and behind the brisket is what Cantonese butchers call *hàahng náahm* 坑腩, a term without an English equivalent. It is located outside of the lower ribs. Further down by the belly is *sóng náahm* 爽腩, which lies outside of the flank and is called the flank meat or outside flank. It has a thin, white lining which also gives the outside flank the Cantonese name *ngàuh baahk náahm* 牛白腩 (literally, the "white" *ngàuh náahm*). Chinese markets in California label the outside flank as "beef plate." Many Cantonese prefer its tender and smooth gelatinous mouthfeel to that of the fibrous brisket. In Hong Kong, the outside flank commands a considerably higher price than the brisket. In the United States, however, the outside flank is treated as scrap and sold alongside other odds and ends as stew meat.

Chinese butcher shops in the U.S. carry both the brisket and the outside flank, while Cantonese restaurants tend to combine the two to give their customers the satisfaction of a rich flavor as well as the smooth tendon-like mouthfeel in every other morsel. The brisket and the outside flank are most often braised and served with greens on top of soup noodles or plain rice, making a complete meal in itself.

Beef Shank (niú jiànzi; ngàuh jín) 牛腱

Beef shanks are the muscles below the knee down to the ankle. They are lean and tough, needing to be cooked for a long time to become tender. Northern Chinese like to braise them with five-spice seasoning and soy sauce, then thinly slice the meat and serve it cold as an appetizer. Beef shank soups with all sorts of vegetable and herb combinations are Cantonese favorites. Chinese butchers remove the bone while U.S. butchers cut the shank in cross sections with the bone in the center.

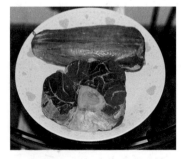

Beef Shank, Cross Cut and Boneless Cut

Beef Tail/Oxtail (níu wěi; ngàuh méih) 牛尾

Beef tail is made up of the last five vertebrae of the ox/cow. It has more fat than meat. Be sure to trim excess fat before cooking.

Braised oxtail with tomatoes, carrots, potatoes, and onions makes a wonderful dish to go with rice. Oxtail is also good for making soups. After boiling, chill in the refrigerator overnight so that excess fat will solidify for easy removal.

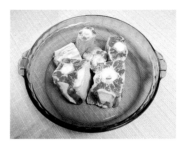

Oxtail

Beef Tendon (niú jīn; ngàuh gàn) 牛筋

Beef tendons are fibrous collagens connecting the muscles to the bones. They become gelatinous after being cooked for a long time. In a soup or stew they are usually paired with beef brisket or outside flank, which adds to its flavor.

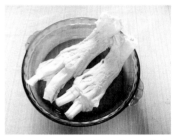

Beef Tendon, whole

Deer Tendon (lù jīn; luhk gàn) 鹿筋

Dried deer tendons, sold with or without the hoof bone attached, are valued for being able to strengthen joints. Warming in nature and slightly salty, they are said to help with rheumatoid arthritis. They require a long pre-soaking period and hours of boiling to become soft and gel-like.

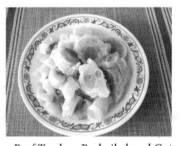

Beef Tendon, Parboiled and Cut

Ham (huǒ tǔi; fó téui) 火腿

Jinhua 金華 ham is to the Chinese what Iberian ham is to the Spaniards. Salty, savory, and chewy, ultra thin slices or shreds of Jinhua ham top many expensive Chinese dishes, including Shark's Fin Soup. While meat products cannot be imported to the U.S. from Asian countries, Spanish Iberian ham (at $30 per pound) would do if you can find a butcher who would shave off a few ounces for you from a whole leg. Virginia or Smithfield ham is also a plausible replacement. Lunchmeat ham is a poor substitute, because it does not even come close to the taste, texture, or dark red color of Jinhua ham.

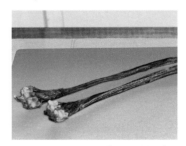

Dried Deer Tendon

Mutton (yáng ròu; yèuhng yuhk) 羊肉

It is rare for Cantonese, or Southerners in general, to include mutton or lamb in their diet. Mutton is used mostly in food therapy to treat vacuity and coldness, by warming the middle burner. In terms of TCM, mutton is sweet and warming and enters the channels of spleen and kidney.

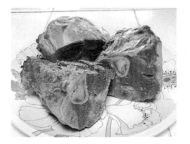

Ham Hock

Pork (zhū ròu; jyù yuhk) 豬肉

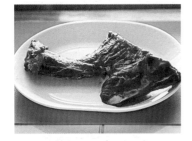

Pork Neck Bone

Pork is arguably the most favored meat of the Cantonese people. It is said to moisten dryness and replenish the yin essence. Pork is high in saturated fat. In one sample, it is found that lean pork contains 16.7 percent protein and 28.8 percent fat, whereas fat pork contains 2.2 percent protein and 90.8 percent fat. The amount of fat will certainly vary from cut to cut. In any case, do not over-indulge.

An anthropological study conducted at Sonoma State University clearly demonstrates the dominance of pork in the Cantonese diet (over 70 percent of total meat consumption) as opposed to that of their Caucasian neighbors (20 percent pork, 20 percent mutton, and 60 percent beef). As shown in the same study, the most common pork cuts consumed were from the shoulder and ham, followed by lower-priced cuts such as belly, ribs, neck, and hock, presumably for making stews and soups.

Nothing goes to waste. Internal organs such as pork liver, lungs, kidneys, spleen (melt), intestines (chitterlings), and stomach are all used. The traditional Chinese diet consisted of so little meat that cholesterol was not an issue. In TCM, emphasis is placed on using corresponding organ meat to treat ailing organs, such as using liver to tonify liver and melt for spleen and pancreas. It makes sense if you consider the iron in the liver and the insulin in the melt.

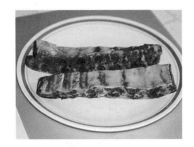

Pork Sparerib

Pork Spareribs (*zhū* pái gǔ; pàah gwāt) 豬排骨、排骨

Pork spareribs, cut in small pieces, are commonly used in soups. While the meat is tender and flavorful, the bones yield minerals and marrow into the soup. For the same reason, pork neck bones are used to make soup stock. After boiling, chill in the refrigerator overnight and then remove excess fat.

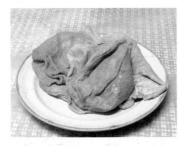

Pork Stomach

Pork Stomach (zhū dǔ; jyù tóu) 豬肚

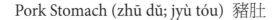

Pork stomach is considered a warming food and a tonic. It is said to combat fatigue and poor appetite. It is cooked with white peppercorns to dispel "wind in the stomach."

Poultry and Eggs 禽類、蛋類

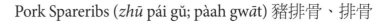

Black-Bone Chicken (wū gǔ jī; jūk sī gāi) 烏骨雞、竹絲雞

This chicken has white feathers with black legs and black feet. Its skin and bones are also black, though the meat looks like that of any ordinary chicken. It is usually sold whole, plucked and cleaned, in Chinese poultry stores. When boiled for hours, the meat yields a superb flavor and is easily shredded with

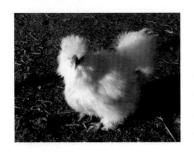

Silkie

a fork, earning the fancy name juk si gai meaning "bamboo-thread chicken." The word "thread" further suggests "silk," hence its nickname "silkie." The shreds blend well in a shark's fin soup.

Chicken Eggs (jī dàn; gài dáan) 雞蛋

In modern-day America, 'eggs' means almost exclusively chicken eggs that come nestled in twelve-count cartons. In rural China, every household raises a few chickens, mostly for eggs. Chicken eggs are a good source of protein and very versatile—they are steamed, scrambled, hard boiled, or made into omelets, custard, pastry, and soups. Eggs are beaten and quickly added last minute to a hot soup to make "Egg Flower" or "Eggdrop" Soup.

Chicken Feet (jī jiǎo; gài geuk) 雞腳

Chicken feet are used in Chinese cuisine after the rough outer skin and toe-nails are removed. What is left becomes gelatinous when stewed and separates easily from the small bones. Rich in collagen, chicken feet are said to strengthen ligaments in the feet and give a luster to skin and hair. Chicken feet are often used to make soup stocks.

Chicken feet can be bought from Asian markets in the meat section. Chicken feet cooked with chile peppers and spices are a popular dim sum dish in Cantonese teahouses.

Chicken Liver (jī gān; gāi yéun) 雞肝、雞膶

Chicken liver is said to strengthen the liver and kidneys while helping treat malnutrition, impotence, and urinary incontinence. Nowadays, chicken giblets can be bought from Asian grocery stores in the meat section. Cantonese like to use chicken liver for making soups and stir-fried dishes. A mixture of chicken liver and chicken gizzard along with morsels of seafood, meat, and vegetables is known as sahp gám 什錦 "the Grand Mix."

Duck (yā; ngaap) 鴨

Ducks come mostly frozen in the market in the United States. They are bigger in size than chickens and take much longer to cook. The Chinese usually make Cantonese roast duck, called siù ngáap 燒鴨, or Peking duck, which is eaten by wrapping the skin (and meat) inside a small bun with hoisin sauce and green onion. In the process of roasting, the fat is allowed to drip off. For a soup, however, it is best to boil the duck and then refrigerate it overnight so that the solidified fat can be skimmed off. Alternatively, you can remove the skin as a first step to minimize the amount of fat in your soup.

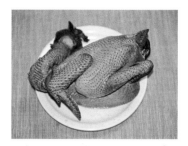

Black-Bone Chicken

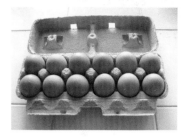

Chicken Eggs

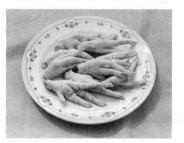

Chicken Feet

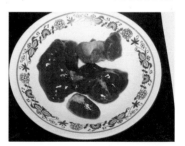

Chicken Giblets

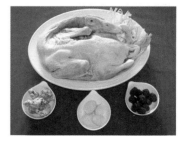

Duck

Duck Eggs (yā dàn; ngaap dáan) 鴨蛋

Duck eggs, which are larger than chicken eggs, can be bought in Asian grocery stores. The eggs are usually made into salted eggs, which are used as an ingredient in soups, congee, moon cakes, and Chinese tamales (júng 粽).

Duck Gizzard (yā zhēn; ngaap sán) 鴨肫、鴨腎

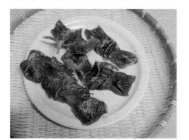

Dried Duck Gizzard

The gizzard of the domesticated duck can be eaten freshly cooked or preserved, salted, and dried. Dried duck gizzards decrease in size and harden, turning purplish in color. They have a chewy texture and are said to help settle an upset stomach. Dried gizzards are available in Chinese grocery stores. Both preserved and fresh duck gizzards are good for soups. Cantonese like to combine both in the same soup, with watercress or bok choy. It is said that they help moisten the system when the air gets very dry as a result of seasonal change or the use of heating.

Partridge (zhè gū; je gū) 鷓鴣

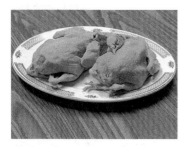

Partridge

The partridge prefers a habitat among bushes and tall grass in hilly areas of Southern China. It is smaller than a chicken but has a similar sweet flavor. A warming food, partridge is said to improve mental energy. This delicate bird is a favorite substitute for chicken in medicinal soups.

Pigeon, Domesticated (gé zi; baahk-gáp/gáp) 鴿子、白鴿/鴿 (See Squab on page 63)

In the United States, many people consider pigeons, especially the feral pigeons found in parks and city squares as scavengers and pests, but by selective breeding, the Chinese have cultivated a breed of white pigeon with tender and flavorful meat. Not only are pigeons raised commercially on large farms, but many rural Chinese families also keep pigeon coops where the pigeons pair up as couples to raise their young in their own nests.

Quail (ān chuān; ām chēun) 鵪鶉

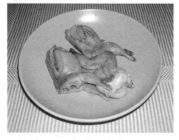

Quail

Judging from the ready availability of quail eggs and quail meat in Asian markets in California, I can safely assume that quails, like pigeons (and squabs), are domesticated. These farm-raised game birds are prized for their sweet flavor and their moistening nature to soothe dry coughs and clear damp-heat. It is a favorite ingredient in tonic soups.

Quail Eggs (ān chūn dàn; ngām cheūn dáan) 鵪鶉蛋

Quail eggs are about the size of the first section of a thumb. They have the most cholesterol among all eggs. They are usually used for vegetarian dishes and sweet soups.

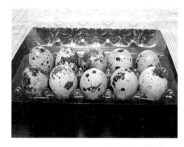

Quail Eggs

Salted Eggs (xián dàn; hàahm dán) 鹹蛋

Salted eggs result from soaking raw, fresh duck eggs in salty water for about thirty days (4 cups of salt to 10 quarts of water with 40 eggs). Cantonese like to make savory jung 粽 (Chinese tamales) with a salted egg yolk for the Dragon Boat Festival and moon cakes for the Mid-Autumn Festival. Previously, salted eggs were imported from China uncooked. Now they are hard-boiled for fear of avian flu and/or spoilage.

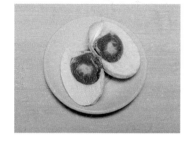

Salted Duck Egg

Squab (rǔ géi; yúh gáp) 乳鴿

Baby pigeons stay in the nest for about twenty-one days and grow to a fairly good size (weighing about one half to three quarters of a pound) before they are fledged and learn to fly. It is at this stage that they are called squabs and are prized as gourmet food. Squabs are farm-raised from a breed of white pigeons. In the United States, fresh and frozen squabs are available in Asian markets.

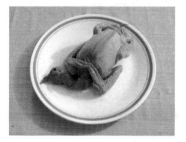

Squab

Swallow's Nest (yàn wō; yin wō) 燕窩

Top quality whole nests come from Indonesia and Vietnam. Southeast Asian swallows or swifts are migratory and feed in flight. After creating a nest with its own saliva, the monogamous bird lays two eggs, which are taken care of by both parents. Once the chicks are old enough, the swallows abandon the nest, which can then be harvested and washed by hand. The prized part is the gel or collagen from the bird's saliva. Whole nests with a light yellow luster can sell for $1,300 a pound or more. Broken pieces sold in bulk are approximately $320 a pound, or $80 for five pieces, enough to make a soup. In Chinese restaurants it is usually referred to as Bird's Nest Soup.

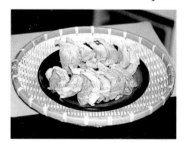

Swallow's Nest, Dried

Thousand-Year Eggs (pí dàn; pèih dáan) 皮蛋

The making of "thousand-year" eggs is a uniquely Chinese culinary invention. Westerners call them "thousand-year" eggs because they assume a fossil-like appearance after being buried in a mud mixture of ashes (from straw, twigs, and charcoal), lime, tea, and salt solution. It only takes thirty days for the eggs to be ready, aged and cooked by the chemical process. The egg white becomes a clear dark brown jelly while the yolk turns into a grayish-green gel

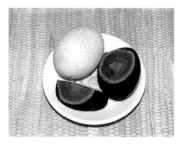

Thousand-Year Eggs

with the consistency of a soft-boiled egg and an alkaline, rather than acidic, composition.

The Chinese prefer making thousand-year eggs with duck eggs. They are served with pickled ginger and fresh coconut as appetizers, or in soups and porridge to get rid of heat from excesses.

Turkey (huǒ jī; fó gāi) 火雞

Not many Chinese warm up to turkey because they consider turkey meat tough, coarse, and bland. However, Chinese-American families serve turkey at Thanksgiving and Christmas, though they may use savory rice stuffing instead of breadcrumbs. Leftovers are adapted to Chinese dishes, especially in soups and porridge made with the carcass.

Fish 魚類

Big Fish (lián yú; daaih yú) 鰱魚、大魚

The big fish Hypophthalmichthys molitrix has no equivalent in America, but it is very common in the Pearl River Delta of China. I suspect that big fish is a variety of the fast-growing grass carp, sharing the similarities of large scales, large size, and color shadings from dark to light on the sides, ending with a white belly. It is imported and available in Chinese fish markets in San Francisco. When a big fish head is called for in a soup recipe, one may substitute a salmon head, though the flavor will be different. When big fish tail is called for, substitute a striped bass tail or a whole black bass or any other white fish.

Black Bass (bái huā lú; màahng chòuh) 白花鱸、 盲鰽

Black bass is native to North America, its habitat ranging from the Hudson Bay basin in Canada to northeastern Mexico. Several species are also found in the Sacramento-San Joaquin Delta. They are popular as a game fish among anglers. The Cathay Club of Stockton used to hold an annual Black Bass Derby. The Cantonese in California call it màahng chòuh 盲鰽.

Firm and sweet tasting, black bass is a ready substitute for grass carp, which is not easily available in the United States. It can be steamed whole. Fresh fillets can be thinly sliced for quick dunking in hot soups or porridges. A bigger variety, the striped bass, is also popular among Delta anglers.

Bonito, Dried (cái yú; chàaih yùh) 柴魚

Dried bonito is hard as a piece of wood, hence the Chinese term "firewood" (cái 柴) in its name. It is a kind of tuna with firm flesh and is the foundation of

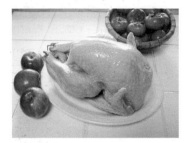

Turkey

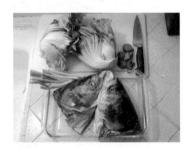

Big Fish Head

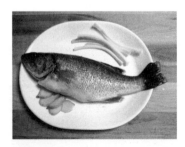

Black Bass

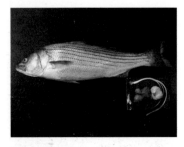

Striped Bass

Japanese fish stock or dashi. In the old days, shavings from the hard dried fish were obtained by using a hand plane, just like shaving wood. Nowadays, both packaged dried bonito shavings and instant dashi are available in Japanese grocery stores.

Chinese and Koreans also use dried flatfish such as flounder to make soup. There seems to be some confusion in the use of the same term, "firewood fish" (*cái yú* 柴魚) to refer to both dried bonito and dried flounder in the stores, even though dried flatfish pieces are usually smaller and not nearly as hard as dried bonito.

Dried flounder fillets come in 4-ounce packages. Dried bonito is considerably more expensive, with shaved bonito from Japan selling for more than twice as much as the flounder.

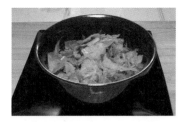

Shaved Dried Bonito

Catfish (táng shì yú; tòhng sāt) 塘虱魚

Most catfish species have prominent barbels resembling cat whiskers, thus giving rise to their common name. Catfish are primarily freshwater fish. They are normally bottom feeders. They do not have scales. Catfish are of considerable commercial importance and are farmed for food in both Asia and the United States. Catfish fillets are available in most supermarkets and provide a good source of protein. The meat is delicate, but may taste like mud if not treated properly. The inside black lining must be thoroughly removed. Before adding to a pot of soup, pan fry the catfish with slices of ginger to brown and remove any unpleasant smell. Catfish meat is traditionally eaten to help with knee and back pain.

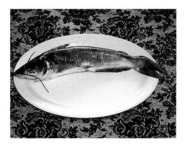

Catfish

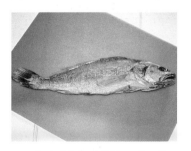

Dried Salted Yellow Croaker

Croaker, Yellow (huáng yú; wòhng yú) 大黃魚、黃魚

What the Chinese call yellow croaker is similar to the white croaker in the Eastern Pacific. The fins are yellow to white in color while the body is brownish to yellowish on the back and silvery at the belly. It varies from 8 to 15 inches in length and weighs up to 1½ pounds. As fishing and catching is good throughout the year, yellow croaker can be made into a year-round soup with pickled vegetables. Frozen yellow croaker, however, loses its sweet flavor and does not fare well in soups. Salted yellow croaker is a common kind of preserved fish in Southern China.

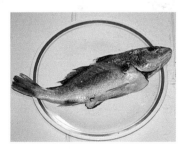

Yellow Croaker

Dace (líng yú; lèhng yú) 鯪魚

Native to the Pearl River Delta, dace feeds on aquatic plants and spends the winters resting in deep areas of the riverbed. Dace is said to relieve bloating and tonify the blood. However, people with a cough as a result of yin deficiency

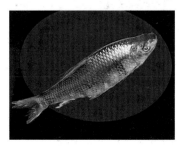

Dace

should avoid it. Dace is bony and, therefore, should be cooked in a gauze bag that can be romoved from the soup before serving.

Flatfish, Dried (dà dì yú; daaih deih yú) 大地魚

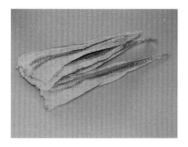
Dried Flatfish

Another common kind of dried flatfish used for making soup is the sole, called daaih deih yú 大地魚 in Cantonese. As dried flatfish pieces are not as hard as dried bonito, and not as big, no shaving is required. Just soak for a couple hours before boiling.

Grass Carp (cǎo yú; wáahn yú) 草魚、鯇魚

The grass carp is a freshwater fish, widely cultivated in China for food. The grass carp grows rapidly, gaining at least 10 pounds a year, attaining nearly 4 feet in length, and weighing 70 to 90 pounds when fully grown. Like the big fish, it is usually cut up and sold in pieces. The torpedo body shape yields thick fillets, perfect for slicing thinly. Grass carp slices are translucent when raw, turning snow white when dunked into hot liquid. The head, which is rich in collagen, and the tail are favorite ingredients for making soup.

Grouper Epinephelinae (shí bān yú; sehk bāan yú) 石斑魚

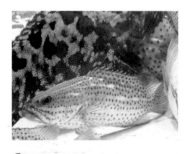
Grouper

Grouper are bottom-dwelling fish found in temperate marine waters by the shore, in bays and lagoons. The English name "grouper" is derived from Portuguese "garoupa" and has nothing to do with groups. As a matter of fact, groupers are loners and do not live in schools. Because of their body markings, which resemble rock patterns, grouper epinephelinae are mistakenly called rockfish or rock cod in Chinese fish markets and restaurants. Like rock cod, grouper have firm and white flesh that forms large flakes upon cooking. The large head of grouper epinephelinae is gelatinous inside, rich in collagen and minerals, and a favorite of the Cantonese for making fish head soup. Some Cantonese restaurants will make you a braised fish dish with the fillets and a delicious soup with the head, tail, and bones together with fresh mustard greens and tofu. But remember to order by its pseudonym: rock cod.

Halibut (qiān díe; hīm dihp/daaih lùhng leih) 鰜鰈、大比目魚/大龍脷

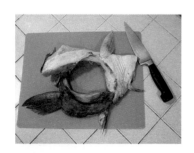
Halibut Collar

The order Pleuronectiformes (meaning "side swimmers" in Greek), includes some four hundred species of flatfish with both eyes lying on one side of the head, a flat body, and an extended dorsal fin as a result of evolutionary adaptation to living on the seabed. Halibut, flounder, sole, plaice, and turbot are all valued food fish. Most smaller flatfish are delicate; only bigger ones like halibut and turbot yield thick enough pieces of fillet to go into soups and chowders. Halibut is mostly available in stores cut up as steaks. Halibut collars are sold as trim or scrap in fish markets in the U.S., but they are treated as a delicacy in Chinese soup-making and Japanese cooking.

Loach (ní qiū; nàih chāu) 泥鰍

Like catfish, the loach is a freshwater fish without scales. Loaches belong to the family Cobitidae while catfish belong to the order Siluriformes, which does not include the loach family. Loaches are capable of burrowing into the mud when a pond or rice paddy dries up and they can survive with just enough moisture to keep their skin slimy. Loaches, unlike the catfish, do not have prominent barbels.

In Asia, loaches are valued for their delicate meat and taste, and are of considerable commercial importance to be farmed for food.

Perch (lú yú; lòuh yùh) 鱸魚

This freshwater fish measures 8 to 12 inches in length and has a coral-colored coat with rough scales and a lateral line system. It has spiny fins. Its flesh is firm, white, and delicate in flavor. Its size is perfect for baking, steaming, or pan-frying whole, as well as for making soup after lightly browning on both sides in a frying pan.

Red Snapper (hóng zhōu yú; hùhng jāu yú) 紅鯛魚

This fish is also known as redfish. Measuring 8 to 12 inches in length, it has a mild flavor. The color of its firm flesh ranges from white to pink. Its size is right for baking, steaming, pan-frying, and making soup. I think it is what the Cantonese would call hùhng sāam yú 紅衫魚 or "red-garment fish," though the orange roughy (sea perch) and coral perch are also likely candidates for that name.

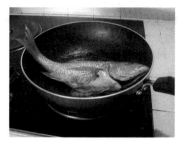

Red Snapper

Salmon (gùi yú; gwai yú/sà màhn yú) 鮭魚、沙文魚

Salmon can grow to be 26 to 30 inches long. Salmon flesh is firm, oily, and moist with a distinct flavor. The orangy-pink color is often referred to as "salmon" color. The big salmon head is used for making fish head soup in Mediterranean cooking. It can be used as a substitute for the big fish head in Cantonese soup recipes, though the color and flavor of the flesh is different. It is rich in calcium, omega-3 essential fatty acids, and other minerals, as well as collagens.

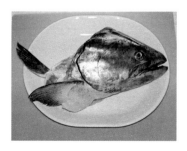

Salmon Head

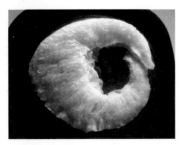

Shark's Fin

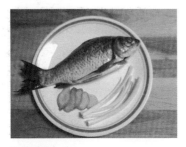

Reconstituted Shark's Fin

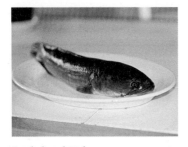

Silver Carp

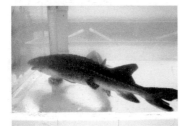

Snakehead Fish

Shark's Fin (yú cì; yùh chi) 魚翅

Shark's fins are the dried and processed dorsal and tailfins of large sharks, such as the white bleeker shark and the gray zebra shark. The hard bones are removed, leaving the golden-colored cartilage in the form of a whole fin or compacted loosely into a 6-ounce block. Depending on size and quality, shark's fin costs, on average, about $110 per pound. To prepare for soup, first soak the dried fin in cold water for 1 hour, before blanching in a pot of boiling water for a few minutes. This process needs to be repeated at least three times. After soaking, it looks like a bundle of translucent gelatin needles. After cooking, the texture of the shark's fin should be smooth and bouncy between the teeth. Shark's fin also comes in quick-frozen packages, which are the easiest to work with. Available in Chinese grocery stores, frozen fin costs about $100 a piece in 2008. Shark's fin soup is a must at Chinese wedding banquets and celebrations, though it is a very expensive ingredient.

Silver Carp (yíng jí; ngàhn jīk) 銀鯽

Silver carp is found in the fresh waters of the Pearl River. Like most fish in the carp family, it is very bony and should be browned on both sides before boiling inside a gauze bag. Commonly cooked with ginger to reduce the strong, earthy taste, silver carp is traditionally used to combat fatigue and tonify the spleen.

Snakehead Fish (shēng yú; sàang yú) 生魚

Snakeheads are popular freshwater fish in Southeast Asia and Southern China, reputed to help heal wounds, such as incisions from surgery. In the United States, frozen snakeheads, whole or in round cutlets, are imported from Vietnam. Frozen snakehead has a strong smell like mackerel, a coarse texture, and is rather tasteless. I wonder if fresh snakehead fish tastes any better. Maybe that is why it was never served in my family, aside from the fact that no one from my family has ever had surgery.

Sturgeon (xún lóng; chàhm lùhng) 鱘龍

This ancient fish of the family Acipenseridae was in existence at the time of the dinosaurs. Sturgeon are the biggest fresh- and saltwater ganoid fish, reportedly growing up to six meters (approximately 20 feet) in length and weighing as much as 3,200 kilograms (over 7,000 pounds). On average, sturgeon take ten to twelve years to mature and travel upstream to spawn. Sturgeon are valued for their flesh, their roe (caviar), and their air bladders prepared into

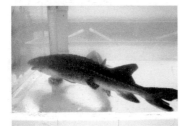

Sturgeon

fish maw. Once threatened with extinction, the Chinese sturgeon is experiencing a comeback in the Yangtze River, thanks to the annual effort to introduce 300,000 newly hatched fry since 1984.

In Chinese fish markets and Chinese seafood restaurants, live sturgeon weighing around 5 pounds are available. On order, the fillets will be carved out for steaming, braising, or stir-fry while the head, tail, and bone go into the soup pot, just the way one would prepare a good-sized grouper for a soup and a dish.

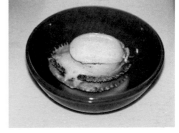

Abalone

Shellfish, Crustaceans, and Other Seafood 海鮮類

Abalone (bāo yú; bàau yùh) 鮑魚

Abalone is an expensive ingredient both fresh and dried, but is considered a must-have delicacy for Chinese feasts and festivities. A full-sized fresh abalone (more than 7 inches in diameter) is easily worth $50 in 2008. Dried abalone goes for about $20 per ounce. Fresh abalone must be pounded before slicing, and dried ones need to be soaked and cleaned. Abalone is a yin food, known for relieving dry coughs and fever.

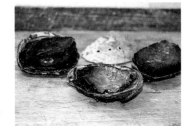

Fresh Abalone

Conch (lúo ròu; lòh tàuh) 螺肉、螺頭

The lustrous apricot-colored conch shell has six tiers, ending in a sharp point. Conch is cooling and said to brighten the eyes.

Conch comes in fresh, frozen, dried, or sliced forms in Asian grocery stores. Fresh or frozen are preferred for stir-frying and steaming. Make sure to get rid of the guts before using. Dried conch meat is good for making soup. It costs about $8.50 per 1-pound package. As the Queen Conch *(Strombus gigas)* is on the list of endangered species and international trade is heavily restricted, dried conch meat is often replaced by whelk meat in recipes.

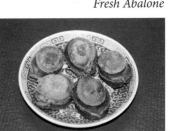

Dried Abalone

Crab (xiè; háaih) 蟹

Crab is sweet and salty. Their meat is ideal for salads, stews, stir-fries, and other dishes. It is always recommended to use high heat when stir-frying crab in the shell. Garlic and fermented black beans or ginger and green onion go well with crab. Crabmeat is used to complement fancy ingredients like fish maw, shark's fin, bamboo pipes and yellow chives in soups.

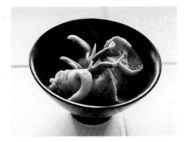

Conch Meat

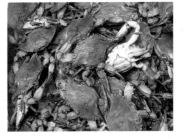

Crabs

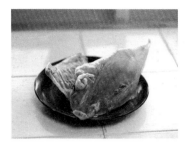

Dried Fish Maw

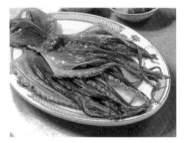

Reconstituted Dried Octopus

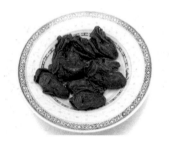

Dried Oysters

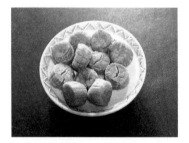

Dried Scallops

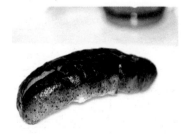

Reconstituted Sea Cucumber

Fish Maw (yú dǔ; yùh tóuh/fā gàau) 魚肚、花膠

Fish maw is the commercial term for the dried swim bladders of large fish like sturgeon. Fish maw has no fishy taste and absorbs the flavors of other ingredients. It is cleaned and dried before being deep-fried to make it puff up into a yellowish, translucent balloon. It must be soaked for hours (often overnight), rinsed, and cut into pieces before being used in a soup. Fish maw is a good source of collagen, which is good for skin beauty. People use fish maw in soups or stews instead of shark's fin and bird's nest, which are sky-high in price, though fish maw itself is not exactly cheap. Depending on size and quality, one piece may cost anywhere from $40 to $100.

Lobster (lóng xiā; lùhng hā) 龍蝦

Literally the "dragon-shrimp" in Chinese, a lobster is indeed the largest crustacean. Chinese people love its flavor but often find its texture a bit too tough. In general, crabmeat and shrimp are preferred in soups.

Octopus, Dried (zhāng yú; jèung yùh) 鱆魚

Dried octopus is considered an energy tonic food and is paired with lotus root in a classic soup recipe. It is traditionally served to the underweight.

Oyster, Dried (háo shì; hòuh sí) 蠔豉

Dark brown in color, dried oysters come in many sizes. They must be soaked in water until soft (2 to 4 hours, depending on quality) and cleaned before being used in soups. The soaking water is commonly saved for its flavor but may have some grit in it, which should be strained out.

Scallop, Dried (gān bèi; gōng yìuh chyúh) 干貝、江珧柱

Scallops turn a golden yellow color when dried. They are expensive, but the budget-conscious can buy broken or quartered dried scallops, which are just as tasty. Soak for 2 hours in cold water and then shred. Traditional Chinese cooks always save the water in which the dried scallops are soaked; it is very flavorful and is used in making soup or sauce.

Sea Cucumber (hǎi shēn; hói sàm) 海參

Found along the coast of Northern China, sea cucumbers are sold dried in Chinese grocery stores and must be soaked in both warm water and boiling water. Repeat several times to remove the chalky taste. They taste like gelatinous seawater and are used to stop bleeding. Sea cucumbers are expensive, fresh or dried.

Shrimp, Dried (xiā mǐ; hà máih) 蝦米

Dried shrimp are salty to the taste. They can be used for cooking and snacking. Fresh dried shrimp are pink or orange in color. They can be kept for months if stored in jars under refrigeration. Stale ones turn grey.

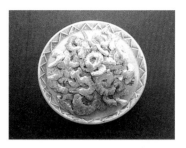

Dried Shrimp

Shrimp/Prawns (xiā; hā) 蝦

Fresh or frozen shrimp and prawns are sweet and available in many sizes. Shrimp are smaller, at 26 or more count to the pound, while prawns are bigger, with 25 or fewer to the pound. Even those at the seafood counter of the supermarket are usually pre-frozen and should not be frozen again. Mixing shrimp or prawns with some salt for 15 to 20 minutes and then rinsing them before cooking will help improve their texture and mouthfeel.

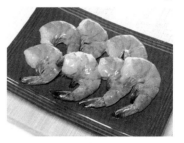

Prawns

Others 其他

Frog (qīng wā; tìhn gāi) 青蛙、田雞

The Cantonese name for frogs is tìhn gāi, literally "chicken of the rice paddies." Frozen frog legs are available in the United States, but Chinese gourmets swear by the fresh frog, claiming that its flavor and texture are superior.

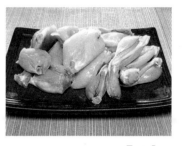

Frog Legs

Pipe-Fish, Dried (hǎi long; hói lùhng) 海龍

Called "sea dragon" in Chinese, the pipe-fish is a small fish encased in bony plates just like the seahorse. It tonifies the Kidneys and strengthens yang for the elderly. Pipe-fish is said to reduce swelling and dissipates nodules from scrofula.

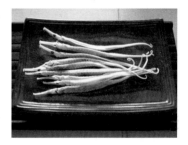

Dried Pipe Fish

Seahorse, Dried (hǎi mǎ; hói máh) 海馬

A seahorse, of the genus Hippocampus of small fish encased in bony plates (at most 5 inches in height), carries its body vertically. With its head angled downward and a curly prehensile tail, a seahorse looks like a miniature horse. The Chinese have used dried seahorses as medicine for centuries and cook them in soups. Dried seahorses can be purchased in Chinese herb stores. Traditionally used to treat asthma and impotence, seahorse soups are also said to help reduce cholesterol. Seahorse is often used with dried pipe-fish, called "sea dragon" in Chinese, in making tonic soups. Seahorse tonifies the Kidneys and fortifies yang. It also invigorates the blood, reducing blood stasis and swelling manifested as sores, boils, and abdominal masses.

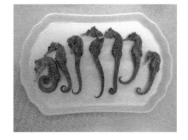

Dried Seahorses

Snake (shé; sèh) 蛇

Snake is considered a tonic for the fall and winter. The Cantonese include a venomous snake such as an agkistrodon or a bungarus to make a popular autumn tonic soup. As snake meat is not readily available in Chinese grocery stores in the U.S., I have not included a recipe.

Softshell Turtles (biē; biht seui yu) 鱉、水魚

Softshell turtles, belonging to the Trionychidae family, are fresh water turtles, though they can adapt to brackish waters. They are basically carnivorous, feeding on aquatic insects, worms, small fish, crustaceans, snails, and amphibians. Their carapace color tends to match the substrate (mud or sand) color of their natural habitat. The underside is of a lighter color.

Softshell turtles are treated as a delicacy in most parts of the world, particularly in East Asia. Turtle soup is also known in European cuisine, though sea turtles are used. In Panama, sea turtles are farmed and their meat is canned and exported to Europe.

The Chinese government has declared Chinese softshell turtles, *Pelodiscus sinensis,* to be Class II endangered species. I chose not to include a turtle soup recipe, in deference to wildlife protection.

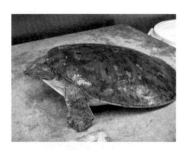

Soft Shell Turtle

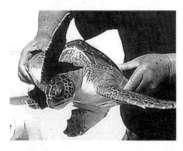

Sea Turtle in Turtle Farm on Cayman Island, Panama

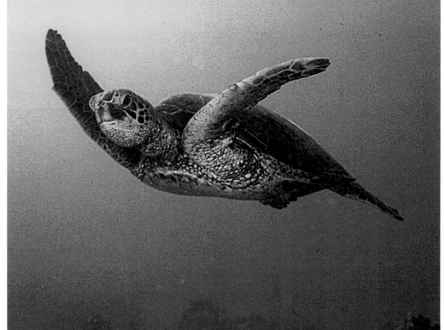

Sea Turtle, Hawaii

PHOTO BY BEN CLARK

8
Plant Sources

~~~~~~~~~~

Vegetables and Fruit 蔬菜、水果

Amaranth (xiàn cài; yihn choi) 莧菜

Also known as "pigweed," amaranth is valued in China as a summer leaf vegetable. The colors of the Chinese varieties are green, purple, or bi-color, the latter two yielding beautiful magenta-colored juice when cooked. Once gathered in the wild, amaranth is now cultivated in arid areas in subtropical regions. Amaranth seeds are abundant and provide a good source of protein, but the Chinese have not yet tapped into this natural resource.

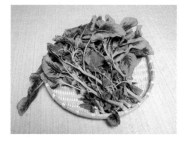

Amaranth

Apple (píng gǔo; pìhng gwó) 蘋果

It's true what they say: "An apple a day keeps the doctor away." Apples are low in calories and high in dietary soluble fibers that help lower cholesterol. A fresh apple is an ideal snack because it is filling. Biting and chewing an apple will stimulate the gum and increase the flow of saliva, helping lower the chance of tooth decay.

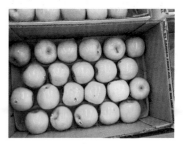

Apple

Arrowhead (cí gū; chìh gū) 慈菇

Sagittaria sagittifolia is commonly called arrowhead due to the shape of its leaves. This aquatic plant grows in shallow water in wetlands, with the arrowhead-shaped leaves rising above water surface at the end of long stems. Its round starchy tuber is edible. In North America, Native Americans used to eat them. Waterfowl, especially diving ducks, feed extensively on the young shoots and tubers, also known as "duck potatoes." Each plant produces twelve to sixteen tubers, which are harvested in the winter. The tuber is roundish with a shoot at the top resembling a phallus.

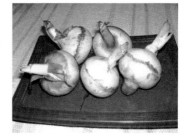

Arrowhead

In Chinese cuisine, the tuber is sliced and used as a vegetable in stir-fries. Crunchy and somewhat bland, the arrowhead tuber is similar to potato in texture as well. The tuber is always included in a Chinese New Year dish or soup, largely because of the tuber's shape, to express the wish of a society that values male offspring.

~~~~~~

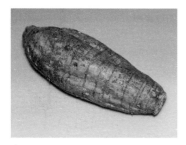

Arrowroot

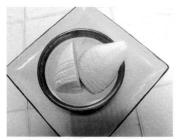

Asparagus

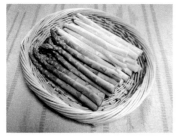

Bamboo Shoot

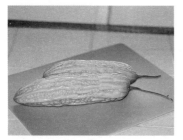

Bitter Melon

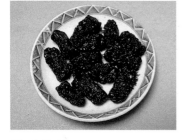

Black Date

Arrowroot (fěn gé; fán gót) 粉葛

The starchy arrowroot is known for alleviating coughs. Its powder is commonly used as a sauce thickener like cornstarch. Fresh arrowroots and dried arrowroot slices are available only in Asian markets, while arrowroot powder may be found in the spice section of any supermarket.

Asparagus (lú sǔn; lòuh séun) 蘆筍

Asparagus belongs to the lily family. Lightly boiled or stir-fried asparagus makes a tasty appetizer or side dish. It is also good in soups. Asparagus should be eaten as soon as it is cut, because it loses half of its vitamin C and its flavor in the first two or three days. Gout sufferers should avoid asparagus because it causes painful attacks. This is probably due to its various degradation products that contain sulfur and ammonia.

The United States is the world's largest asparagus producer, yielding 90,200 tons on 54,000 acres in 2005. The U.S. is also the world's largest asparagus consumer, importing 92,405 tons in 2004. Asparagus production in California's Sacramento-San Joaquin River Delta region is significant enough for the city of Stockton to hold an annual Asparagus Festival every April.

Bamboo Shoots (zhú sǔn; júk séun/dùng séun) 竹筍、冬筍

Bamboo shoots can be obtained young and fresh in Chinese grocery stores, but in the U.S. they are most available in cans. The fresh ones have layers of brownish-white skin that need to be peeled off. The center is crunchy in texture and is delicious in soups and stir-fry dishes. If fresh bamboo shoots are not available, canned ones can serve the same purpose. High in fiber, bamboo shoots are good for weight loss and cleansing.

Bitter Melon (kǔ guā; fú gwā) 苦瓜

The unique taste of this aptly named vegetable comes from quinine, an anti-malarial mineral also found in tonic water. The greener the ridged, elongated melon, the more bitter the taste. It is especially refreshing in hot weather and makes a good summer soup.

Black Date, Dried (hēi zǎo; haak jóu) 黑棗

Black dates are derived from red jujube dates with special processing. They are considered more warming than the red ones and more effective in female tonics. Black dates should always be pitted before use.

Black Moss (fǎ cài; faat choi) 髮菜

A hair-like moss, its name sounding like fat choy, which means "prosperity" in Cantonese, is a favorite in New Year's dishes. Because of the insatiable demands of gourmets, the black moss is now an endangered species. Gathering and exporting it is prohibited by the Chinese government. It costs about $10 per ½-ounce package and, even at this price, one must beware of fakes, which might be nothing more than dyed cornsilk.

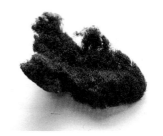

Black Moss

Bok Choy (See Chinese Cabbage) 白菜

Broccoli (lü cài huā; sài làahn fā) 西蘭花

Broccoli is one of the most nutritious vegetables. It is rich in beta carotene, potassium, calcium, iron, and vitamins C and E. It is also low in calories. Broccoli is believed to play an important role in cancer prevention by removing carcinogens before they damage cells and trigger the growth of tumors. Broccoli is available year-round and can be eaten raw. Steaming or stir-frying broccoli will retain most of the nutrients. Its florets are good in a quickly cooked summer soup. Overcooking will produce an unpleasant earthy taste.

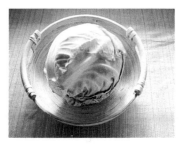

Bok Choy

Cabbage (juǎn xīn cài; yèh choi) 卷心菜、椰菜

Cabbage is rich in potassium, vitamin C, and fiber and low in calories. It is said to prevent colon cancer and its juice to heal peptic ulcer. Cabbage is good in salads, soups, and stir-fries. It is not advisable to cook cabbage in an aluminum pan, which will alter its color and flavor.

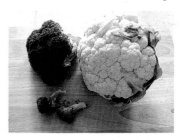

Cabbage

Cauliflower (bái cài huā; yèh choi fā) 椰菜花

Cauliflower is a cancer-fighting vegetable that is low in calories, high in fiber, and rich in potassium and vitamin C. A white head with crisp green leaves signifies a fresh cauliflower. They are good for stir-fries, salads, and soups. Cauliflower is recommended as a substitute for potatoes in a low carbohydrate diet.

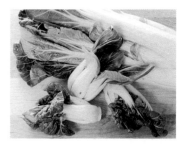

Broccoli and Cauliflower

Cereus Flower (bà wáng huā; ba wòhng fā) 霸王花

These are the edible blossoms of the night-blooming cereus, also known as the "triangular cactus" (hylocereus undatus, san jiao lian 三角蓮), and of the broadleaf cactus (epiphyllum oxypetalum, tan hua 曇花). They both originate in Brazil. The colossal white flowers turn yellow when dried. They are edible and sour in taste. Sold in packages in Chinese grocery stores, cereus

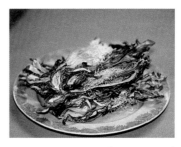

Cereus Flowers, Dried

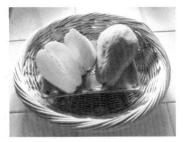

Chayote

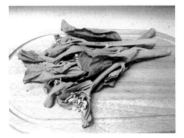

Chinese Broccoli

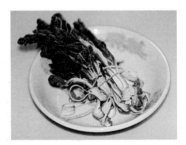

Chinese Cabbage, Dried

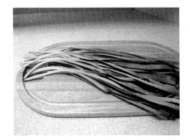

Chinese Chives

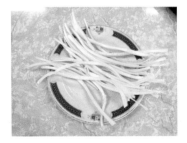

Yellow Chives

flowers should be soaked before cooking in soup. They are traditionally used to clear phlegm and strengthen the lungs. The fresh blossoms can also be used in soups.

Chayote (hè zhǎng guā; hahp jéung gwā) 合掌瓜

The chayote belongs to the gourd family with cucumbers, melons, and squash. Not a native plant of China, it has become a favorite of Chinese-Americans because of its soothing and lubricating qualities that tonify the lungs. Chayotes are harvested in the fall.

Chinese Broccoli (jiè lán; gaai láan) 芥蘭

Chinese broccoli has narrow stems, small flower heads, and a slightly bitter taste. They are used stir-fried or simply blanched. Adding some sugar and oil into the water during boiling will help give it a bright green color. The tender tips are quickly boiled and served with soup noodles.

Chinese Cabbage (bái cài; baahk choi) 白菜

Also known as bok choy, this leafy vegetable has white stalks and dark green leaves. It is rich in calcium and best in winter and spring. It is also available in dried form known as choi gon 菜乾 in Cantonese.

Chinese Cabbage, Dried (cài gān; choi gōn) 菜乾

Before cooking, choi gon needs to be soaked overnight until soft. It should be rinsed thoroughly to get rid of grit. The dried and fresh versions of bok choy are frequently paired in soups, called the "gold (yellow) and silver (white) cabbage" (gàm ngàhn choi 金銀菜).

Chinese Chive (jiǔ cài; gáu choi) 韭菜

Also known as garlic chive, Chinese chive belong to the allium family with garlic, onion, leek, and scallion. It has a pungent flavor. All year round we can snip off the green leaves for food. Toward the end of summer, flower stalks will shoot up. Before the cluster of small white flowers open, the tender stalk with the bud sac can be cut for stir-fries. It is a seasonal delicacy.

When Chinese chive plants are covered up and deprived of sunlight, tender new shoots that come up become yellowish and whitish in color. These yellow chives (gáu wòhng 韭黄) are a delicacy available mostly during the spring and summer growing season.

Cilantro (yuán xū; yùhn sāi) 芫荽

Cilantro looks like Italian parsley, so it is sometimes called Chinese parsley. Chinese use cilantro for garnishing as well as in soups with specific anti-pyretic purposes.

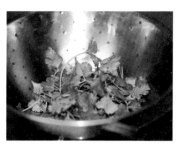

Cilantro

Cucumber (huáng guā; wòhng gwā) 黃瓜

Cucumber belongs to the same family as melons, pumpkins, and squash. Besides using as a salad ingredient or as pickles, people put cucumber slices on the face as a remedy for skin blemishes. The Cantonese people also stir-fry or quick-boil sliced cucumbers in summer soups.

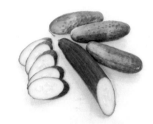

Cucumber

Dragon-Eye Fruit, Dried (lóng yǎn; lùhng ngáahn/lùhng ngáahn yuhk) 龍眼肉

Within a thin, brown shell lies a layer of sweet white flesh covering a black pit, hence the name dragon-eye, which is lùhng ngáahn in Cantonese. In the West it is referred to as the longan fruit. The fruit can be eaten raw like a lychee. When dried, the meat turns reddish brown. It is sold in packages already shelled and pitted. Its shelf life is short. Keep refrigerated in a jar and use before the meat turns dark. Each pitted fruit is counted as one piece in the recipes.

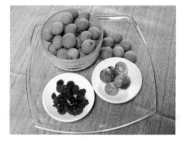

Dragon-Eye or Longan Fruit

Figs, Dried (wú huā guǒ; mòuh fà gwó) 無花果

Unlike Western dried figs, Chinese dried figs are pale in color and not very sweet. Figs have many tiny edible seeds inside. If necessary, substitute with Western dried figs, but use less as Western dried figs are significantly sweeter.

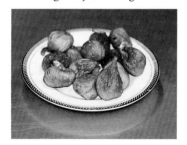

Figs, Dried

Fuzzy Melon (máo guā; mòu gwā/jit gwā) 毛瓜、節瓜

This summer squash, covered with short prickly fuzz, comes in two varieties. The readily available kind in the U.S. is shaped like a fat cucumber. The other variety, grown mostly in Southern China, is shorter and more globular in shape. The Chinese prefer the shorter kind, claiming that it tastes sweeter. Specialty farmers in California grow them locally. It is the favorite summer squash of the Cantonese people.

Garland Chrysanthemum (tóng hāo; tòhng hōu) 茼蒿

The edible chrysanthemum green is a leaf vegetable known as tóng hāo 茼蒿 in Chinese and as shungiku 春菊 in Japanese. It is popular in Cantonese cuisine, especially in hot pot cooking. It is used similarly in Japanese hot

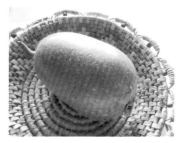

Fuzzy Melon

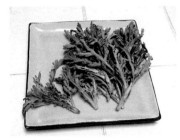

Garland Chrysanthemum

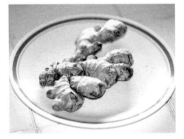

Garlic

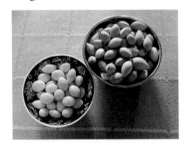

Ginger Root

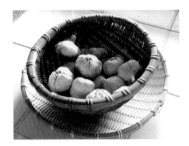

Gingko Nuts

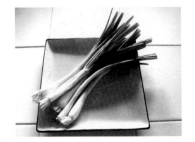

Green Onion

pot, referred to as nabemono. Chrysanthemum coronarium goes quickly into flowering in warm spring weather so the vegetable is at its best during mild and slightly cold winter months in Southern China.

Garlic (suàn; syun) 蒜

Garlic is one of the most important seasonings in Chinese cooking. It improves the flavor of both meat and vegetables. Garlic is a must for braising beef, mutton, and liver. Some vegetables, like eggplant and water spinach, actually require cooking with garlic to deactivate allergens that some people are sensitive to. Peeled garlic can be saved for a long time, dropped into a jar of hot oil and then kept in the refrigerator after the oil cools.

Ginger Root (shēng jiāng; sàang gèung) 生薑

Ginger root is a warming food. Fresh ginger helps eliminate the fishy smell in seafood and improve the flavor of meat. A ginger tea also helps with nausea and chills. Young ginger, which is pale yellow with pink-tipped shoots, is mild in flavor and usually pickled in sweet vinegar. The more commonly available ginger has rough, dry skin and is more fibrous. It is available year-round. When an herbal formula or a soup recipe calls for fresh ginger, never substitute with ginger powder. Cleaned fresh ginger can be kept in a jar of dry sherry in the refrigerator for up to six months. The soaking wine is great for cooking.

Gingko Nut (yín xìng; baahk gwó) 銀杏、白果

Not to be confused with gingko biloba, which is derived from the leaves of the gingko tree, gingko nuts are the fruit from the female tree. Before cooking, fresh gingko nuts have to be shelled. The hard shell is cracked and the inner skin is removed by placing the nuts in boiling water for a few minutes. Remove the embryo as well. The yellow nut is slightly bitter and toxic and should not be eaten raw. Do not eat a lot at one time.

Goji Berries (See Wolfberries)

Goji Leaves (See Wolfberry Leaves)

Green Onion (cōng; chūng) 蔥

Green onion belongs to the onion family. It is pungent and mildly bitter in flavor, and, paired with ginger, is one of the main seasonings in Chinese cuisine.

Steamed fish and chicken simply do not taste right without them. In combination with ginger or unsalted fermented black bean, green onion helps to treat flu or cold at the incipient stage. It is a remedy for diarrhea and abdominal discomfort as well. Green onion can be cut in sections, in shreds, or finely chopped for cooking or as garnish in soups.

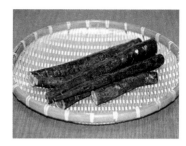

Greater Burdock Root

Greater Burdock (níu bàng; ngàuh bong) 牛蒡

Greater burdock is cultivated for its root. Given the proper conditions of full sun and loosened soil rich in humus and nitrogen, the fleshy taproot can reach 3 feet in length. It tastes somewhat like the artichoke to which it is related. In the last fifty years, the burdock root has become increasingly popular because of the advocacy for the macrobiotic diet. It is low in calories but high in dietary fiber, calcium, potassium, and amino acids.

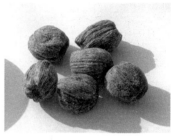

Honey Date

Honey Date (mì zǎo; maht jóu) 蜜棗

The sweet, brown date is the result of preserving fresh jujube dates in honey. Its pit does not need to be removed before cooking. In Chinese grocery stores, honey dates are commonly sold prepackaged. They are said to lubricate the lungs and stop coughing.

Jujube Date (dà zǎo; hòhng jóu) 大棗、紅棗

The jujube date is not really a date. The fresh fruit is crunchy like an apple and can be eaten raw. Upon drying, the skin reddens and the fruit shrivels. They are commonly sold pitted. A mild sedative, they are added to potent soups, such as ginseng soup, to slow down absorption into the body.

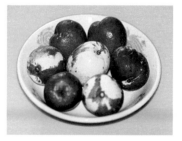

Jujube Date, Fresh

Kabocha Pumpkin (nán guā; fāan gwā) 南瓜、番瓜

An Asian variety of the pumpkin, the kabocha is rich in beta-carotene, vitamin C, potassium, and dietary fiber. It is good for soup, stew, and dessert. The seeds are edible and are a good source of protein. Kabocha pumpkins can be saved for more than a month if stored in a cool, dry place.

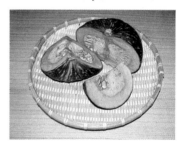

Kabocha Pumpkin

Lily Bulbs (bǎi hé; baak hahp) 百合

The scaly bulbs of fragrant Easter lilies and other oriental lilies are harvested in late fall. Once separated and dried, the scales turn ivory in color. Available in Chinese grocery stores and herb shops, they should be added to soups in the last 30 minutes of cooking if you want them to retain their shape. When in season, fresh lily bulbs are wonderful in stir-fries and soups.

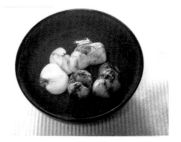

Lily Bulb, Fresh

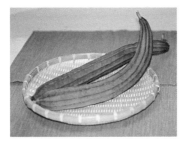

Loofah Squash

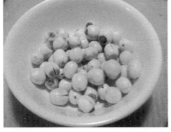

Lotus Root

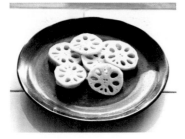

Cross-section of Lotus Root

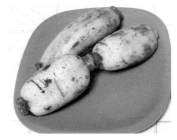

Lotus Seeds

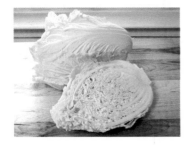

Napa Cabbage

Longan Fruit (See Dragon-Eye Fruit)

Loofah Squash (sī guā; sī gwā) 絲瓜

The loofah squash has dark green skin and prominent ribs that must be peeled. It is sweet tasting and has a tender texture like zucchini. It makes wonderful summer soups and stir-fry dishes. The loofah squash has to be picked when tender. Upon maturity, the inside fiber hardens to the loofah we use for scrubbing.

In some Cantonese dialects, *si* sounds like *syu,* which means "to lose." Gamblers euphemize the name of loofah squash to *sing gwa* 勝瓜, with *sing* meaning, "to win."

Lotus Root (lián ǒu; lìhn ngáuh) 蓮藕

The lotus is a perennial aquatic plant, cultivated in lakes and ponds. It is farmed on acres of marshy land in the Pearl River Delta. The root is long, with multiple sections. When cut into thin slices, the lotus root reveals a beautiful pattern of holes. It has a cooling nature when used raw, but is slightly warming when cooked. When intended for soup or stew, it is best to choose more mature roots.

Lotus Seeds (lián zǐ; ìihn jí) 蓮子

When in season, fresh lotus seeds are available in the pod. The rest of the year, they are available dried, either whole with a dark green embryo inside, or halved. Dried lotus seeds are cream colored. Slightly sweet, they are used to treat an upset stomach and are said to tonify the heart, kidney, and spleen. They are also said to treat impotence.

Lycii Berry (See Wolfberry)

Lycii Leaves (See Wolfberry Leaves) 枸杞葉

Napa Cabbage (dà bái cài; wòhng ngàah baahk) 大白菜、 黄芽白

Napa cabbage is a variety of Chinese cabbage, Napa being the Japanese name for this Chinese cabbage. It is big and oval with ruffled, pale green leaves and firm white stems. It is available year-round in California and can be bought in supermarkets. It is excellent for soups, stir-fries, and many Chinese vegetarian dishes.

Onion (yáng cōng; yèuhng chūng) 洋蔥

Onions come in many sizes, colors, and flavors. They should not be stored near potatoes, which give off moisture and a gas that causes onions to spoil. Onions are good for stir-fries, soups, and stews in Chinese cooking. For best results, always sauté onion before adding it to a soup or stew.

Papaya (mù guā; muhk gwā) 木瓜

Both ripe and green papayas are used in fish soups. Papaya aids digestion and is said to increase milk production in nursing mothers. Sun-dried green papaya powder is used as a meat tenderizer, as well as a medicine to treat intestinal worms.

Pear (lí zi; léi) 梨

Pear is a good source of vitamin C and dietary fiber. Most of the Vitamin C is concentrated in the skin, so pears should be eaten unpeeled. It has a smooth texture, and is ideal for snacks and dessert. A pear steamed with fritillary bulbs is effective for soothing sore throats and to stop coughing.

Potato (yáng shān yù; syùh jái) 洋山芋、 薯仔

The Mandarin term for potatoes, yang shan yu 洋山芋, tells of its origin across the ocean from the Americas, probably as early as the sixteenth century when Portuguese and Spanish ships arrived at Asian shores. Potatoes must be cooked before eating and are good for salads, soups, and stews. Old potatoes with buds coming up become toxic and must be discarded.

Rue (chòu cǎo; chau chóu) 臭草

Rue is an herb with a strong disagreeable odor, though its foliage is rather attractive. People grow rue in the garden as an insect and pest repellant. A sweet mung bean soup with kelp and a few sprigs of rue cleanses the system and acts as a remedy for acne. Dried rue is sold in herb stores, if fresh rue is not available.

Shepherd's Purse (qí cài; chàih choi) 薺菜

This is a common wild herb found in the Yangtze River delta in springtime. As the leaves are tiny, they are usually chopped up and mixed in with other minced ingredients to make filling for wonton and buns. These goodies belong to Shanghai cuisine, but have become popular in Hong Kong and, recently, in the United States. Now cultivated varieties are grown in China and available frozen (liked chopped spinach) overseas.

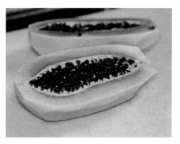

Papaya

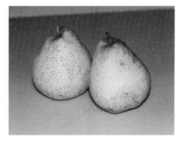

Pear

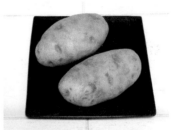

Potato

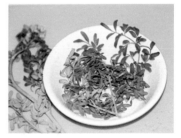

Rue

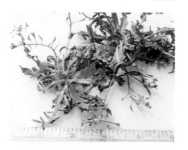

Shepherd's Purse

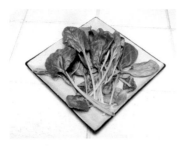

Spinach

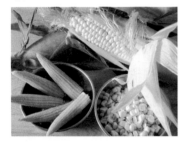

Sweet Corn

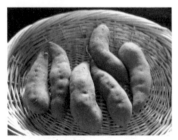

Sweet Potato

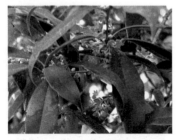

Sweet Osmanthus in Bloom

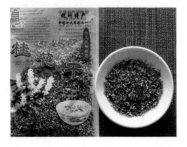

Sweet Osmanthus Flowers, Dried

Spinach (bō cài; bō choi) 菠菜

Spinach is rich in iron and potassium. It can be eaten raw in salads or cooked in soups and stir-fries. Like all dark leafy vegetables, spinach is believed to be beneficial in preventing cancer. Avoid overcooking to preserve color, texture, and flavor and to minimize the loss of nutrients and vitamins.

Sweet Corn (yù mì; yuhk máih/sūk mái) 玉米、粟米

Sweet corn is the only variety of maize used in Cantonese soups. Dent corn, also called field corn, from which cornmeal is made, is never adopted in Cantonese cuisine. Corn kernels are cut from the cob and made into a thickened sweet corn soup. Or, the corn on the cob may be cut into 2-inch sections to boil in a soup. Tender baby corncobs are used whole in stir-fries and in soups. As sweet corn begins to lose its flavor soon after it is picked, use the ears right away.

Sweet Potato (fān shú; fàan syú) 番薯

The sweet potato (Ipomoea batatas) is commonly called a yam in some parts of the United States, causing confusion with the true yam (Dioscorea) native to China and Africa. In Chinese, sweet potatoes are called faan syu 番薯, literally "yam of foreign origin," because they are native to the tropical Americas. Sweet potatoes are an excellent source of beta-carotene, an antioxidant precursor to vitamin A, and a good source of starch and potassium. The tender leaves and shoots are eaten as greens. The tuberous root is long and tapered, with flesh color ranging from white, yellow, or orange to purple. During hard times sweet potatoes are cooked alone or mixed with rice as main staple. They are also made into a sweet soup, with or without added sugar.

Sweet Osmanthus Flowers (gùi huā; gwai fā) 桂花

The Sweet Osmanthus (also known as sweet olive) is an evergreen shrub or small tree that grows to five to twelve meters (between 16 and 40 feet) tall. The Latin name is Osmanthus fragrans. Sweet osmanthus is native to southwestern parts of China, where more than twenty cities claim it as their city flower. It has small, shiny oval leaves and tiny flowers that grow in clusters, with colors ranging between white, yellow, and orange. The flowers (also called "cassia flowers" by tour de force translation) are tiny (one centimeter long), with a four-lobed corolla and a delicious fragrance, even when dried, somewhat like the scent of ripe peaches or apricots. They bloom around mid-autumn. In Chinese cuisine, fresh and dried sweet osmanthus flowers are used in teas and soups with dumplings. They are also used to flavor pastry, candies, and wine. Dried osmanthus flowers come in packages, available in some choice Asian markets.

Taro Root (yù tóu; wuh táu) 芋頭

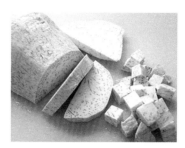

Taro Root

There are two types of taro root in Asian grocery stores. One is the size of a football while the other, the size of an egg. The large taro is good for stews. The small taro has a more delicate texture and is good for sweet soups. Some people have to wear gloves when peeling taro roots because raw taro may cause itchiness.

Tigerlily Buds (jīn zhēn; gām jàm) 金針

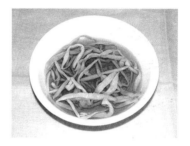

Tigerlily Buds

Dried tigerlily buds are golden or light brown in color. They have bumps at their ends, which should be removed after soaking. For presentation, they may be tied in knots before cooking.

Tomato (fān qié; fāan ké) 番茄

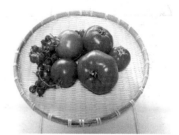

Tomato

Tomatoes are one of the world's leading vegetable crops. Tomatoes can be eaten raw or cooked and are wonderful in salads, soups, stews, and sandwiches. The most popular commercially prepared condiment is probably the tomato-based ketchup. The lycopene in tomato sauce is cancer preventing.

Turnip, Chinese (lúo bó; lòh baahk) 蘿蔔

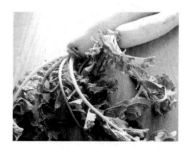

Chinese Turnip/Daikon

Technically a radish, the Chinese turnip is similar to the Japanese daikon. Both are white and approximately the same texture and size. They can be used interchangeably, though some insist that the Chinese turnip is more flavorful. It is also called the white turnip (bái lúo bó; baahk lòh baahk) 白蘿蔔 to distinguish it from the green one and from the carrot, which is called hùhng lòh baahk 紅蘿蔔 in Cantonese, literally the "red turnip."

The Chinese do not have a taste for real turnips. Fresh turnip, specifically the round knobby rutabaga, is made into Sichuan-style preserved turnip (see Sichuan Preserved Turnips on page 114).

Turnip, Green (qīng lúo bó; chèng lòh baahk) 青蘿蔔

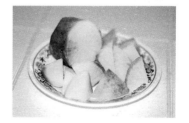

Green Turnip

About half the size of a daikon, this chubby root is distinguished by its dark green skin and bright green flesh. Technically a radish, it tastes more like a radish than a turnip. It can be used interchangeably with daikon or Chinese turnip. Its bright green color is used to create colorful soups in the company of carrot and/or white turnip.

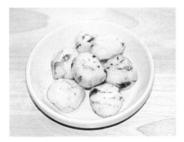

Peeled Water Chestnuts

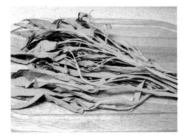

Water Spinach

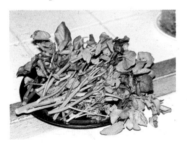

Watercress

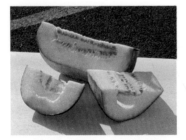

Winter Melon

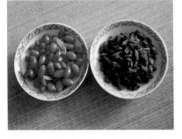

Wolfberries, Fresh and Dried

Water Chestnuts (bí qí; buht chàih/máh tái) 荸薺、馬蹄

Water chestnuts come to the market fresh or in cans. They are chestnut brown and about the size of walnuts. Fresh water chestnuts should be firm when pressed and the meat should not have turned yellow. They have a mild sweet taste. They are used mostly for soups and stir-fries. Most of the time, water chestnuts are peeled before using, but they can be boiled whole. The skin comes easily off a boiled water chestnut, like the shell of a cooked prawn.

Water Spinach (kōng xīn cài; ung choi) 空心菜、蕹菜

Water spinach is sweet in flavor and slightly cold in nature. Cantonese always cook water spinach with garlic, even in soups.

Watercress (xī yáng cài; sài yèuhng choi) 西洋菜

This popular Chinese vegetable, with long stems and small rounded leaves, is sold in bunches. Watercress is rich in vitamin A, chlorophyll, sulphur, and calcium. Watercress grows in flowing water sources as far north as the hot springs in the Canadian Rockies. Watercress is cooling and pungent, sweet, and bitter. It influences the lungs, kidneys, and bladder. It helps dissolve yellowish phlegm due to heat condition of the lungs. Watercress is also diuretic and cleansing, clearing facial blemishes, and improves night vision.

Watercress can be eaten raw in a salad, slightly cooked, or slow-cooked for hours in a soup. In the latter case, cooking reduces the herb's cleansing properties, making it more digestible and nurturing, especially good for lung and qi deficiencies. The concentrated flavor of watercress in a louhfo soup is simply gastronomical.

Winter Melon (dōng guā; dūng gwā) 冬瓜

The most desirable winter melons are the mature ones. Look for a heavy dusting of white powder on the rind. They are mostly hollow with seeds attached to an inch-thick layer of flesh. When cooked, this flesh becomes translucent and is said to have a soothing effect on the body.

Wolfberries (gǒu jì zi; gáu géi jí/géi jí) 枸杞子、杞子

Wolfberries are also known as lycii berries and, more recently, as goji berries. The plant that bears fruit is a different variety from that grown for its nutritious leaves. Unless you grow them yourself, it is unlikely that you will find fresh wolfberries or goji berries in the U.S. (please see the entry for wolfberries under Medicinal Herbs on page 106 to learn more).

Wolfberry Leaves (gǒu jì; gáu géi) 枸杞葉、枸杞

Also known as lycii or goji leaves, the plant of the Chinese wolfberry is very thorny. The leaves are rich in iron and traditionally known to enhance liver function and improve eyesight. Wash and strip the leaves off the cut branches. Cook only briefly to retain its green color. This variety of wolfberry plant does not bear fruit and is propagated by cuttings only.

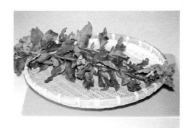

Wolfberry Leaves

Yam, Dried (fān shú gān; jyū jái syú) 豬仔薯

Commonly sold in oval slices, dried yams have a light tan peel and resemble flattened pieces of chalk. Instead of pre-soaking, dried yam can be directly reconstituted in soups during the cooking process. It is rather bland in taste. Like sweet potatoes, yams are used as meal stretchers.

Grains 穀類

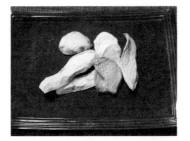

Dried Yam Slices

Brown Rice (zaò mǐ; chou máih) 糙米

Brown rice is obtained from the seeds of the rice plant by hulling or removing the outer husk of the grain. Nutritionally it is superior to white rice, which is the result of milling one step beyond brown rice and removing the bran with the germ, leading to the loss of many of the nutrients found in the whole grain.

Glutinous Rice (nuò mǐ; noh máih) 糯米

This is a variety of short-grain rice. It is sweet and sticky when cooked. Often, cooked sweet rice is pounded with wooden pestles into rice cakes. Glutinous rice powder is used to make dumplings. Glutinous rice also comes in a black variety. Black glutinous rice turns purple when it is cooked, hence its two interchangeable Chinese names: hei mi 黑米 "black rice" and zi mi 紫米 "purple rice." I like to regulate the shade of purple by mixing in some white rice to lighten and brighten it.

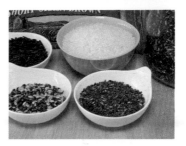

Rice: Brown, Red, Black, White

Job's Tears (See Pearl Barley)

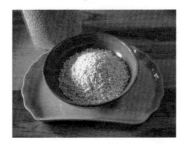

Glutinous Rice

Pearl Barley (yì yǐ rén; yi máih) 薏苡仁、薏米

The pearl barley commonly found in the United States is smaller and milder in flavor than Chinese pearl barley, but the two can be used interchangeably, and regular barley is also an acceptable substitute. Pearl barley is high in protein and is also available fermented into a liquor. A diuretic, pearl barley is used to reduce swelling. Both raw and roasted pearl barley are available in Chinese grocery and herb stores. I use only the raw variety for my soups.

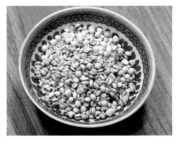

Pearl Barley

Rice (dà mǐ/mǐ; máih) 大米、米

Rice is a cereal crop, a grain belonging to the poaceae ("true grass") family. Rice is the main staple of many people in the world. The earliest cultivation or domestication of rice is placed at 3000 BCE in India and at 4500 BCE in China. Archaeologists also claim that dry-land rice farming predated rice growing in the wet alluvial plains of the Yangtze Delta by 1500 to 2000 years.

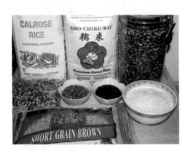

Ear of Rice Plant

Rice can be grown practically anywhere, even on a steep hillside, as long as there is water. To feed China's population, terraced fields have been developed to fully utilize every inch of arable land. The traditional method of flooding the fields or paddies reduces the growth of weeds, though it requires damming up and channeling the water for irrigation. Rice growing is very labor-intensive and requires plenty of water.

The major varieties of rice are long-grain and short-grain. Long-grain rice is less starchy than the short-grain variety. The long grains do not stick together, and they keep their form after cooking. This makes long-grains most suitable for making fried rice. Short-grain rice, on the other hand, is moist and sticky, more suitable for making rice porridge (juk 粥), food served to the sick, plain or mixed with a decoction of medicinal herbs. Juk is also a common breakfast food, served with Chinese pastry and dim sum, or with small side dishes, like pickled vegetables, nuts, XO sauce, and salted egg. Such a breakfast is called *ching juk siu choi* 清粥小菜, meaning "clear rice porridge with small dishes." A medium-grain rice is cultivated in Taiwan and Eastern China. The Taiwanese call it "Paradise Rice" (*Penglai mi* 蓬萊米). Though I am not sure where the medium-grain originated, it has become the favorite choice in China, Japan, and Korea. The medium-grain rice is ideal for making Japanese sushi. Rice can be ground into rice powder for making pastry and pasta.

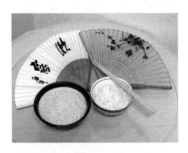

Varieties of Rice

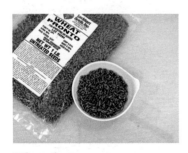

Rice, Raw and Cooked

Wheat (xiǎo mài; siú mahk/mahk) 小麥、麥

Wheat originated in the Fertile Crescent of Southwest Asia and reached China about 4000 years ago. In Northern China wheat grain is a staple food used to make flour, which in turn is made into noodles and other forms of pasta and pastry. Chinese vegetarians get gluten, a protein, from wheat and make it into various forms of imitation meat. For some unknown reason, one in every 100 or 200 persons in the United States is allergic to gluten. The white powder left behind after the gluten has been extracted is called dang mihn 澄麵 in Cantonese. It is used as a dim sum dough. The Cantonese also like to make wheat germ candy and a sweet soup with wheat berries and sweet rice.

Wheat Grains

Legumes 豆類

Aduki Beans (chì xiǎo dòu; chek síu dáu) 赤小豆

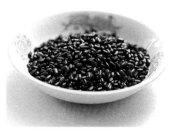

Aduki Beans

Also known as the adzuki bean, the aduki bean is not the same as the Chinese red bean, though they are similar in color and taste. Aduki beans are elongated in shape while Chinese red beans are round. Examine the beans instead of relying on the English label which may be misleading, as the term "red beans" is indiscriminately used to describe both types. In Japan, aduki beans are frequently sweetened and used in pastry. In China, aduki beans are used in soups with arrowroot to help with sore throat due to inflammation of the tonsils. Aduki beans strengthen the spleen and help dispel dampness manifested as edema in the lower limbs.

Black Beans (hēi dòu; haak dáu/wù dáu) 黑豆、烏豆

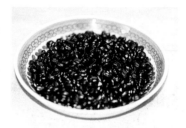

Black Beans

Chinese black beans are different from South American black beans. Chinese black beans are the mature black seeds of the soya plant. Chinese black beans are said to detoxify the kidney. As a soybean, undercooked black beans inhibit the digestive enzyme trypsin. It is advisable to pan-fry (without oil) black beans until they crack before cooking in a soup or stew. When black beans are fermented, they can be used as medicine, besides being made into soy sauce (also called soya sauce), black bean sauce, and other condiments.

Black-Eyed Peas (méi dòu; mèih dáu) 眉豆

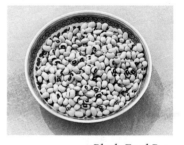

Black-Eyed Peas

Though originally from Africa, black-eyed peas have been cultivated in China since ancient times. They may be added directly to soup, but fare better if soaked overnight to eliminate flatulence-causing gas. Black-eyed peas are an excellent source of fiber and iron.

Hyacinth Beans (biǎn dòu; bín dáu) 扁豆

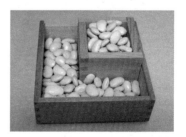

Hyacinth Beans

The hyacinth bean is sweet and neutral in properties. It helps to improve poor appetite and stop diarrhea and vomiting caused by summer heat. Dried hyacinth beans are available in Chinese grocery stores while fresh ones are in season only in late spring and early summer.

Mung Beans (lü dòu; luhk dáu) 綠豆

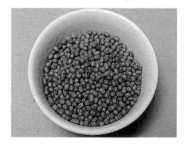

Mung Beans

Green mung beans are yellow when hulled. Mung beans are slightly sweet and especially popular in the summer, when their cooling properties help combat irritability and thirst. Mung bean paste can also be used for treating burns. The

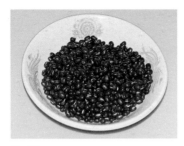

Red Beans

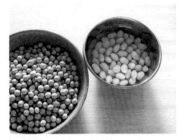

Soybeans, Dried and Soaked

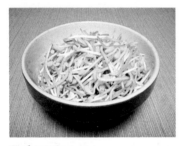

Soybean Sprouts

Chinese make noodles out of mung bean powder. The dried noodles come in sheets, flat, or thread-like (see Mung Bean Pasta on page 113). When reconstituted, mung bean noodles turn translucent.

Red Beans (chì dòu/hóng dòu; hùhng dáu) 赤豆、紅豆

The red bean is a more common variety of Phaseolus Calcaratus Roxb. While the elongated aduki bean is preferred for medicinal purposes, the rounder red bean is used for sweet dumplings and dessert soups in Chinese cuisine.

Soybeans (dà dòu; daaih dáu/wòhng dáu) 大豆、黃豆

The soybean is a legume. According to Traditional Chinese Medicine classification, soybean and soybean products have a heat-clearing nature. Soybeans moisten conditions of dryness. Soybeans have a high protein content (38 percent), more than cow's milk and without its saturated fat and cholesterol, making soy milk a superior substitute for cow's milk, especially for people who are lactose intolerant.

Raw soybeans are impossible to digest due to the inhibition of a digestive enzyme. Therefore, all soybeans, whether green and tender or mature and dried, yellow or black, have to be cooked. The processes for making soup and tofu, as well as the fermentation process for making bean paste and soy sauce, eliminate the trypsin-inhibiting effect.

Soybeans are rich in essential fatty acids (EFAs), including omega-3, which plays an important role in balancing the levels of low-density lipoproteins (LDLs) and high-density lipoproteins (HDLs). Unlike cholesterols, EFAs are not produced by the human body and must be obtained from dietary fats and oils. Soybean is also rich in isoflavones. Soy protein and isoflavones have been shown to protect the arteries, balance cholesterol, and aid in the prevention of breast and uterine cancer. Isoflavones also help with bone density, and maintaining libido and heart health. Soybeans and tofu are also desirable foods for people with diabetes.

Nuts and Seeds 硬殼果、果仁

Apricot Kernels (xìng rén; hahng yàhn) 杏仁

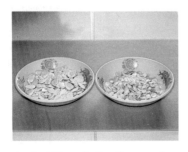

Apricot Kernels, Southern and Northern

Two kinds of apricot kernels are available in Chinese grocery and herb stores. The larger, longer kernels are from the South. The smaller, rounder kernels are from the North. Northern apricot kernels are mildly toxic and bitter and should be used sparingly. Throughout the text and recipes, I repeatedly use the descriptive label "small, Northern" to issue a warning. Please heed. When both the Southern and Northern varieties are called for in the same recipe, use in a ratio of four to one.

Chestnuts (lì zǐ; leuht jí) 栗子

The chestnut is a shelled seed, sweet in flavor and warm in nature. It can be eaten raw or cooked. According to TCM, chestnuts act to nourish the stomach, strengthen the spleen, and tonify the kidneys. Chestnuts ripen in late autumn. Dried chestnuts are available in Chinese grocery stores.

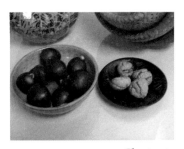
Chestnuts

Foxnuts (See entry under Medicinal Herbs on page 100)

Peanuts (huā shēng; fā sāng) 花生

In Chinese soups, peanuts are used shelled and blanched. They become very soft after boiling and are said to combat insomnia. Peanuts also help with lactation in nursing mothers.

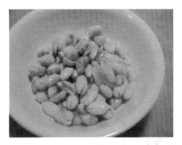
Peanuts, Shelled and Blanched

Pine Nuts (sōng zǐ; chùhng jí) 松子

In terms of TCM, pine nuts are sweet in flavor and warm in nature. They help to moisturize the lungs and lubricate the large intestine. Pine nut kernels may be eaten whole or ground into powder.

Sesame Seeds (zhī má; jì màh) 芝麻

Sesame seeds are one of the most common condiments in Asian cooking. They can be bought in supermarkets in the spice section. There are white and black varieties. They help tonify the liver and kidneys, and are said to be effective for blurred version, ringing ears, dizziness, and numbness of the arms and legs.

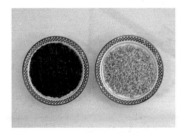
Sesame Seeds

Walnuts (hé táo; hahp tòuh) 核桃

Walnut kernels can be eaten raw or cooked. Walnuts are traditionally said to improve brainpower because the kernel resembles a human brain. In terms of modern nutrition, walnuts do contain a number of nutrients for the brain.

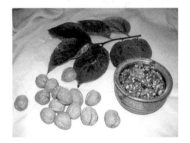
Walnuts and Kernels

Sea Vegetables 水藻類

Kelp (hǎi dài; hói daai) 海帶

The ribbon-like fronds of this giant seaweed or sea vegetable are especially popular in Japan (where it is known as kombu 昆布), and are air-dried after being collected from the sea. A common ingredient in lipstick and other cosmetics, kelp has a salty flavor and has a cooling effect on the body. Cantonese

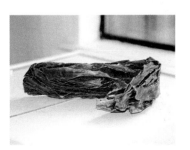
Dried Kelp

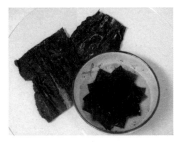

Kelp, Reconstituted and Sliced

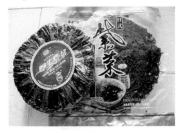

Purple Laver

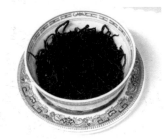

Brown Seaweed, Reconstituted

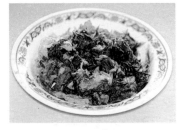

Green Seaweed, Reconstituted

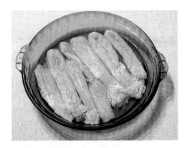

Bamboo-Pipe Fungus,
Reconstituted

people often cook kelp with mung beans in a sweet soup for treating acne. Like all seaweeds, kelp is a great source of iodine and helps the body eliminate heavy metals.

Purple Laver (zǐ cài; jí choi) 紫菜

Laver, or the fronds of porphyra tenera, is a sea vegetable rich in mineral salts, especially iodine and iron. Because of its high iodine content, it is good for people with thyroid disorders. Purple laver is called nori in Japanese. Laver can be cultivated along rugged coastlines and harvested during the warmer months. It has a sweet and salty taste. Laver makes good soups, especially with tofu, dried shrimp, sliced pork, and/or eggs.

Seaweed, Brown (hǎi zǎo; hói jóu) 海藻

Brown seaweed is small, with bunches of round stems and thin branches. It is found on rocks at low tide along the seashore. Once dried, it turns black and is similar in taste and appearance to the Japanese wakame. It is cooling and salty, and detoxifies the body by helping eliminate heavy metals.

Seaweed, Green (kūn bù; kwàn bou) 昆布

This leafy, green seaweed shrivels and turns brown when dried. It should not be confused with kelp, which is called kombu in Japanese and written the same way in Chinese characters. Be sure to rinse out fine sand before adding to soups. Available in Chinese grocery or herb stores under the Latin name sargassum, it is an excellent source of iodine and has antibiotic properties. Green and brown seaweeds are often paired in soups. Ask for them together in the Chinese store, so you won't get the Japanese kelp instead. Upon rehydration, this seaweed turns light yellowish green.

Fungi 菌蕈類

Bamboo-Pipe Fungus (zhú sūn/zhú shēng; juk syùn/juk sàng) 竹蓀、竹笙

Bamboo-pipe is a fungus that grows inside the hollow part of bamboo stems. Bamboo-pipe fungus grows among bamboo groves in the southwestern province of Yunnan. It is called zhu sun 竹蓀, or zhu sheng 竹笙 in Chinese because the fungus resembles the reed pipe. The English term "bamboo pith" is a misnomer. Good quality bamboo-pipe fungus should be yellowish-white with a pleasant smell. It is valued as a delicacy mainly for its texture. The bamboo-pipe fungus has no taste. It gets its flavor from other ingredients. Before using, the dried bamboo-pipes have to be soaked and rinsed thoroughly. Bamboo-pipe fungus is eaten as a vegetable. It is good for soups and many other vegetarian dishes.

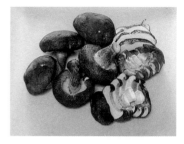

Fresh Shiitake

Black Mushroom (xiāng gū; dūng gū) 香菇、冬菇

Fresh and dried black mushrooms are very fragrant. In terms of warming and cooling properties in foods, black mushrooms are neutral in nature. A Japanese variety is the shiitake mushroom. Research has shown that shiitake mushroom extract (from both the cap and the mycelium) can be used for treating rickets, high cholesterol, liver inflammation, gastric cancer, and cervical carcinoma. Fresh shiitake is now available in the U.S. Chinese dried black mushrooms are preferred for making soups and stews because of their stronger aroma and flavor.

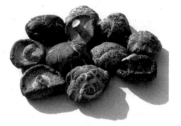

Dried Black Mushroom

Cordeceps (please see the entry under Medicinal Herbs on page 98)

Golden Needle Mushroom (jīn zhēn gū; gām jām gu) 金針菇

This mushroom is long like the tigerlily bud, which is also referred to as jin-zhen "golden needle" in Chinese. Golden needle mushrooms were previously available only in cans in the U.S. Now they are cultivated and known by the Japanese name enoki; fresh enoki is white in color. When the stems are cut into ¾-inch sections, they resemble dried scallop shreds and make a favorite addition to vegetarian soups.

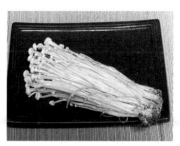

Fresh Enoki

Poria Cocos (please see the entry under Medicinal Herbs on page 103)

Straw Mushroom (cǎo gū; chóu gū) 草菇

Used extensively in Asian cuisines, straw mushrooms are available only in canned form in the U.S. They are cultivated on beds of rice straw. Dried straw mushrooms are preferred to the stronger black mushroom for making vegetarian soup stock in China because, in a soup base, their subtle and pleasingly sweet taste goes well with other ingredients.

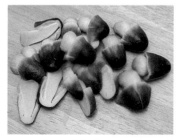

Straw Mushroom, Canned

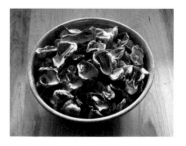

Dried Straw Mushroom

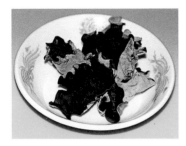

Dried Black Woodear

Woodear, Black (hēi mù ěr; haak muhk yíh/wàhn yíh) 黑木耳、雲耳

The black woodear has a rough exterior and a tan underside. Soak and remove the hard knob before adding to soup. Almost flavorless, woodears are instead prized for their crunchy texture and medicinal value, and are used traditionally in soups for post-partum women to encourage blood production and circulation. Black woodears are also said to help lower blood pressure in hypertensive people.

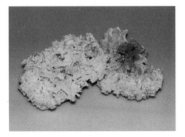

Dried White Woodear

Woodear, White (bái mù ěr; baahk muhk yíh/syut yíh) 白木耳、雪耳

White woodears look like pale, yellowish dried flowers. They become silky and snowy white and expand in size upon being soaked in cold water for 2 to 3 hours. Added to soup, this bland ingredient either retains its crunchiness or, with longer cooking time, becomes smooth and gelatinous.

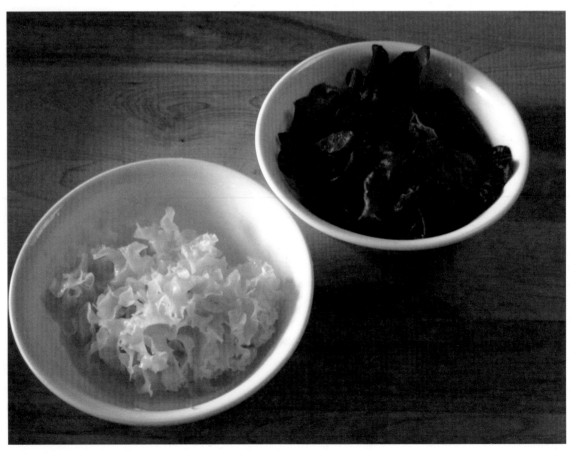

Reconstitued Woodears, Black and White

9
Medicinal Herbs

Selection and Storage

Most dried ingredients, including common medicinal herbs, are available in Asian grocery stores. Exotic items like fish maw, sea cucumber, swallow's nest, shark's fin, cordeceps, and hasmar are found only in specialty stores. Chinese herb shops also carry expensive herbs like dendrobium knots, fritillary bulbs, American ginseng, panax ginseng, and seahorse.

A rule of thumb for selection is freshness, even for dried herbs. Herbs kept past their shelf life become dry and brittle. Colors darken. Jujube dates and Chinese wolfberries are ready examples. Old eucommia bark (*du zhong* 杜仲) and beef steak plant (*zi su* 紫蘇) leaves will crumble. If the herbs are sealed inside plastic wrapping, examine carefully for any sign of bugs or insect eggs. Starchy items like dried Chinese wild yam, poria cocos, grains, beans, and lotus seeds are all susceptible to infestation.

Loose and bulk herbs should be kept in airtight jars, not in brown paper bags or plastic bags. Keep the jars in a cool, dry place, preferably in a pantry. Label each jar with the name of the herb and acquisition date. Herbs with sweet contents like chrysanthemum flowers, Chinese wolfberries, jujube dates, figs, and ginseng slices are best kept moisture-proof in the refrigerator. Seeds and nuts turn rancid within a year. It helps to keep raw peanuts, walnuts, almonds, apricot kernels, and pine nuts in the refrigerator.

Dried seafood like scallops, shrimp, octopus, abalone, and flatfish fare well in airtight jars and kept in cool dark places. It is very hard to reconstitute dried seafood items like shark's fin, fish maw, abalone, and conch meat after they have been kept in the freezer for a long time. That may not be your doing. When these items are being shipped and warehoused, they are kept frozen to avoid spoilage.

It is important to pay attention to the shelf-life of each food and herb item.

Healing Properties

There are 5,767 herbal entries in China's definitive compilation of Materia Medica published in 1977 entitled *Zhong Yao Da Ci Dian* 中藥大辭典 (Encyclopedia of Traditional Chinese Medicinal Substances). The abridged English translation by Bensky and Gamble included only 470 entries, arranged in eighteen categories by their action or indication in TCM terms. The majority of herbs used in food therapy are tonics to supplement deficiencies of yin and yang, and for invigorating qi and blood. Then come the herbs to correct conditions of excessive heat or cold, dampness or dryness, wind or stagnation. Least used are the purgative herbs. In general, herbs that build up the body's vitality and immunity with few side effects are superior herbs most suited for food and beverage. The fifty or so medicinal herbs chosen here are either tonics or regulators. Even those known for draining dampness and clearing heat are regulators, not abrasive purgatives.

Each food or medicinal herb has its own individual properties that can be described in TCM terms according to taste, temperature, tendency, and meridian(s) entered. The healing properties are listed as indications, while side effects are listed as counter-indications. As this is a cookbook, I describe the healing properties of the herbs in the soups the way a traditional home cook would, in terms of their synergistic function. If further understanding is sought, please consult *Chinese Herbal Medicine Materia Medica* by Bensky and Gamble.

A group of herbs used in a recipe or formula demonstrates synergistic healing properties by enhancing positive effects or canceling out side effects or toxicity. It is a futile, if not downright dangerous pursuit to single out one herb or food item and use it repeatedly because its indications appeal to you. Take sea vegetables, for example. While seaweeds are good for cleansing/chelating the body of heavy metal and radiation pollutants, they are cold in nature. Repeated consumption will throw the body off balance. Also, while kelp and mung bean soup helps with acne in teenagers, the coldness of this soup interferes with the menstrual flow of young women, thus warming Mandarin orange peel needs to be added to the recipe.

A second example involves ginseng. Known as an energy booster in the West, ginseng is added to many power drinks, including orange juice. However, ginseng and vitamin C cancel out each other's effects. Besides, with "rising" and yang tendencies, ginseng is really not for young people whose yang energy is high. I recoiled in horror when a soccer mom wanted to give her daughter and mine some ginseng so they could help win the upcoming tournament. The girls would probably have collapsed on the field with vertigo instead. Because of this quick-fix mentality, I have grown wary over the years and reluctant to answer the seemingly harmless question: "What is this herb good for?"

A beneficial herb used in the wrong context can be harmful and even deadly. Ephedra or *mahuang* 麻黃 suffered its undue notoriety in the hands of manufacturers of weight-loss teas who were both ignorant and too eager to tap into its power to promote sweating and urination and reduce edema. While normal dosage per decoction in TCM is between three and nine grams, the amount of *mahuang* in unregulated weight-loss tea is more than tenfold that, raising blood pressure and causing profuse sweating and cardiac arrhythmia.

Dosage

Traditional Chinese doctors or herbalists are specific about the amount of each herb used in a formula. The toxicity in certain herbs can be tolerated if only a small amount is used. As seen in the case of ephedra, an unwarranted high dosage can be fatal.

An example of dosage sensitive food is the apricot kernel. The small, bitter Northern apricot kernel should be used in proportion of one-to-four to the bigger, sweeter Southern apricot kernel. And the amount should not exceed ten whole Northern kernels (about a teaspoon) for each pot of soup (for two to six people). Do not increase the amount proportionately. While we like the soothing benefit for a cough, we can do without the cyanide in the kernels. Unfortunately, the packaging of the two different kinds of apricot kernels looks exactly the same, leading some to mix them together in a one-to-one proportion. Fortunately, nobody dies from using too much Northern apricot kernels because a natural warning is issued by its bitter taste.

There are also those who think that, especially when it comes to expensive ingredients, the more the better. If you can afford it, then the more the merrier. Of course, this is not true.

I have mentioned earlier that ginseng, the potent yang tonic, is not for everyone. For older people, the tonic soup can be made with higher frequency, but not with higher dosage. Many years ago, on a trip to China, Bob Hong, one of the soup recipe contributors for this book, came across some ginseng at very reasonable price. He presented it to his father. Learning that the ginseng was "cheap," his mother doubled the dosage in the soup. Bob, who drank the first bowl, was taken to the emergency room. Subsequent tests of the ginseng run by the School of Pharmacy at the University of the Pacific showed no toxicity. This was a case of overdose.

Common Medicinal Herbs

Bensky and Gamble, after the TCM textbook classification of medicinal herbs by their properties of taste and temperature, the meridians or channels they enter, and their therapeutic actions singly and in combination, present Chinese herbal medicine Materia Medica in eighteen categories. Only twelve of these eighteen categories are represented in this cookbook.

For soup recipes, herbs from the category of Substances for External Application are excluded. Also not used in soups are the Aromatic Herbs that Transform Dampness and those Aromatic Substances that Open the Orifices such as musk, benzoin, and borneol. Downward Draining Herbs, including hemp seed and morning glory seeds, are excluded as food due to their higher content of toxicity. Herbs that Dispel Wind-Dampness (associated with arthritis) constitute a popular category in food therapy, but these herbs or substances including tiger bone, quince fruit, and the bark of acanthopanax root (or Siberian ginseng) are best preserved in alcohol. Herbs that Expel Parasites are also poorly represented in our inventory. Only garlic is mentioned but not specifically used in a soup for that purpose.

The descriptions in this section follow Bensky and Gamble, though much shorter and modified. For detailed information, please consult the source.

Quite a few ingredients in the previous chapter, especially grains, legumes, sea vegetables, and fungi, are also listed in Bensky and Gamble as medicinal herbs. The overlapping is inevitable as both food and medicine carry health benefits and fit into similar taxonomy.

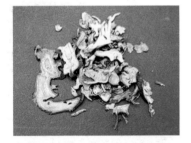

Niu Xi, Achyranthes Aspera

Achyranthes Aspera (niú xī; ngàuh sāt) 牛膝

This root herb is said to improve circulation and dissolve clots. It is traditionally used for injuries, stiffness, lower back pains, and weak legs and feet.

Adenophora Tetraphylla (shā shēn; sā sàm) 沙參

Slightly sweet and known to be demulcent to lungs, this herb helps ease dry coughing. It is also good for stomach-yin deficiency symptoms such as parched lips. It partners with Solomon's Seal to combat internal dryness.

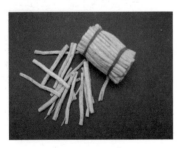

Sha Shen, Adenophora Tetraphylla

Alisma (See Water Plantain)

Alpinia Oxyphylla Fruit (See Black Cardamon)

Angelica Dahurica (bái zhǐ; baahk jí) 白芷

Acrid and warm in nature, angelica root enters the lung and stomach channels. It acts to expel wind and alleviate externally-contracted wind-cold symptoms, especially headache and nasal congestion. In combination with chuan xiong 川芎 (Ligusticum Root), it helps wind-cold induced headaches, especially orbital headache, sinus headache, and headache at the vertex.

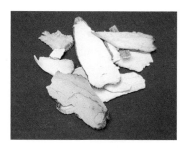

Bai Zhi, Angelica Dahurica

Angelica Sinensis (dāng gūi; dòng gwài) 當歸

This herb is best identified by its unique, strong aroma. It is rather tasty with a bitter element. Both men and women may drink a soup with dang gui to tonify the liver and spleen and to promote blood circulation. However, as dang gui is well known for treating menstrual disorders and menopausal syndrome, and because it is frequently mislabeled a "female hormone substitute," many men are embarrassed to take it. As angelica sinensis is a hormone regulator, it should be recommended to men as well.

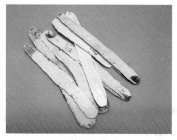

Dang Gui, Angelica Sinensis

Astragalus or Yellow Vetch (huáng qí; wòhng kèih/bāk kèih) 黃芪、北芪

Dried astragalus roots are cut into long slices that resemble tongue depressors. Said to improve circulation, lower blood pressure, lower blood sugar, and combat fatigue, astragalus is used as a qi tonic to build up immunity. The cooked pieces are hard and unpalatable and, therefore, should be removed from the tea or soup before serving.

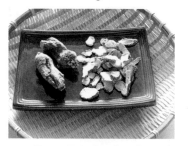

Huang Qi, Astragalus

Atractylodes Macrocephala (bái zǔ; baak seut) 白朮

Like ginseng, this tonic herb is said to restore strength and accelerate recovery from chronic ailments. It is frequently paired with poria cocos.

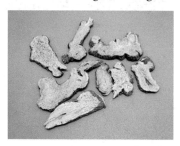

Bai Zu, Atractylodes

Black Cardamom (yì zhì rén; yīk ji yàhn) 益智仁

This herb's Chinese name literally translates as the "benefit intelligence kernel" in English. It warms the kidneys and the spleen. The fruit is actually brown. It is aromatic and must be crushed before using. This herb grows in Southern China.

Caltrop (cì jí lí; lak jat làih) 刺蒺藜

Caltrop fruits are sweet and warming. They are tiny and prickly and must be picked out of the soup and discarded after cooking. Known for strengthening

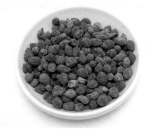

Yi Zhi Ren, Black Cardamom

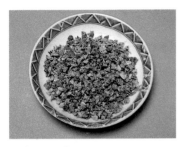

Ci Ji Li, Caltrop

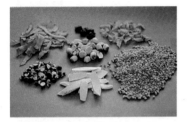

Ching Bo Leung Mix

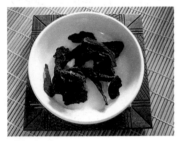

Rou Cong Rong, Cistanches Deserticolae

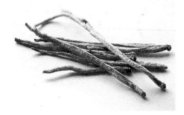

Dang Shen, Codonopsitis

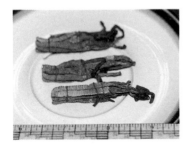

Dong Cong Xia Cao, Cordeceps

the bones and tonifying the kidneys, caltrops are said to tonify the liver and improve vision as well. It is paired with tian ma 天麻 (Gastrodiae Elatae) in a fish head soup to ease headache on the side and back of the head, including the temples.

Ching Bo Leung (qīng bǔ liáng; chìng bóu léung) 清補涼

Ching Bo Leung is such a popular soup that its ingredients are pre-packaged and available in Chinese grocery stores worldwide, even though all seven dried ingredients are regulars in a Chinese home pantry. The seven ingredients and their proportions are: pearl barley (3 ounces), Chinese wild yam (¼ ounce), lotus seed (½ ounce), lily bulb scales (½ ounce), longan meat (0.1 ounce), fox-nuts (½ ounce), and Solomon's seal (½ ounce). Many of these ingredients are identified as antioxidants.

Cistanches Deserticolae (ròu cóng róng; yuhk chùhng yùhng) 肉蓯蓉

This herb is sweet and salty in flavor and warm in nature. It helps to tonify the kidneys and moisten the intestines. Cooked with warming meat like mutton and beef, it is said to invigorate and correct impotence.

Cnidium (See Lovage Root)

Codonopsitis Root (dǎng shēn; dóng sàm) 黨參

Aiding with chronic fatigue and lack of appetite, codonopsitis roots are sweet and warming in nature. Codonopsitis roots are hard and should be removed and discarded before serving.

Cordeceps (dōng chóng xià cǎo; dùng chùhng chóu) 冬蟲夏草、冬蟲草

The Chinese name literally translates as "winter worm, summer plant" because it is a rare parasitic fungus that grows inside the body of moth larvae. This fungus is found on the Tibetan highlands of China, at altitudes of 3,000 to 4,000 meters. Cordeceps are harvested in the early summer. These fungi are known to aid a variety of symptoms, including impotence and chronic coughing. However, too large of a dose can be tranquilizing, hypnotic, or even fatal. As with all other herbs, do not exceed the amount recommended in the recipe. Highly prized in Chinese traditional and folk medicine for treatment of ailments, including fatigue, impotence, and cancer, the herb was valued at $650 per pound in 2002.

Cornbind (hé shǒu wū; hòh sáu wū) 何首烏

Considered an anti-aging herb, these bitter roots, stems, and leaves are said to counter premature graying, high blood pressure, and the hardening of blood vessels.

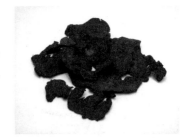

He Shou Wu, Cornbind

Cornelian Cherry Fruit (shān zhū yú; sàan jù yùh) 山茱萸

This Asiatic Cornelian cherry fruit, also known as cornus, is sour, astringent, and slightly warm. It tonifies and stabilizes the kidneys and retains the essence, correcting excessive urination, incontinence, and profuse sweating, and helping such symptoms as lightheadedness, sore and weak lower back and knees, or impotence due to chronic disease or old age. Cornus goes well with Astragalus (huang qi) and Codonopsitis (dang shen) for treating yang or qi deficiency, and with Angelica Sinensis (dang gui) and treated Rehmannia (shu di huang) for treating yin deficiency.

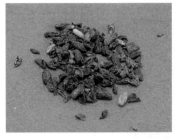

Shan Zhu Yu, Cornelian Cherry

Dendrobium (shí hú; sehk hohk) 石斛

Though it may be used fresh, this orchid stem is mostly available in dried form. A diuretic and expectorant, it is sweet, slightly salty, and cooling in nature. The knotted herb costs at least $25 per ounce, but the loose herb is cheaper. It can be used in place of or in conjunction with American ginseng. Dendrobium is treasured by singers because it protects the vocal cords from irritation and fatigue.

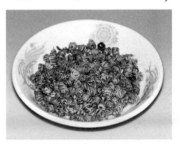

Shi Hu, Dendrobium

Dispel Dampness Soup Ingredients (qù shí zhóu liào; heui sāp jūk líu) 去濕粥料

The ingredients for Dispel Dampness Soup are not pre-packaged, as most of them are readily found in a Chinese home pantry, but any clerk in a Chinese herb store can quickly assemble them for you for about $2. The soup consists of eight ingredients: rush pith, kapok flower, hyacinth beans, tokoro (chyun taai or bei haaih), poria cocos, aduki beans, foxnuts, and pearl barley. Despite the name juk, we do not add rice to the ingredients. It is basically a bean soup.

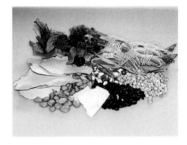

Dispel Dampness Soup Ingredients

Eucommia (dù zhòng; douh juhng) 杜仲

A tree bark, eucommia is sweet and warming. It is said to strengthen the bones, sinews, and cartilage, and is also used traditionally to prevent miscarriages.

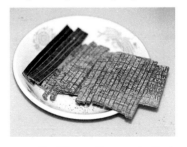

Du Zhong, Eucommia Bark

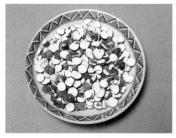

Qian Shi, Foxnut

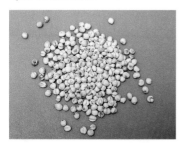

Chuan Bei Mu, Fritillary Bulb

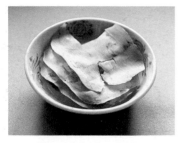

Tian Ma, Gastrodiae Elatae

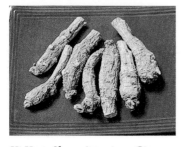

Xi Yang Shen, American Ginseng

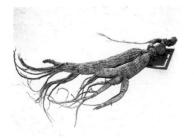

Ren Shen, Panax Ginseng

Foxglove Root (See Rehmannia)

Foxnut (qiàn shí; chìh saht) 芡實

A mild, neutral herb, the foxnut is a seed with a reddish skin and a white starchy interior, rather like a grain. One of the main ingredients in Ching Bo Leung, foxnuts are said to strengthen the kidneys and spleen.

Fritillary Bulb (chuān bèi mǔ; chyùn bui móuh) 川貝母

Fritillary bulb, bei mu, is both sweet and bitter in taste and slightly cold in temperature. It tonifies the heart and lungs. It helps to clear heat and stop coughing. It is a tonic herb for people with lung and bronchial ailments. Chuan bei mu is from Sichuan province; hence, Sichuan fritillary bulb.

Gastrodiae Elatae (tiān má; tìn màh) 天麻

Gastrodiae elatae or tian ma is a perennial plant with a large central root and twelve smaller surrounding tubers that are edible raw or steamed. When dried, the tubers are sold in yellowish-brown thin slices that turn translucent white upon boiling. Tian ma is said to help calm headaches, vertigo, and nervous exhaustion.

Ginseng, American (xī yáng shēn; fà kèih sàm) 花旗參

American ginseng grows mainly in Wisconsin and comes whole in gift boxes or in bulk. Both the wild and cultivated forms are available in Chinese herb stores. The cultivated kind is less expensive and milder in taste (it is also said to be less potent). American ginseng differs from Korean and Chinese panax ginseng in its cooling properties. When American ginseng is specified in a recipe, do not substitute with Korean or Chinese ginseng.

Ginseng, Panax (rén shēn; yàhn sàm) 人參

Ginseng is an energy tonic, said to help rejuvenate the body after convalescence from an illness. Unprocessed ginseng is white in color, fresh or dried. Red ginseng is Korean ginseng, which has been steamed until it turns from white to red. It is extremely potent and should be avoided by people with high blood pressure. In Traditional Chinese Medicine guides, it is also advised to strictly avoid eating turnips or radishes while taking ginseng.

Hasmar (hā shì mā yóu; syut gap gōu) 哈士蟆油、雪蛤膏

A unique and expensive ingredient, hasmar is collected from female frogs found in Northeastern China. Hasmar is obtained after a multi-day process in which the frog's female reproductive organs are carefully removed and air-dried. High in protein, hasmar also contains a multitude of vitamins, minerals, and beneficial hormones. Hasmar is said to be especially good for maintaining a dewy complexion and smooth skin.

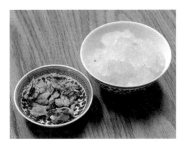

Hasmar, Dried and Reconstituted

Hawthorn Berry (shān zhā; sàan jà) 山楂

Hawthorn berries have a sweet and sour taste. They are warm in nature. They enter into the liver, spleen and stomach meridians. They are good for lowering blood pressure as well as improving poor appetite and indigestion. They are available in dried pitted form in Chinese grocery stores.

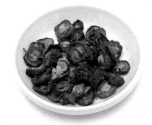

Shan Zha, Hawthorn Berry

Honeysuckle Flower (jīn yín huā; gàm ngàhn fā) 金銀花

Honeysuckle flowers come in two colors, yellow and white, growing on the same vine, hence the name meaning "gold and silver." Honeysuckle is sweet and cold in nature. It enters into the large intestine, lung, and stomach meridians. The honeysuckle flower is used to treat warm-febrile diseases with symptoms of fever, sore throat, and headache. A brew helps with boils and rashes. It is also good for painful urinary dysfunction.

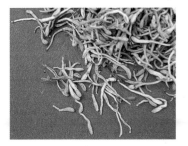

Jin Yin Hua, Honeysuckle Flower

Kapok Flower (mù mián huā; muhk mìhn fā) 木棉花

Also known as the "hero flower," the kapok flower is bright red and is the city flower of Guangzhou. Dried for cooking, the flower shrivels to about half of its original size and becomes brown with stamens intact. This ingredient promotes the flow of liquid out of the body. It also soothes stomach discomfort from excess heat. It is one of the ingredients for Dispel Dampness Soup.

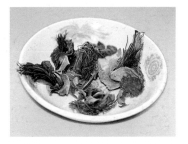

Mu Mian Hua, Kapok Flower

Kudzu Root, Pueraria (gé gēn; got gàn) 葛根

This sweet, acrid, and cool herb enters the spleen and stomach meridians. Kudzu root relieves stiffness in the neck and upper back, and headache at the base of the head due to wind-cold. It is also used in combination with other herbs to alleviate thirst due to stomach heat, and treat diarrhea due to stomach and spleen deficiency. Kudzu root is often used with chrysanthemum flower to relieve intoxication or hangover.

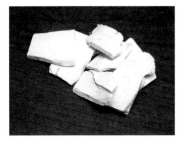

Ge Gen, Kudzu Root

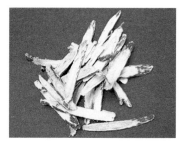

Gan Cao, Licorice

Licorice (gān cǎo; gàm chóu) 甘草

Licorice is sweet and neutral. It is often used to harmonize the taste as well as the therapeutic actions of other herbs because licorice is said to enter all twelve channels, principally the spleen, stomach, heart, and lung. It can moderate hot and cold herbs, and mitigate extreme properties that may cause violent allergic or toxic responses. Licorice and mung beans are used widely as an antidote for many toxins including cocaine, arsenobenzol, and urethane. Licorice root can be combined with white peony root for treating abdominal pain due to disharmony between liver and stomach, and also for treating muscle cramps, especially of the calf, due to blood deficiency.

Ligusticum Chuanxiong (See Lovage Root)

Lovage Root (chuān xiōng; chyùn gùng) 川芎

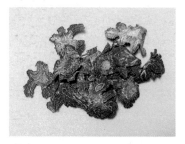

Chuan Xiong, Lovage Root

Lovage root, also known as cnidium, is acrid in flavor and warm in nature. It helps to promote qi movement and correct blood deficiency. It has a strong smell and is almost always paired with Angelica Dahurica (baahk jí 白芷) in food and formula. Its botanical name is Ligusticum Chuanxiong.

Loquat Leaf (pí pá yè; pèih pàh yihp) 枇杷葉

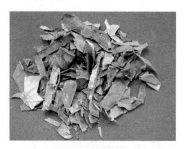

Pi Pa Ye, Loquat Leaf

The loquat fruit is one of the most delicious summer fruits while its leaves can be harvested year-round. Loquat leaf is bitter and cool in nature. It can help to lubricate the lung, clear hardened phlegm, and stop coughing. The hairy leaves need to be treated before using. Dried and shredded loquat leaves are available in Chinese herb stores.

Luo Han Guo (See Momordica Fruit)

Mandarin Orange Peel, Dried (guǒ pí; chàhn pèih) 陳皮

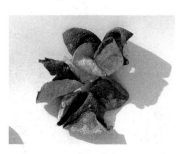

Guo Pi, Mandarin Orange Peel

The Mandarin orange is a citrus fruit with a thin, loose peel. After being dried in the sun, the peel becomes brown and brittle. It is bitter and said to help with digestion. Peels from Xinhui 新會 are more fragrant and thus more expensive. Do not soak in water for more than 30 minutes, or it may lose flavor. The white coating inside is usually scraped off. Its warming nature is used to balance the cooling qualities of tofu, shellfish, sea vegetables, and mung beans.

Momordica Fruit (luó hàn gǔo; lòh hon gwó) 羅漢果

Round, brown, with a thin smooth hard shell, luo han guo is the size of a golf ball. It is said to help the body expel hardened phlegm. The momordica fruit is ripe in the fall, but sold dried year-round in Chinese grocery and herb stores. It is traditionally used for treating chronic bronchitis and coughs.

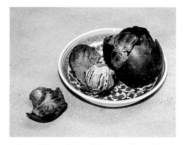

Luo Han Guo, Momordica Fruit

Mulberry Leaf, Dried (sāng yè; sōng yihp) 桑葉

Mulberry leaf expels wind and clears heat from the lungs and liver. It helps clear symptoms of red and dry eyes, headache behind the eyes, and sore throat.

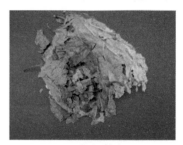

Mulberry Leaf, dried

Notoginseng Root (tián qī; tìhn chāt) 田七

Aptly named, notoginseng is not really a ginseng. However, like ginseng, it is warm in nature and slightly bitter. It is traditionally used to combat bleeding and swelling, and also helps lower high blood pressure and cholesterol. Notoginseng is available whole (hard as a stone), pounded into small chunks, or powderized.

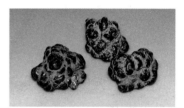

Tian Qi, Notoginseng

Pseudostellaria (tài zǐ shēn; taai jí sàm) 太子參

Literally translated as "prince ginseng," taizishen looks like a miniature ginseng. Look for those that are thick, moist, yellowish-white, and free of small rootlets. Slightly bitter, it is traditionally used to alleviate fatigue and is served to help feverish children. Like ginseng, taizishen tonifies qi and strengthens energy, only at a fragment of the cost of ginseng.

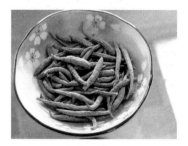

Tai Zi Shen, Pseudostellaria

Poria Cocos (fú líng; fuhk lìhng/wàhn lìhng) 茯苓、雲苓

A pinecone-sized fungus found near tree roots, poria cocos is slightly sweet, and diuretic. It helps combat bloating and is used in the treatment of damp heat. The pinkish variety is called red poria (chì fú líng, chehk fuhk lìhng) 赤茯苓. It is also referred to as hoelin (due to dialect variation). Poria is sold sliced, diced, powdered, and in rolls.

Rehmannia, Raw (shēng dì huáng; sàang deihdaaih sàang deih) 生地黃、生地、大生地

In TCM terms, Chinese foxglove root is both sweet and bitter in taste, and cold in temperature. If it is of good quality, it will be thick and reddish in color. It helps to clear heat and nourish yin deficiency.

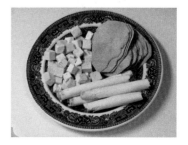

Fu Ling, Poria Cocos—diced, sliced, and rolled

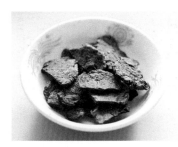

Di Huang, Rehmannia

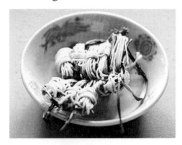

Deng Xin Cao, Rush Pith

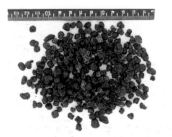

Wu Wei Zi, Schisandra Fruit

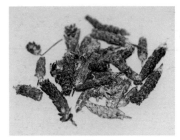

Xia Ku Cao, Selfheal

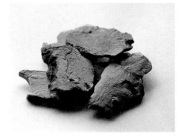

Tu Fu Ling, Smilax Glabra

When used with seaweed, this cooling, slightly bitter root dispels internal heat. To enhance the cooling effect of this herb, it is best to make the stock for a summer soup with pork and not chicken, which has a reverse, warming effect.

Rehmannia, Treated (shóu dì húang; suhk deih) 熟地黃、熟地

After harvesting in autumn, the root is cooked in wine. Its properties are sweet and slightly warm. It is used to tonify the essence and blood and to nourish kidney yin. It helps with symptoms of dizziness and insomnia, tinnitus, and low back pain. It is also used with other herbs like Angelica Sinensis (dang gui) and Chinese wild yam (shan yao) in food and formula to treat forgetfulness.

Rush Pith (dēng xīn cǎo; dāng sàm chóu) 燈芯草

Sold in small lightweight bundles, the rush pith is also known as the wick herb for its resemblance to candle wicks. It combats painful, scant urination and bloating by leaching out dampness and promoting urination. The rush pith is also said to clear the heart channel that causes restless sleep. It is an ingredient of Dispel Dampness Soup. Rush pith is also referred to as juncos.

Schisandra Fruit (wǔ wèi zǐ; ńgh meih jí) 五味子

The schisandra is the small fruit of the Chinese magnoliavine (schisandra). Its Chinese name means "a fruit with five flavors," so named because its skin and flesh are mixtures of sweet, sour, and salty flavor while its kernel tastes pungent and bitter. The five-flavored fruit enters the lung and kidney meridians and helps conditions of tuberculosis, asthma and cough, night sweats, and diarrhea.

Selfheal/Prunella (xià kū cǎo; hah fù chóu) 夏枯草

The dried flower spike of selfheal helps in treating hypertension, clearing liver heat, and brightening the eyes. To capitalize on its cooling property, do not cook with chicken or warming meat.

Smilax Glabra (tǔ fú líng; tóu fuhk lìhng) 土茯苓

The root of this vine is harvested from autumn to early winter. It relieves toxicity and eliminates damp heat, therefore helping to reduce joint pain, jaundice, and skin lesions. Though sharing a similar Chinese name as Poria Cocos (fu ling 茯苓), Smilax Glabra (tu fu ling 土茯苓) is not a fungus.

Solomon's Seal (yù zhǔ; yuhk jūk) 玉竹

Sold in long, thick, yellowish-white slices, this cooling herb can be used to combat internal dryness. It is one of the Ching Bo Leung ingredients. It is also used in combination with Adenophora Tetraphylla (sha shen 沙參) to deal with stomach-yin deficiency.

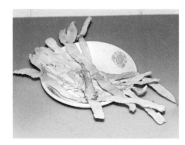

Yu Zhu, Solomon's Seal

Tai Zi Shen (See Pseudostellaria) 太子參

Tian Ma (See Gastrodiae Elatae) 天麻

Tokoro (bēi xiè; bèi háaih/chyùn taai/chyùn bèi háaih) 萆薢、川太、川萆薢

A rhizome sliced paper-thin, tokoro is commonly used to combat cloudy urine or skin ailments, such as eczema and adult acne, caused by damp-heat. It is one of the ingredients in Dispel Dampness Soup.

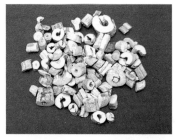

Mu Dan Pi, Tree Peony Bark

Tree Peony Bark (mǔ dān pí; máuh dāan pèih) 牡丹皮

Tree peony grows throughout China and is greatly appreciated for its large, vibrant-colored flowers. The bark of its stems is acrid, bitter, and cool, good for treating warm-febrile disease with such symptoms as nosebleed, sores, and abscess associated with ascending liver fire.

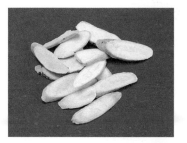

Bai Shao, White Peony Root

Tuckahoe (See Poria Cocos) 茯苓

White Peony Root (bái sháo; baahk cheuk) 白芍

White peony root enters liver and spleen channels. It tonifies the blood, retains the yin, and pacifies the liver. White peony root is commonly used for treating women's disorders, during menstruation and at menopause, associated with yin deficiency and floating yang that causes night sweats.

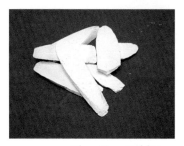

Shan Yao, Wild Yam

Wild Yam (shān yào; wàaih sàan) 山藥、淮山

Chinese wild yam is sold in its dried, sliced form. The smooth white pieces are about one-eighth of an inch in thickness. One of the seven ingredients in Ching Bo Leung and one of the four ingredients in Four Flavor Soup, wild yam is often paired with Chinese wolfberry in recipes. Once boiled, wild yam slices become slightly translucent and are said to tonify the spleen. Fresh wild yam is known as nakaimo or yamaimo in Japan. It is commonly used in soups and for steaming, sliced or diced, with fish or meat in Cantonese cuisine. Of course, it is great for vegetarian soups and dishes.

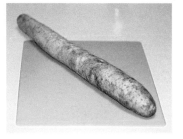

Fresh Wild Yam

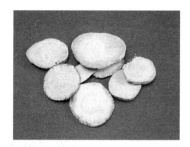

Ze Xie, Water Plantain

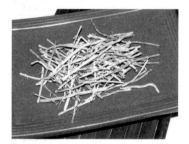

Bai Mao Gen, Woolly Grass Rhizome

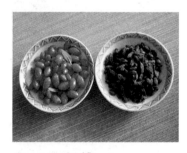

Gou Ji Zi, Wolfberries

Water Plantain Rhizome (zé xiè; jaahk she) 澤瀉

This herb promotes urination and is useful with a damp-heat condition in the lower burner. It has less of a tendency to harm kidney yin than other draining herbs. Actually, it protects kidney yin by preventing kidney fire from flaring up as a side effect of tonification.

Woolly Grass Rhizome (bái máo gēn; maàoh gàn) 白茅根、茅根

The rhizome of woolly grass, also known as white grass or imperata, is a sweet and cold herb. It clears heat from the stomach and lungs and aids nausea and thirst due to stomach heat or wheezing due to lung heat. It is often paired with fresh sugarcane to make a heat-clearing beverage or soup. It is used in combination with aduki beans (chi xiao dou) for edema from damp-heat and with astragalus (huang qi) for edema due to qi deficiency.

Wolfberries, dried (gǒu jì zi; géi jí) 枸杞子、杞子

Wolfberries grow on a low thorny bush. The dried berries are the size and consistency of raisins. They are available in Chinese grocery stores and herb shops, and are frequently paired with the Chinese wild yam in soups and stews. Also known as goji berries, wolfberries are growing in popularity in recent years as a tonic. The fruit-bearing wolfberry plant is a separate variety from the leafy wolfberry plant, though both belong to the lycii family.

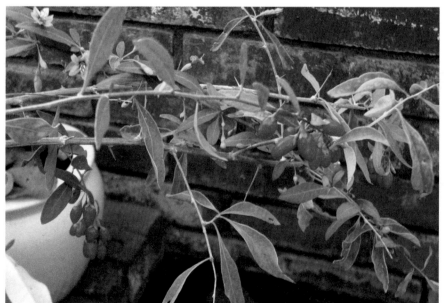

Wolfberry Plant with Flowers and Fruit

10
Other Food Products

Tofu and Soybean Products 大豆製品

Bean Curd (dòu fù; dauh fuh) 豆腐

Bean curd, widely known as tofu, is made from soybean milk. Three kinds are available in the U.S.: soft, regular, and firm. Package sizes vary. The soft kind is silky smooth in texture and is used in gang 羹 soups. The regular kind can be cooked quickly in gwan soups or for over 2 hours in louhfo 老火 soups, giving rise to a honeycomb texture. The firm type can be shredded and cooked in Hot and Sour Soup. Both firm and regular tofu can be frozen. It becomes spongy and assumes a meaty texture when it is defrosted.

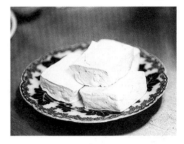

Bean Curd/Tofu

Bean Curd Puffs (dòu fù pào; dauh fuh pōk) 豆腐泡

Fresh bean curd may be cut into cubes or pieces resembling mahjong tiles and deep-fried into bean curd puffs. In Japanese, it is called age-toufu. Bean curd puffs are white and soft in the inside and golden brown and lightly crispy on the outside. Also known as tofu puffs, they are sold in packages in Asian grocery stores. Chinese cooks like to cut the bean curd puffs diagonally or into strips and cook them in vegetarian soups or dishes.

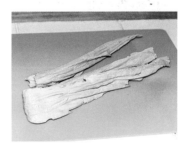

Deep-fried Tofu

Bean Curd Stick (fù zhú; fuh jūk/jī jūk) 腐竹、枝竹

In the process of making bean curd, a thin film is formed on the surface of the cooling soybean milk. This thin layer is carefully lifted off. Instead of laying it flat to dry on a bamboo mat, as with bean curd skin, the sheet is gathered on one end, twisted like a wet towel, and then line-dried. Reconstituted bean curd sticks are a favorite meat substitute in vegetarian dishes and stews.

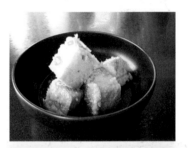

Dried Bean Curd Stick

Bean Curd Skin (dòu fù pí; fuh pèih/fuh jūk) 豆腐皮、腐皮、腐竹

During the process of making soybean milk and bean curd, a filmy layer is formed when the soybean milk cools off. This layer is carefully lifted off the surface and dried into a brittle yellow sheet called "bean curd skin." Conceptually, it is really the skim of the soybean milk, but the name has long been established and I'll just go along with it.

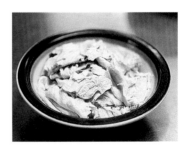

Reconstituted Bean Curd Stick

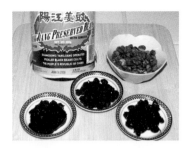

Fermented Black Beans

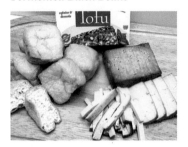

Tofu Puffs and Pressed Bean Curd

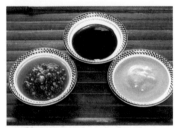

Chile Sauce, Oyster Sauce, and Chinese Mustard

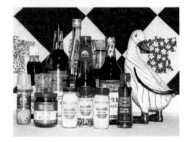

Chinese Spices and Condiments

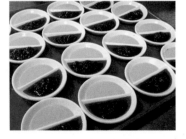

Chinese Mustard and Chile Sauce

Fermented Black Soybean (dòu shì; dauh sih) 豆豉

Black soybean becomes more digestible after undergoing a fermentation process. Unsalted fermented black soybean (dan dou shi 淡豆豉) is made into a soup or tea that is used as a cold medicine with ginger and the white part of green onions, while the salted kind is a pungent seasoning that is never used in soups or teas.

Pressed Bean Curd (dòu fù gān; dauh fuh gōn) 豆腐乾

When fresh bean curd is placed under a big piece of board with weights, such as bricks, on top, it becomes firm and compact as liquid is pressed out of it. It assumes a meat-like texture ideal for vegetarian dishes. Pressed bean curd is available marinated or plain.

Seasonings and Condiments 調味品

Only a few basic herbs are used for seasoning soups. The most common are fresh ginger and green onions. Honey dates, momordica fruit, or licorice are used along with carrots to sweeten the pot. White pepper is sprinkled over fish soup, congee, and thickened soup (gang) according to individual taste. The Chinese do not use table salt as a condiment. Rather, salt is handled as a seasoning in the kitchen.

Strong sauces and pastes are never used in Cantonese soups. They are served as condiments for side dishes.

Chinese Mustard (jiè mò; gaai laaht) 芥末、芥辣

Chinese mustard is derived from horseradish. It is hot and pungent like Japanese wasabi, but is yellow in color, similar to American mustard. It is prepared by mixing dried powder with cold water. It can deliver a spicy bite to open up your sinuses. Chinese mustard is never directly put into a soup. It is included here because it is a condiment to accompany meat—beef or pork—that has been boiled in the soup to be served as a side dish. Chinese mustard sauce also goes well with roast pork (chā siū 叉燒) and braised beef (ngàuh náahm 牛腩) served with soup noodles.

Cooking Wine (jiǔ; jáu) 酒

Chinese cooks are rather flexible with their cooking wine. Though traditional rice wine is preferred, dry sherry, dry vermouth, or vodka can be used. If you use the Japanese sweet cooking sake, be sure to adjust the amount of sugar in your recipe.

Ground Pepper (hú jiāo fěn; wùh jiù fán) 胡椒粉

Black or white ground pepper is readily available in the spice section of all markets. Black and white peppercorns are also available. Some people prefer using a pepper mill to grind the peppercorn as needed. Cantonese people normally use white pepper for fish and seafood, and for sprinkling over gang (thickened soup) and juk (rice soup). Black pepper is mostly used for marinating meat and making stews (see White Peppercorn on page 113).

Hot Chile Sauce or Paste (là jiāo jiàng; laaht jiù jeung) 辣椒醬

Most Chinese hot chile pastes are made from a blend of fresh and dried chiles with vinegar, with various degrees of hotness. Some are mixed with minced garlic, ginger, sesame oil, soybeans, and/or fermented soybean paste. Cantonese use hot chile paste mostly as a condiment to accompany dim sum or sliced meat. The only occasion for its use in a soup is in Hot and Sour Soup, which is a newly introduced exception.

Oil and Fats (shí yóu; sihk yàuh/yàuh) 食油、油

Cooking oil for the Chinese means vegetable oils like peanut oil, canola oil, safflower oil, and soybean oil. Sesame oil is used mostly for seasoning, not for cooking. All these oils contain mono- and polyunsaturated fatty acids. Traditionally the Chinese do not use olive oil or flax seed oil. The Chinese also cook with lard and chicken fat, but not butter or ghee. Chinese and Chinese-Americans did not learn to cook with trans-fats or hydrogenated oils until they became fashionable in the 1950s.

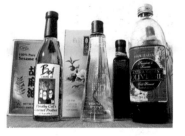

Oils

As high heat destroys beneficial fatty acids and creates toxic ones, deep-frying is not a cooking method we would endorse. According to Finnegan, author of *The Facts About Fats,* peanut oil and soybean oil should be ruled out from our diet because they are subjected to high temperature during the manufacturing process. Omega-3 stays intact under 320°F; so with a boiling point at around 220°F, soup-making is compatible with the omega-3 in, say, salmon and canola oil.

Canola oil with its mild flavor is our best bet where health benefits are concerned. Fresh pressed canola (from the mustard family) contains omega-3, -6, and -9 fatty acids in the unrefined organic state. They are antioxidants that strengthen cellular membranes and the immune system and protect us against cancer, heart disease, arthritis, allergies, and candida. Safflower oil is also good for light sautéing and stir-frying because its flavor is lighter than that of sesame oil.

Macrobiotic cooking highly recommends the use of sesame oil because sesame oil is rich in both monounsaturated and polyunsaturated fatty acids. Besides, it is a stable oil that does not easily turn rancid.

Oyster-Flavored Sauce (háo yóu; hòuh yàuh) 蠔油

This thick, flavorful sauce is made from oyster extracts mixed with cornstarch, salt, and seasoning. It is smooth in texture and dark brown in color. Oyster sauce is never used in soups. It is included here because it is a favorite condiment of the Cantonese to accompany poached chicken, pork, and abalone that are served as side dishes with the broth.

Salt (yán; yìhm/sihk yìhm) 鹽、食鹽

Salt is arguably the most popular food seasoning. It is also the most important food preservative. Salt comes either from the evaporation of sea water or from mineral deposits in rocks. In the former case, it is called sea salt. Natural sea salt that is harvested by hand is called fleur de sel, meaning "flower of the sea," and is popular among the gourmet and the health-conscious. Sea salt is recommended over and above regular or even iodized table salt, which has lost all other trace minerals during the refining process. Refined or table salt widely in use in the U.S. is obtained from rock salt via stages of purification that beget pure sodium chloride crystals. To make table salt free-running, a small amount of anti-caking agents such as sodium silicoaluminate are added. A small quantity of iodine is also added to prevent goiter. Still, our table salt is 99 percent sodium chloride.

Sodium is one of the primary electrolytes in the body. While insufficient intake may lead to muscle cramps, dizziness, or electrolyte disturbance, too much sodium gives rise to a possible array of health problems, including hypertension, left ventricular hypertrophy (cardiac enlargement), edema, and hypernatremia. The recommended amount of daily sodium (or salt) intake varies from country to country. The *Dietary Guidelines for Americans 2005* suggests the consumption of less than 2.3 grams of sodium (or 5.8 grams of salt) per day. That includes sodium (or salt) already contained in salt-laden food like ham, pastrami, potato chips, salsa, and soda, and in condiments like soy sauce, oyster sauce, fish sauce, and fermented bean paste. Read your food labels and you will be surprised how quickly the sodium adds up.

Satay Sauce or Paste (shā chá jiàng; sà chàah jeung) 沙茶醬

This sauce is a blend of garlic, shallot, chile, peanut powder, sesame seed powder, coconut powder, ground dried shrimp, salt, and peanut oil. It is grainy in

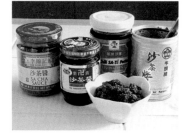

Satay Sauce or Paste

texture. Satay sauce is also known as a barbecue sauce because it is used in Indonesia to marinate thin strips of meat for grilling on a skewer. It is indispensable as a dipping sauce for hot pots. Vegetarian satay sauce is available without the dried shrimp as an ingredient. In its place, wheat germ is added.

Soy Sauce (jiàng yóu; sih yàuh) 醬油、豉油

Soy sauces are made from soybeans and wheat through natural fermentation. A lighter color soy sauce, called sāang chāu 生抽 in Cantonese, is thinner and saltier than regular soy sauce, whereas a darker and thicker soy sauce is called lóuh chāu 老抽. Low- or reduced-sodium soy sauces are also available. Soy sauce is never used directly in a soup, but a small amount can be used to marinate the meat that goes into a gwan or quickly boiled soup. Soy sauces are standard condiments in Asian restaurants.

Sugar (táng; tòhng) 糖

Sugar is the common name for sucrose, also called saccharose. Sugar has its origin in plants such as sugarcanes and sugar beets. In its natural form, sugarcane provides a rich source of vitamins and minerals. Fresh pressed sugarcane juice and boiled sugarcane are favorite beverages of the Cantonese people. Sugar is most often prepared as a fine, white, granulated, odorless powder. Large sugar crystals, called rock crystal sugar (bìng tòhng 冰糖), are formed by allowing a supersaturated solution of sugar to settle for several days. In China, rock crystal sugar is used for sweet soups and sweet teas. Both brown sugar and molasses come from late stages of sugar refining. The later into the process, the stronger the color and taste will be. Between the true raw sugar found in unheated sugarcane juice and refined sugar are specialty "raw" sugars that are part sugar and part molasses poured into molds to dry. This results in brown sugar cakes or sugar slices called bìng pin tòhng 冰片糖 or simply pin tòhng 片糖 in Cantonese. This specialty sugar is preferred in Chinese cuisine for braising and stews.

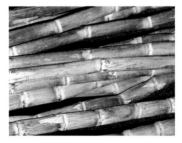

Sugarcanes

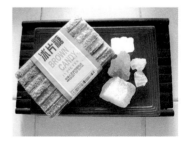

Brown Sugar Cakes and Rock Crystal Sugar

Refined sugar is devoid of nutrients. Over consumption of refined sugar can cause tooth decay, contribute to obesity, and adversely affect people with diabetes, damaging eyes, kidneys, nerves, heart, and blood vessels. It is also known to cause hyperactivity in some children. Research shows that refined sugar may also cause growth-hormone deficiency and deplete the body of potassium and magnesium. In view of the possible health hazards, it is best to read all food labels to find out about the sugar content of each food item, including candy bars, chips, ice cream, soft drinks, fruit juice, jam, peanut butter, yogurt, and breads, because sugar and high-fructose corn syrup are generously used by food manufacturers in food products. A World Health Organization (WHO) Technical Report, "Nutrition and the Prevention of Chronic Diseases," recommended against the consumption of all monosaccharides and disaccharides added to foods. Instead, WHO approves only of natural sugars—the unrefined sugar found in fruit, grains, vegetables, pure honey, and maple syrup—for unrestricted consumption.

Sugar Substitute (dài táng; doih tòhng) 代糖

In view of the various health problems linked to excessive carbohydrate intake with refined sugar consumption, the search is on for a sugar substitute, natural or artificial, that mimics the pleasant sweet taste of real sugar. Saccharin, the first artificial sugar substitute, was synthesized in 1879. Of the many artificial sweeteners approved by the FDA, aspartame is perhaps the most commonly used in the food industry, especially since the expiration of the Monsanto patent in 1992, which was accompanied by a significant price drop. Rising in popularity is sucralose (Tate and Lyle's patent), known as Splenda. Sucralose is great for baking because it is stable in heat. It is said to be harmless to the body because it passes through with minimal absorption.

Stevia, a natural sugar substitute, imported from northern Paraguay and southern Brazil, is said to offer the healthiest alternative to sugar and artificial sweeteners because it is calorie-free (sugar carries 109 calories per ounce) and stable in heat up to 392°F. As stevia is 300 times sweeter than white sugar by volume, a dash (0.16 teaspoon) is equivalent to 1 cup of white sugar.

Vinegar (cù; chou) 醋

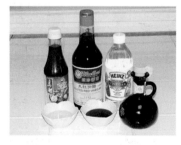

Vinegar

Vinegar is the product of a natural oxidation process, acting on wine, cider, or fermented fruit juice, and resulting in acetic acid. Examples are wine vinegar, apple cider vinegar, balsamic vinegar, rice vinegar, and white vinegar. In East and Southeast Asia, rice vinegar is the most popular, with colors ranging from pale yellow or red to brown and black. Traditionally, colored vinegars are products of aging as well as added ingredients. Red vinegar results from the use of red yeast rice, whereas brown and black vinegars may contain added malt and spices. The Cantonese use many kinds of vinegar for cooking—white, golden, red, brown, and black—that vary in degrees of sourness and sweetness.

Regular white vinegar, with 100 percent pure acetic acid is the most pungent and tart. Rice vinegar is less pungent and sweeter. Black vinegar, made from a fermentation of a mixture of rice, wheat, sorghum, and/or millet, is dark in color and more flavorful than other vinegars. Sweetened black vinegar is primarily used for cooking pig's feet and ginger or eggs in their shells to replenish calcium for a new mother. Brown vinegar, a specialty of Zhenjiang of the Jiangsu Province, is well known as a dipping vinegar for the famous hairy crabs, also from that region. Red vinegar from China's Zhejiang Province is as pretty as it is smooth, making it the favorite as a table condiment to accompany shark's fin soup and the Shanghai steamed buns called *xiao long bao* 小籠包.

White Peppercorn (bái hú jiāo lì; baahk wùh jiū lāp) 白胡椒粒

When the grayish-black outer shell of the peppercorn is removed, the more delicate white peppercorn is revealed. Used both whole and ground, white peppercorn is a traditional antidote to food poisoning and is also said to stimulate metabolism and dispel stomach wind.

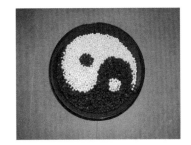

Peppercorn, Black and White

Noodles 粉麵

Mung Bean Pasta

The most common form of noodle made from mung bean powder is the thin thread or vermicelli, fán sī 粉絲 in Cantonese, also known as cellophane noodle, though broad and sheet mung bean noodles are also available. The long clear noodle is used for soups and vegetarian dishes throughout East and Southeast Asia. It is readily available in Asian grocery stores. It can easily be reconstituted soaking in cold water for 15 minutes.

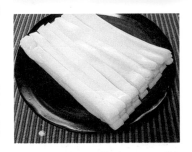

Mung Bean Pasta

Rice Noodles

The Cantonese have created many forms of pasta from rice powder. The most famous is the flat, broad rice noodle known in Cantonese as sà hòh fán 沙河粉 or hòh fán 河粉. We also have round noodles called laaih fán 瀨粉, and sheet noodles, that are rolled up, called jù chèuhng fán 豬腸粉.

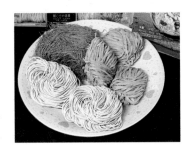

Rice Noodles

Wheat Noodles (miàn; mihn) 麵

Chinese wheat noodles come in different shapes and sizes. Some are round and some are flat. Some are thick and some are thin. Some are fresh and some are dried. Some are raw and some are cooked. They are mostly store-bought, as making noodles from wheat flour is not the forte of Cantonese housewives. Wheat noodles are simply referred to as noodles, as the Chinese character for noodles, 麵, contains the wheat radical 麥 and the ingredient is implied. The

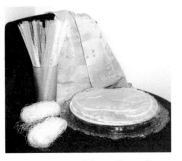

Wheat Noodles

Cantonese in general are innovative with food. By adding eggs to the dough, Cantonese noodle-makers created egg noodles. The chef of the Yi family invented the long life noodle by wrapping a single strand into the shape of a cake and lightly deep-frying it.

Pickles or Preserved Vegetables 醃菜

Pickled Mustard Heart (suān cài; syùn choi) 酸菜

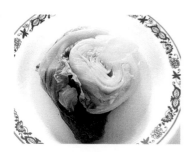

Suan Cai, Pickled Mustard Heart

One kind of mustard green has fleshy stems around a round base. After peeling off a few outer layers, we get the globular core, which the Cantonese would call the gall (choi dáam 菜膽), while Westerners call it the heart. Fresh mustard hearts are favorites at banquets. Exquisitely flavored with vinegar and spices, pickled mustard hearts go well with meat dishes or soups, and are especially good for cutting the smell of innards like pork stomach and beef tripe.

Preserved Potherb Mustard Green (xǔe lǐ hóng; syut leúi hùhng) 雪裡蕻

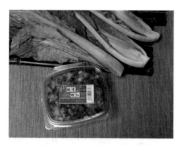

Xue Li Hong, Preserved and Fresh Potherb Mustard Green

This variety of mustard green, with long narrow stems, is preserved by adding salt, wringing out the liquid, and packing the greens into earthenware to ferment. It tastes sour and salty and smells like sauerkraut. The preserved vegetable turns greenish-brown in color but retains a certain crunchiness. It is a popular ingredient for noodle soup with shredded pork. It is also a favorite in fish soups. Rinse to remove its pickling brine before using.

Sichuan Preserved Turnip (zhà cài; ja choi) 榨菜

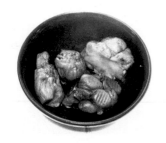

Zha Cai, Sichuan Preserved Turnip

Rutabaga (the root of a turnip) is preserved in salt, pressed and dried, then treated with a hot chile paste and packed into earthenware to ferment. The taste is at once salty, sour, and spicy. The texture is tender and crunchy.

Zha cai needs to be washed before using to get rid of the extra chile and salt coating the preserved vegetable. Only a small amount is needed, thinly sliced or finely shredded, to season stir-fry dishes or soups. It is especially good in noodle soup with shredded pork.

Miscellaneous 其他

Pre-Packaged Soup Ingredients

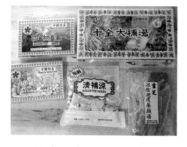

Pre-Packaged Soup Ingredients

Some established recipes of tonic soups find their way to international marketplaces with the help of enterprising Chinese merchants. The herbal ingredients are measured out and packaged. Each package weighs three to six ounces. These include the classic Ching Bo Leung 清補涼 and the Four Items 四物湯.

The Big Ten Tonic 十全大補湯 is conveniently wrapped and boxed. Then there are the assorted herbs to cook with black-bone chicken and to cook with pork stomach and guts; and assorted herbs with fancy fungi like *lingzhi (reishi)* mushroom 靈芝 and *hericium erinaceus* 猴頭菇.

Commercially Packaged Soup Stocks

In stores, we can find chicken consommé and beef bouillon cubes. Canned chicken and beef broth and bottled clam juice are also available. Recently, organic chicken broth and other organic soups in cartons have become widely available. These modern conveniences allow for easy soup making. Be sure to read the nutritional information labels, paying special attention to saturated fat, trans fat, and sodium content.

Mock Meats

Chinese vegetarian cuisine distinguishes itself with a great variety of mock or imitation meats made out of bean curd skin, gluten, and koniyaku powder. Mock meats imitate their real counterparts in shape, color, and texture. Some even mimic the taste by using similar seasonings. Dishes made with mock meat appear to be just like those cooked with real meat, so vegetarians can still enjoy gourmet food. You can find mock chicken, mock duck, mock goose, mock fish, mock abalone, mock prawn, mock beef, mock pork, mock ham, mock pork kidney, mock squid, mock sea cucumber, and even mock shark's fin. I don't know, however, if the Chinese have ever made any "mock turtle" or if it is just a figment of Lewis Carroll's imagination.

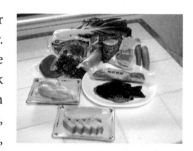

Mock Meat Sampler

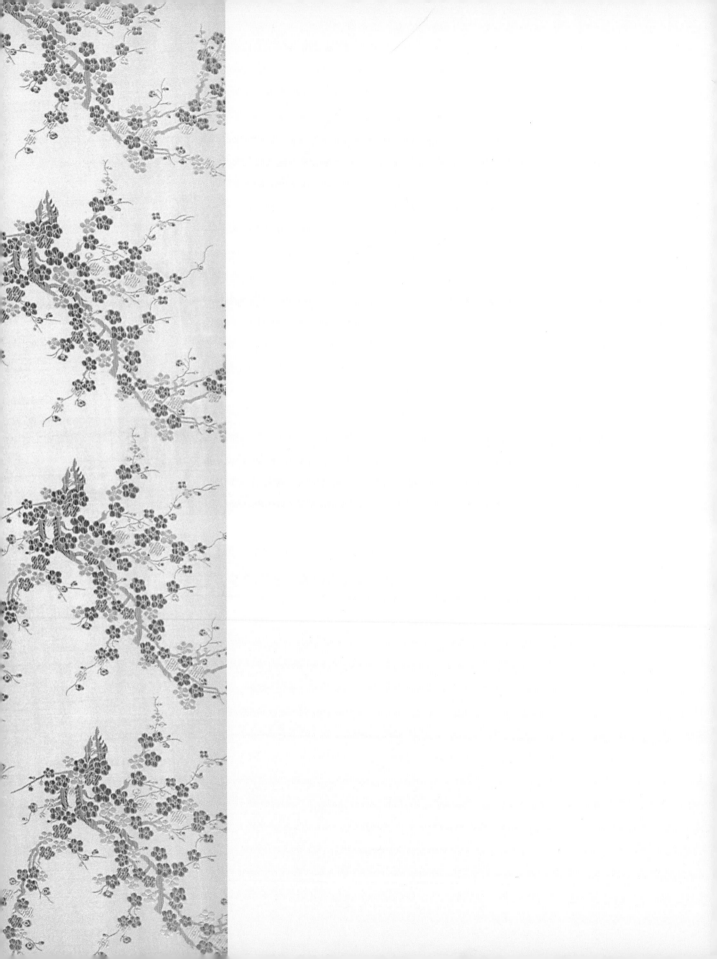

PART FOUR

Soup Recipes

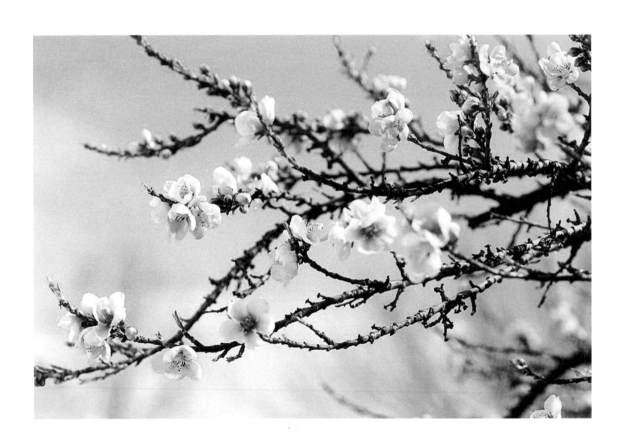

11
Healthful Soups for the Four Seasons

To eat in harmony with the seasons is an important consideration in menu planning. A trip to your vegetable garden or the farmers' market will give you an idea of what is in season and the freshness of seasonal produce will entice you to make the right choice.

What I have included in the recipes should never be regarded as the absolute combination. Rather, you are free to substitute zucchini or summer squash for cucumber, or add slices of it to enhance a tomato and beef soup. There should be no limit to your creativity.

Spring Soups

Spring is a time of growth, but it is also a time dominated by wind. The weather is unstable in spring and it is easy to catch a cold or become affected by external pathogens. To protect and nourish the liver, the spring viscera, opt for green leafy vegetables, food with sour flavors like schisandra, and food that enters into the liver meridian like chrysanthemum, Chinese wolfberries (lycii berries), pork liver, and green leafy vegetables like lycii leaves and watercress.

Spring wind also causes allergies and headaches. The Cantonese have several soup recipes that use fish heads to dispel or quell the wind in the head.

SPRING SOUP RECIPES	春天湯水
Two-Tone Bok Choy and Tofu Soup	金銀莢鹹魚頭豆腐湯
Cereus Blossom and Lean Pork Soup	霸王花煲豬肉
Fermented Black Bean and Tofu Soup	薑蔥淡豆豉豆腐湯
Two-Color Turnip and Beef Shank Soup	青紅蘿蔔牛腱湯
Halibut Collar and Daikon Soup	蘿蔔魚腮湯
Arrowroot, Aduki Beans, and Dace Soup	粉葛赤小豆煲鯪魚
Watercress and Gizzard Soup	西洋菜煲鮮陳腎湯
Chrysanthemum, Lycii Leaves, Lycii Berry, and Pork Liver Soup	菊花杞子枸杞葉豬肝湯
Ligusticum and Angelica Dahurica with Fish Head Soup	川芎白芷燉魚頭湯

Two-Tone Bok Choy and Tofu Soup 金銀莢鹹魚頭豆腐湯

To Round Up the Heat and Moisturize the System from the Inside-Out

One of the most popular and abundant Chinese vegetables, bok choy is eaten both for its delicious taste and its ability to counter internal dryness. When both dried bok choy and fresh bok choy are used in the same soup, they are called gam ngahn choi 金銀莢 to reflect the yellow (gold) and white (silver) tones. The tofu, after cooking for hours, becomes spongy and honeycomb-like. It is known as louhfo tofu.

> 1 ounce dried bok choy
> 1½ pounds pork neck bone
> 1 tablespoon vegetable oil
> 5 thin slices (about ⅛-inch thick) peeled fresh ginger
> 1 12-ounce package firm tofu, cut into 2- x 2- x 1-inch pieces
> ¼ cup dried mussels, cleaned
> 3½ ounces salted fish head, cleaned
> ½ piece dried Mandarin orange peel
> 1¾ pounds fresh bok choy, trimmed and cut into 3-inch pieces

Reconstitute the dried bok choy by soaking it for at least 3 hours in warm water. Drain and rinse clean of grit and cut into 3-inch pieces.

Feiseui: In a pot large enough to hold the pork bones, bring 2 quarts of water to a boil over high heat, add pork bones, and boil for 5 to 10 minutes. Drain and rinse bones with cold water.

In a skillet, heat the vegetable oil and add the ginger. Cook for 1 or 2 minutes, until slightly browned. Add 1 cup of water and set aside.

Put pork bones, tofu, mussels, salted fish head, orange peel, browned ginger along with the liquid, reconstituted bok choy, and 4 quarts of water into a large pot. Bring to boil over high heat, reduce heat to medium, and cook for 2 hours. Add the fresh bok choy and continue to cook, covered, over medium heat for 30 minutes more.

Serves 6.

SUGGESTIONS AND VARIATIONS:

Dried bok choy can be used alone off-season when fresh bok choy is not available.

If salted fish head is not available, use dried oysters instead. Half a pound of lean pork, salted overnight with 1 tablespoon of sea salt, may also substitute for the salted fish head. Rinse salted pork before using.

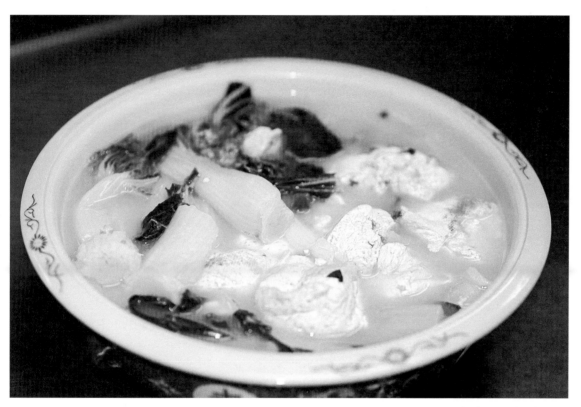

Two-Tone Bok Choy and Tofu Soup

Cereus Blossom and Lean Pork Soup 霸王花煲豬肉

To Soothe a Dry Throat

A beautiful white succulent flower that can grow up to 1 foot in diameter, the cereus blossom blooms at night in warm, semi-tropical climates and tastes a bit like artichoke. Boiled cereus bloosom is softer than dried bok choy and less chewy.

3 ounces (approximately 12 blossoms) dried cereus blossoms
6 brown or honey dates, rinsed
¼ cup large, Southern apricot kernels, rinsed
1 tablespoon small, Northern apricot kernels, rinsed
1 luo han guo
1½ pounds lean pork, cut into chunks

Soak dried cereus blossom in cold water overnight or in warm water for 1 hour, then drain.

Feiseui: In a large pot, bring 2 quarts of water to a boil and add pork. Cook over high heat for about 10 minutes, until foam forms on the top. Drain, discarding cooking water, and rinse pork in cold water.

In a large pot, bring 4 quarts of water to a boil. Add cereus blossoms, dates, apricot kernels, and luo han guo, and cook over high heat for 15 minutes. Add pork, reduce heat to medium, and cook for 2 hours more. To avoid boiling over, raise the lid with a pair of bamboo chopsticks set across the rim of the pot. Remove luo han guo pieces. Salt to taste.

Serves 6.

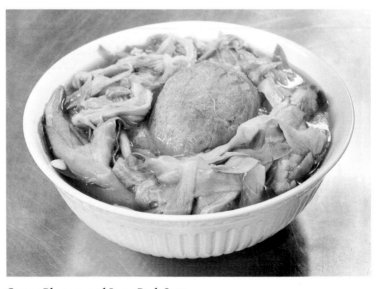

Cereus Blossom and Lean Pork Soup

Fermented Black Bean and Tofu Soup 薑蔥淡豆豉豆腐湯

Preventive and Curative of Colds

A decoction of fresh ginger, green onion, and unsalted fermented black beans has been used for generations to treat the common cold. It is recorded among the classical formulas in *Essential Prescriptions of the Golden Chest* (Jin-Gui Yao-Lue Fang-Lun) 金匱要略方論, by Zhang Zhong-Jing, circa 220 AD. This soup disperses cold and helps with itchy throat, nose, and eyes. Taken regularly in early and mid-spring, it can build up the body's resistance. It also beats the cold-like symptoms of a hangover.

> 1 tablespoon vegetable oil
> 5 green onions, white parts only, cut into 1-inch lengths
> 1 12-ounce package firm tofu, cut into 2- x 2- x 1-inch pieces
> 4 thin slices (about ⅛-inch thick) peeled fresh ginger
> ¼ cup unsalted fermented black beans, rinsed

Heat vegetable oil in a wok or large, heavy skillet over medium-high heat. Add the tofu and cook until lightly browned on one side, about 5 minutes, then turn over and brown the other side.

In a separate pot, combine the browned tofu, fermented black beans, and ginger with 1½ quarts (6 cups) of cold water. Bring to a boil, then reduce heat and cook for 30 minutes. Add white part of green onions, return to a boil, and serve immediately. Strain, discard the solids, and serve the liquid.

Serves 4.

Two-Color Turnip and Beef Shank Soup 青紅蘿蔔牛腱湯

This soup gets its good looks from green turnip and carrot, which is called hùhng lòh baahk (literally "red turnip") in Cantonese. You may want to add white daikon to make the soup even more colorful. Cooked beef shank can be sliced and served as a cold plate along with oyster-flavored sauce or soy sauce seasoned with thinly sliced fresh garlic for dipping. Green turnips are best in early spring.

> 10 slices ginger
> 1 long beef shank piece or 3 crosscut pieces of beef shank (approximately 2 pounds)
> 3 green turnips (approximately 2 pounds), peeled and roll-cut into 1½-inch pieces
> 4–5 carrots (approximately 2 pounds), peeled and roll-cut into 1½-inch pieces

Feiseui: If using crosscut pieces of beef shank, bring 2 quarts of water, along with the ginger slices, to a boil in a large pot. Cook for 5 to 10 minutes, until a foamy residue rises to the top. Drain, discard water, and rinse thoroughly. If using whole shank, you may skip this step as the whole shank will not yield scum; just rinse it and use directly in soup, bypassing the feiseui step.

In a large pot, combine the beef shank, green turnips, and carrots with 4 quarts of water and bring to a boil. Reduce heat to medium and cook for 3 hours. Salt to taste. Serve hot.

Serves 6.

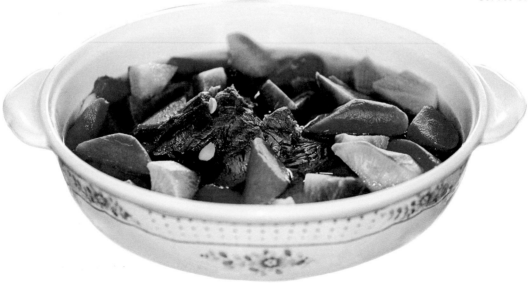

Two-Color Turnip and Beef Shank Soup

Halibut Collar and Daikon Soup 蘿蔔魚腮湯

The collar part of any good-sized fish can be used for this soup. I personally prefer halibut collar or salmon collar because of their meatiness.

3 tablespoons vegetable oil

7 thin slices (about ⅛-inch thick) peeled fresh ginger

2 pieces halibut collar (approximately 1½ pounds), rinsed and patted dry

2 large daikon (approximately 4 pounds), peeled and roll-cut into 1½-inch pieces

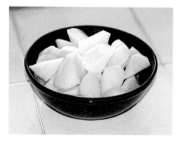

Heat vegetable oil in a deep frying pan over medium-high heat. Add 4 slices of the ginger and cook until browned. Add halibut collar and brown on both sides. Discard the ginger pieces.

In a large pot, combine the daikon, halibut collar, and remaining fresh ginger with 4 quarts of water. Bring to a boil, reduce heat to medium, and simmer for 2 hours. Salt to taste. Serve hot.

Cut Daikon

Serves 6.

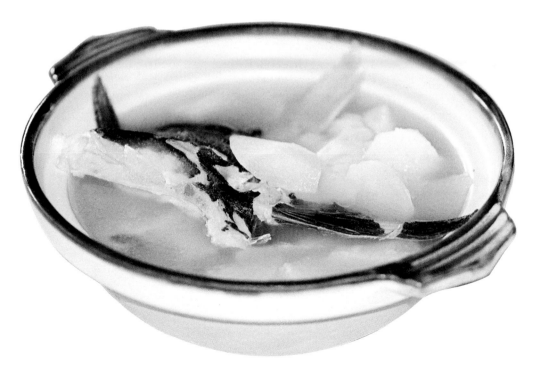

Halibut Collar and Daikon Soup

Arrowroot, Aduki Beans, and Dace Soup 粉葛赤小豆煲鯪魚

To Soothe a Cough

Arrowroot and aduki beans help replenish the body when it is recovering from a cold or hangover. The small bones of the dace-carp are sharp and forked, so some prefer to place the fish in a bag made of cheesecloth. Vegetarians may omit the fish entirely, along with the dried oysters, dried scallops, and pork bones.

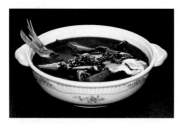

Arrowroot, Aduki Beans, and Dace Soup

1½ pounds pork bone
2 dace-carp (approximately 1½ pounds), cleaned and patted dry
2 whole arrowroots, peeled and cut into ¼-inch slices
5 ounces aduki beans
9 honey dates
1 whole piece dried Mandarin orange peel
1 luo han guo
1½ cups dried oysters, rinsed
8 dried scallops
4 tablespoons vegetable oil
4 thin slices (about ⅙-inch thick) peeled fresh ginger

Feiseui: Place pork bone into a pot of boiling water and cook for 10 minutes. Drain pork bone, discarding water, and rinse off fat and residue.

In a large skillet, heat the oil over medium-high heat, add the ginger and carp and cook fish, turning once, until it is browned on both sides, about 5 minutes per side. Place the fish in a mesh bag.

Fill a large pot with 4 quarts of cold water and add pork bone, browned fish, arrowroot slices, aduki beans, dates, orange peel, luo han guo, dried oysters, and dried scallops. Bring to a boil, lower heat to medium, and simmer for 3 hours. Remove the fish bag. Salt to taste and serve hot.

Serves 6.

Watercress and Gizzard Soup 西洋菜煲鮮陳腎湯

With the slow-cooking method, the minerals in watercress are well dissolved in the soup, making them easier for our bodies to absorb.

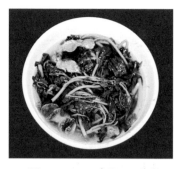

2 pounds pork bones
2 ounces dried duck gizzards
9 ounces fresh chicken or duck gizzards
6 honey dates
4 bunches watercress (approximately 1½ pounds)

*Watercress and Gizzard Soup
(cooked only 1 hour)*

Feiseui: Place pork bones in a large pot of hot water. Bring to a boil and cook for 10 minutes. Drain pork bones, discarding water, and rinse thoroughly.

Place both dried and fresh gizzards in 4 quarts of water, together with the rinsed pork bones, and bring to a boil. Add watercress and dates and bring to a boil again. Lower heat and simmer for 3 hours. Serve hot.

Serves 6.

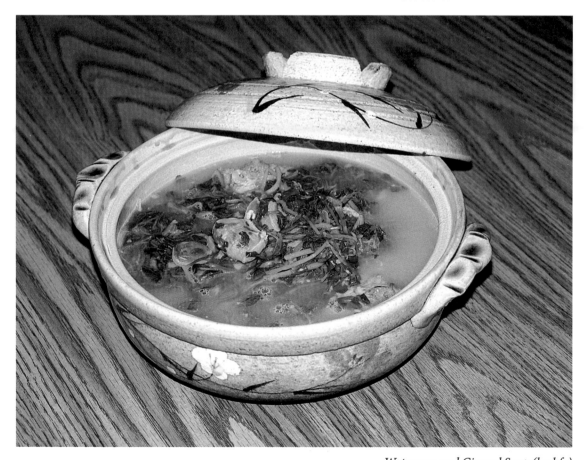

Watercress and Gizzard Soup (louhfo)

Chrysanthemum, Lycii Leaves, Lycii Berry, and Pork Liver Soup 菊花杞子·枸杞葉豬肝湯

Eyebright Soup

Lycii is also known as Chinese wolfberry or goji berry. The dark green lycii leaves are rich in iron and are good for tonifying the blood. Lycii leaves help dispel wind and brighten the eyes. Pork liver reputedly has similar functions. When the two are boiled together, however, a dark, murky and somewhat bitter soup results. The situation can be improved by marinating and coating the liver with cornstarch. To sweeten the pot and brighten its color, I have taken the liberty of adding some red goji berries and a few dried white chrysanthemums to the classic recipe. This soup tonifies the liver.

> 7 ounces pork liver, thinly sliced
> 1 teaspoon cornstarch
> ¼ teaspoon salt
> ¼ teaspoon sugar
> ¼ teaspoon ginger powder
> 2 tablespoons lycii berries
> 2 tablespoons dried white chrysanthemums (about 7 blossoms)
> 5 ounces lycii leaves, removed from stems and rinsed

In a bowl, combine pork liver, cornstarch, salt, sugar, and ginger powder. Marinate for at least 30 minutes.

Soak the lycii berries and chrysanthemum separately in hot water for 10 minutes. Do not drain.

In a stainless steel or clay pot, bring 2½ quarts of water to a boil. Add lycii leaves and bring back to a boil. Stir in the pork liver and add the lycii berries and chrysanthemums along with their soaking liquid. Reduce heat to medium and continue to cook for 15 minutes more. Serve hot.

Serves 4.

SUGGESTIONS AND VARIATIONS:

If you have an issue with the cholesterol in the liver, use lean pork and/or egg white instead.

Chicken liver, which can be purchased in smaller quantity, may be substituted for the pork liver.

You'll get a vegetarian liver tonic by simply eliminating the use of liver and adding eggdrops to the soup.

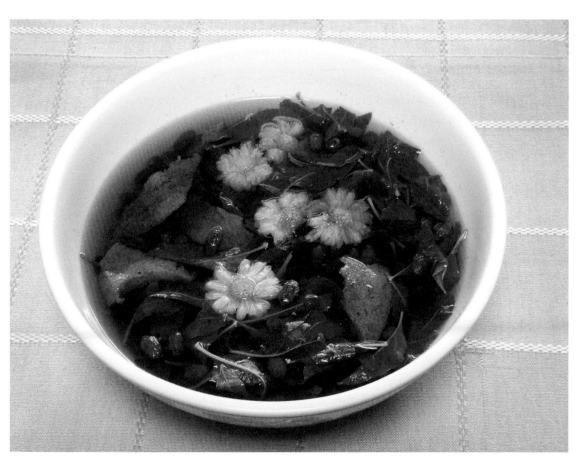

Chrysanthemum, Lycii Leaves, Lycii Berry, and Pork Liver Soup

Ligusticum and Angelica Dahurica with Fish Head Soup
川芎白芷燉魚頭湯

Helping with Sinus Headache

Headaches caused by sinus problems or blood and qi obstruction can be helped with this medicinal soup. Angelica dahurica is the herb for dispelling wind-cold, while ligusticum moves the qi and blood as well. This soup helps open up the sinuses and reduce headaches on the forehead, around the eyes, and on top of the head.

Traditional Chinese food therapy uses fish heads to treat dizziness and headaches. Cantonese cooks favor the head of the grass carp or the Big Fish which is rich in gelatin. Because of the rich minerals therein, the use of fish head to cure headaches is more than tapping into the power of suggestion.

> 6 thin slices (about ⅙-inch thick) peeled fresh ginger
> 1 large fish head (about 2 pounds), rinsed and left whole or
>   chopped into large chunk, patted dry
> 3 tablespoons vegetable oil
> ½ ounce ligusticum, rinsed
> ⅓ ounce angelica dahuria, rinsed
> 10 red jujube dates, pitted
> Dash ground white pepper

Heat vegetable oil in a deep frying pan or wok over medium high heat. Add 4 ginger slices and cook until browned. Add fish head and cook until browned. Discard ginger.

Place ligusticum, angelica dahuria, dates, remaining ginger, and fish head in a porcelain pot. Fill with enough hot water to just cover the ingredients. Cover the pot and boil for 2 hours over medium heat. Season to taste with salt and white pepper. Serve hot.

Serves 4.

SUGGESTIONS AND VARIATIONS:

For headaches at the temples, side and back of the head, replace ligusticum and angelica dahurica with tian ma (½ ounce) and caltrop (1/3 ounce). For headaches at the lower part and base of the head, use kudzu root (½ ounce) instead.

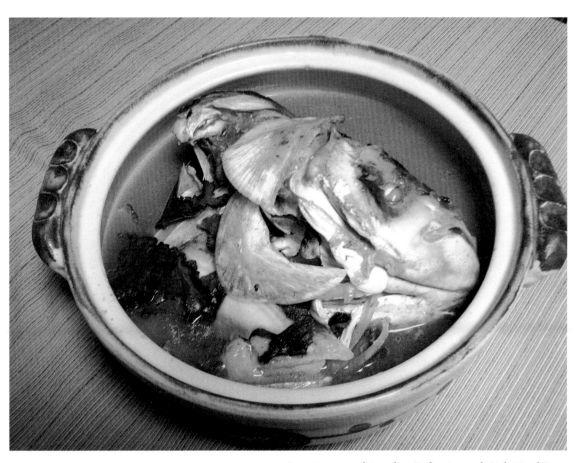

Ligusticum and Angelica Dahurica with Fish Head Soup

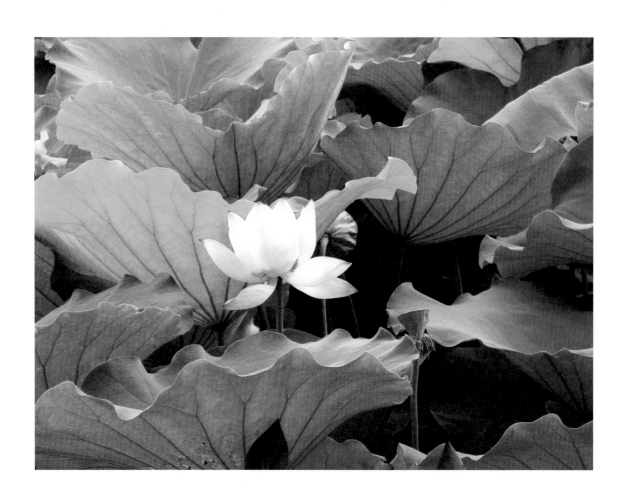

Summer Soups

Summer belongs to the Fire element. The heat rises and affects the heart. During this season, we should avoid heavy and greasy food. Eat light and clear. Cooling and cleansing food is in order. Sea vegetables are great for this time of year. The favorite taste of the season is bitter. Among all the wonderful summer squashes, bitter melon is arguably the favorite.

The Chinese also recognize the Long Summer, known in the U.S. as "Indian summer." This is the fifth season corresponding to the Earth element. Like summer, the food should also lean on the clear and light side. The internal organs involved, however, are the pivotal spleen and stomach, and we should aim to clear heat and dispel dampness. Tonify the body with foods that are helpful to the spleen and stomach, such as whole grains and Ching Bo Leung.

SUMMER SOUP RECIPES	夏日湯水
Winter Melon, Pearl Barley, and Sparerib Soup	什錦冬瓜湯
Ching Bo Leung Soup	清補涼
Salted Egg and Mustard Green Soup	鹹蛋芥菜湯
Bitter Melon and Fish Soup	苦瓜魚湯
Cucumber and Lean Pork Soup	黃瓜瘦肉湯
Tomato and Beef Soup	番茄牛肉湯
Purple Laver and Tofu Soup	紫菜豆腐湯
Seaweeds, Rehmannia, and Pork Sparerib Soup	昆布海藻大生地湯
Fuzzy Melon, Dried Scallop, and Sparerib Soup	節瓜干貝排骨湯
Soybean Sprouts and Kelp Soup	黃豆芽菜海帶湯

Winter Melon, Pearl Barley, and Sparerib Soup 什錦冬瓜湯

Radiant Skin

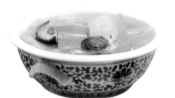

Winter Melon, Pearl Barley, and Sparerib Soup

Winter melons keep well throughout the year, though they mature in early winter. A soup made with winter melon clears internal heat and helps with edema. Pearl barley helps improve appetite and skin complexion.

> 1½ pounds winter melon
> 1½ pounds pork spareribs, cut into medium-sized pieces
> 4 dried scallops
> 1 piece dried Mandarin orange peel
> 3 ounces pearl barley, rinsed
> 1 set chicken giblets (one of each chicken liver, heart, and gizzard)
> 3 thin slices (about ⅛-inch thick) peeled fresh ginger (the old
>   stringy kind is preferred)

Scrub the skin of the winter melon, remove seeds and pulp, and cut into 2-inch cubes.

Feiseui: In a pot of boiling water, add spareribs and cook for 10 minutes. Drain, discard water, and rinse ribs.

Feiseui: In a small pot of boiling water, add rinsed chicken giblets, cook for 10 minutes. Drain, discard liquid, and rinse. Crisscross-cut the gizzard.

Soak dried scallops in warm water for 2 hours, retaining liquid.

Soak dried Mandarin orange peel in cold water for 30 minutes and scrape off and discard the white pith inside.

Place spareribs, chicken giblets, scallops along with their soaking liquid, pearl barley, orange peel, ginger, and winter melon in a large pot along with 4 quarts of cold water. Bring to a boil over high heat. Reduce heat to medium, cover, and boil for another 2½ to 3 hours. The melon will turn translucent. Salt to taste. Serve hot.

Serves 6.

SUGGESTIONS AND VARIATIONS:

Instead of cutting the winter melon and meat into big chunks, finely dice the melon and meat (½-inch cubes) and use other finely diced ingredients such as bamboo shoots, bamboo pipe, black mushroom, fresh mushroom, ham, gizzard, shrimp, and chicken breast. This will make for a fancier recipe fit for feasts. (see Eight Treasure Diced Melon Soup on page 199).

Ching Bo Leung Soup 清補涼

A Cleansing and Cooling Tonic

Ching means "to clear or cleanse," bo means "to tonify," and leung means "to cool" in the Cantonese dialect. This herbal combination is so popular that the combined herbs are available pre-packaged in Asian markets. Ching Bo Leung can also be made into a sweet soup by omitting the meat and adding a cup of rock crystal sugar.

> **8 ounces lean pork**
> **1 6-ounce package of Ching Bo Leung, rinsed**

Feiseui: Place pork in a large pot along with 2½ quarts of cold water. Bring to a boil over high heat and skim off any residue that rises to the surface.

Add the herbs and return to a boil. Reduce heat to medium and simmer for 2 hours. Salt to taste. Serve hot.

Serves 4.

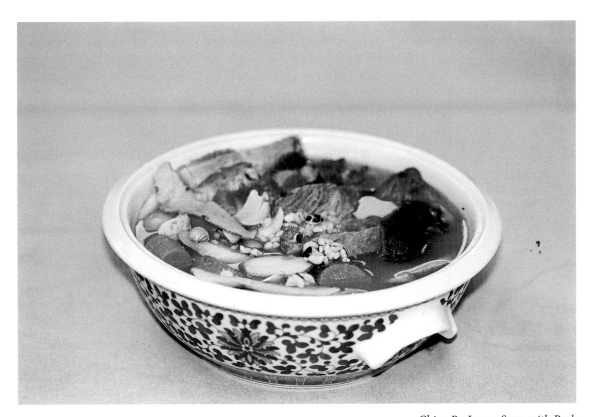

Ching Bo Leung Soup with Pork

Salted Egg and Mustard Green Soup 鹹蛋芥菜湯

A Refreshing Summer Soup

With its bitter taste, mustard green is a cooling vegetable to combat summer heat.

¾ pound lean pork, thinly sliced
¼ teaspoon salt (optional)
¼ teaspoon sugar
1 teaspoon soy sauce
1 teaspoon cornstarch
1 teaspoon vegetable oil
1½ pound pounds mustard greens, cut into 2-inch pieces
1 salted duck egg, diced
3 thin slices (about ⅛-inch thick) peeled fresh ginger

In a bowl, combine pork, salt (if using), sugar, soy sauce, constrach, and oil. Marinate for 30 minutes.

Place mustard greens and ginger along with 2½ quarts of cold water in a large pot. Bring to a boil and add marinated pork and salted egg. Return to a boil, reduce heat, and simmer for 5 to 10 more minutes. Serve hot.

Serves 6.

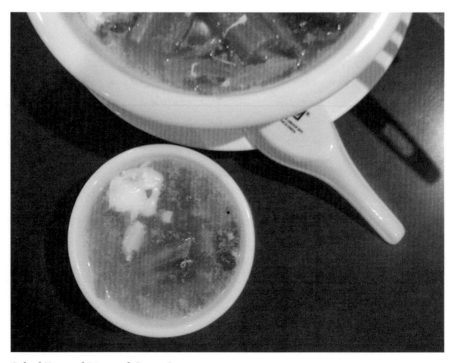

Salted Egg and Mustard Green Soup

Bitter Melon and Fish Soup 苦瓜魚湯

A Cooling Summer Soup

The bitter melon is also called leung gwa, "the cooling melon," in Cantonese.

Bitter melons are in season in the summer. They are dried for off-season use. Using both fresh and dried bitter melons in the same soup gives it a very interesting taste, at once green and earthy. Bitter melon soup is good for parched lips and parched mouth resulting from eating too much fried and spicy food. It quenches thirst from the summer heat.

Recently, some old formulas with bitter melon as a major ingredient have been rediscovered for the treatment of diabetes. Bitter melon tea is available these days in health food stores.

½ ounce dried bitter melon
2 fresh bitter melons (approximately 1 pound)
6 red jujube dates
1 piece Mandarin orange peel (about ⅓ of a whole peel)
4 tablespoons vegetable oil
3 thin slices (about ⅛-inch thick) peeled fresh ginger
1 black bass or silver carp (approximately 1½ pounds), scales, gills,
    and black belly lining removed
2 tablespoons cooking wine
½ luo han guo, rinsed

Rinse and soak dried bitter melon in warm water for 30 minutes.

Halve fresh bitter melon lengthwise, scrape out the seeds and pulp, and cut into 2-inch pieces.

Rinse and soak red jujube dates in warm water for 30 minutes, drain, and remove pits.

Rinse and soak Mandarin orange peel in cold water for 20 to 30 minutes, scrape off the white inside part.

Heat the oil in a deep frying pan, add the ginger, and cook until browned. Add the fish and cook, turning once, until both sides are golden brown. Remove ginger. Add wine and 2 cups of hot water to the fish. Cover and cook for 5 to 10 minutes over medium heat.

In a large pot, bring 4 quarts of water to a boil. Add the cooked fish and liquid, along with the fresh and dried bitter melon, luo han guo, dates, and Mandarin orange peel. Bring to a boil. Reduce heat to medium, and cook for 2 hours. Remove luo hau guo pieces. Salt to taste. Serve hot.

Serves 6.

If you like the fresh bitter melon to retain its green color, do not put the lid on. If you do, the bitter melon will become soft and yellowish. It is only a matter of personal preference.

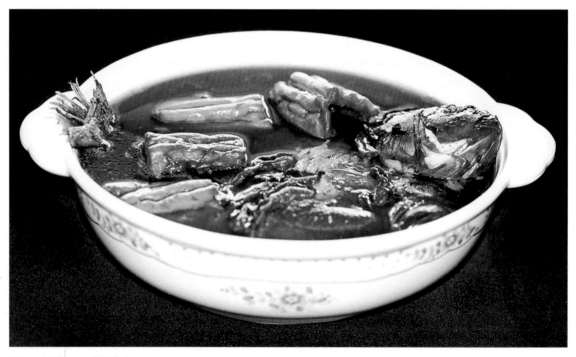

Bitter Melon and Fish Soup

Cucumber and Lean Pork Soup 黃瓜瘦肉湯

The Western simile "cool as a cucumber" holds true even after the cucumber is cooked. Cucumbers can be stuffed and steamed, sautéed, or boiled in a soup. They are favorite Cantonese summer cuisine.

> 4 dried scallops
> 1 piece Mandarin orange peel (about ⅓ of a whole peel)
> 1 pound lean pork
> ¼ cup large, Southern apricot kernels, rinsed
> 1 tablespoon (½ ounce) small, Northern apricot kernels, rinsed
> 3 thin slices (about ⅛-inch thick) peeled fresh ginger
> 3 honey dates, rinsed
> 1½ pounds cucumber, peeled, seeded, and cut into 1½-inch pieces

Rinse and soak dried scallops in warm water for 2 hours, retaining liquid.

Soak Mandarin orange peel for 30 minutes, scrape off and discard the white inside pith.

Feiseui: Cook pork in boiling water for 5 to 10 minutes. Drain and rinse with cold water.

In a large pot, combine soaked dried scallops along with their soaking liquid, orange peel, both types of apricot kernels, ginger, dates, and pork with 4 quarts of water and bring to a boil over high heat. Reduce heat to medium and cook for an hour.

Remove the pork and chill for 1 hour in the freezer.

Add cucumber to the soup. Bring to a boil and then simmer uncovered over medium-low heat for 20 minutes. Salt to taste.

Thinly slice the chilled pork and serve on the side along with any desired condiments.

Serve the soup hot or at room temperature.

Serves 6.

SUGGESTIONS AND VARIATIONS:

Some varieties of cucumber such as English cucumber or Japanese cucumber do not require peeling. Tender seeds need not be removed.

You may use any summer squash in place of cucumber for this soup, including bitter melon, loofah squash, zucchini, and fuzzy melon.

Tomato and Beef Soup 番茄牛肉湯

Tomatoes are refreshing. Their flavor is enhanced by fresh vegetables like onions, carrots, celery, and cabbage.

> ¾ pound beef (round or flank steak)
> ¼ teaspoon salt
> ¼ teaspoon sugar
> 1 teaspoon soy sauce
> 1 teaspoon cornstarch
> 1 teaspoon vegetable oil, for marinating
> 1 medium yellow onion, sliced
> ¾ pound tomatoes, cut into wedges
> ½ pound carrots, peeled and cut into 1-inch pieces
> ½ pound celery, cut into 1-inch pieces
> 2 tablespoons vegetable oil, for sautéing

Thinly slice the beef against the grain into ⅛-inch (2 to 3 mm) slices.

In a bowl, combine sliced beef with salt, sugar, soy sauce, cornstarch, and vegetable oil. Marinate for 1 hour in the refrigerator.

In a large skillet, heat vegetable oil over medium-high heat, sauté the onion.

In a large pot, bring 4 quarts of water to a boil, then add sautéed onion along with the tomatoes, carrots, and celery. Return to a boil, reduce heat to medium, and cook for 1 hour.

Return soup to high heat. Add beef and cook for and additional 5 to 10 minutes. Serve hot or at room temperature.

Serves 6.

SUGGESTIONS AND VARIATIONS:

I like to use beef shank cut the Chinese way in a tomato soup. Simply boil the beef with all the other ingredients. Take the beef shank out and chill. Thinly slice the beef and arrange on a plate or on the soup.

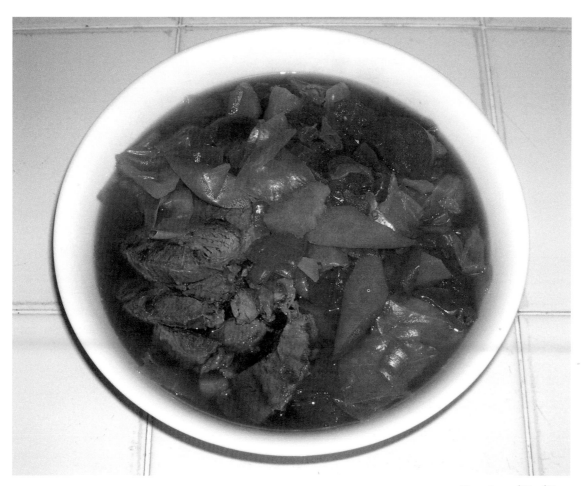

Tomato and Beef Soup

Purple Laver and Tofu Soup 紫菜豆腐湯

Purple laver, known as nori in Japanese, is rich in iodine and other minerals.

¼ pound purple laver
1 tablespoon dried shrimp (about 1 ounce)
¾ pound lean pork, sliced
½ teaspoon salt
1 teaspoon soy sauce
¼ teaspoon sugar
1 teaspoon vegetable oil
1 teaspoon cornstarch
1 12-ounce package silken tofu, cut into 1-inch cubes
2 teaspoons finely minced ginger
3 green onions, finely chopped

Rinse purple laver and soak in cold water for 30 minutes. Rinse again to get rid of grit and drain.

Soak dried shrimp in cold water for 1 hour, retaining liquid.

In a bowl, combine pork, salt, soy sauce, sugar, vegetable oil, and cornstarch and marinate for 30 minutes.

In a large pot, combine 2½ quarts of hot water and purple laver and bring to a boil. Add dried shrimp along with their soaking liquid, pork, and tofu and return to a boil. Stir in minced ginger and chopped green onion and serve immediately.

Serves 4.

SUGGESTIONS AND VARIATIONS:

You may leave out the pork and dried shrimp and enjoy this as a vegetarian soup. Add one or two beaten egg whites at the end, if desired.

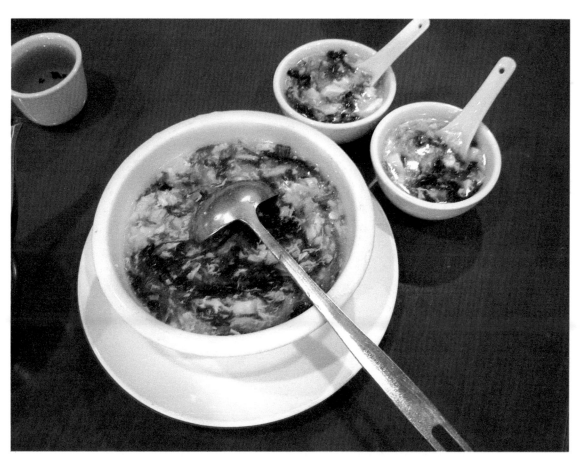

Purple Laver and Tofu Soup with Eggdrop

Seaweeds, Rehmannia, and Pork Sparerib Soup
昆布海藻大生地湯

Chelating Heavy Metal and Radioactive Material

This soup is recommended for people exposed to X-rays or radiotherapy. In our polluted environment, it is desirable to serve seaweed soup once in a while to cleanse the system, as seaweeds are known for their ability to dispel heavy metals such as lead and radioactive materials from our bodies. Usually, it is not recommended for women in their menstrual period because it may induce heavy discharge.

In this traditional recipe, the brown seaweed *kwan bou* and the green seaweed *hoi jou* are always used together.

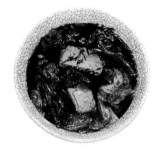

Seaweeds, Rehmannia, and Pork Sparerib Soup

1 piece Mandarin orange peel (about ⅓ of a whole peel)
½ ounce *kwan bou* (brown seaweed)
½ ounce *hoi jou* (green seaweed)
1 pound pork spareribs, cut into narrow strips
1 ounce untreated rehmannia root, sliced

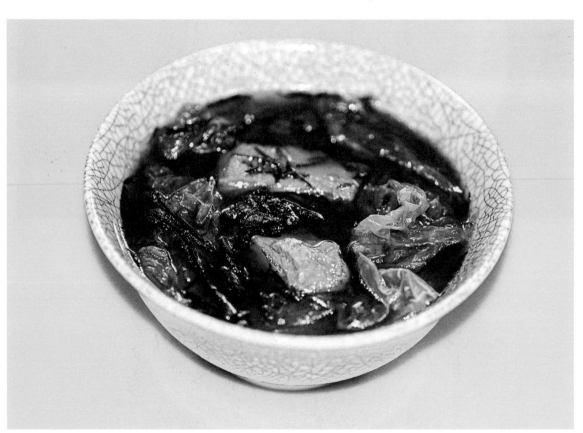

Seaweeds, Rehmannia, and Pork Sparerib Soup

Soak Mandarin orange peel in cold water for 30 minutes. Scrape off and discard the white inside pith.

Rinse and soak brown seaweed in cold water for 1 hour.

Rinse and soak green seaweed repeatedly to get rid of sand.

Feiseui: In a large pot, cook spareribs in boiling water for 5 to 10 minutes. Drain and rinse with cold water. Cut into approximately 1-inch pieces between bones.

In a large pot, combine the pork, seaweeds, Mandarin orange peel, and rehmannia root with 4 quarts of cold water. Bring to a boil, and then reduce heat to medium-low and simmer for 2 hours. Add additional hot water to the soup as needed. Serve hot.

Serves 6.

SUGGESTIONS AND VARIATIONS:

Some people use a whole pound of pork shoulder, probably to balance the "lean-ness" of sea vegetables. For a richer flavor, dried scallops or dried shrimp may be added.

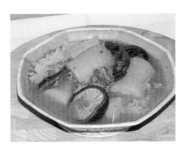

Fuzzy Melon Soup with Black Mushroom

Fuzzy Melon, Dried Scallop, and Sparerib Soup
節瓜干貝排骨湯

A Refreshing Soup to Right the Qi

Squashes and melons are in season in the summer. A soup made with fuzzy melon quenches thirst and calms the qi from the summer heat.

3 fuzzy melons (approximately 1½ pounds)
1½ pounds pork spareribs, cut into 1-inch pieces
4 dried scallops
6–8 dried black mushrooms (optional)

Peel fuzzy melons, halve lengthwise, then into 2-inch sections crosswise, and then cut into domino-sized pieces.

Cook spareribs in boiling water for 5 to 10 minutes. Drain.

Rinse and soak dried scallops in cold water for 2 hours, retaining liquid.

Rinse and soak dried black mushrooms, if using, in hot water for 30 minutes, or until soft, retaining liquid. Cut big ones into halves or quarters.

In a large pot, combine spareribs, scallops along with their soaking liquid, black mushrooms along with their soaking liquid, and fuzzy melon with 4 quarts of cold water. Bring to a boil. Reduce heat to medium, cover, and simmer for another 2 hours. Serve hot.

Serves 6.

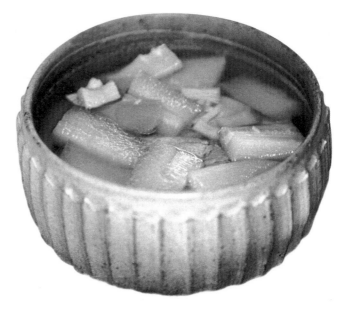

Fuzzy Melon, Dried Scallop, and Sparerib Soup

Soybean Sprouts and Kelp Soup 黃豆芽菜海帶湯

Kelp is the cosmetic sea vegetable. It opens the pores for people with oily skin and helps with acne. Soybean sprouts are tasty and rich in fiber. As they come from the hard-to-digest soybean, however, they need to be cooked 45 minutes or more for good digestion.

½ pound kelp
1 pound pork spareribs, cut into 1-inch pieces
2 carrots, peeled and cut on the diagonal into ¼-inch slices
½ pound soybean sprouts, rinsed, drained, and with stringy ends
     pinched off
3 slices ginger

Wash and soak kelp overnight until soft. Rinse and cut into 1-inch strips.

Feiseui: Cook spareribs in boiling water for 5 to 10 minutes. Drain and rinse in cold water.

In a large pot, put spareribs, carrots, kelp, soybean sprouts, and ginger in 4 quarts of water and bring to a boil. Reduce heat to medium and cook for 1½ hours. Serve hot.

Serves 6.

SUGGESTIONS AND VARIATIONS:

Just the soybean sprouts and kelp make a great vegetarian soup, which can double as a soup base with other ingredients. Use the above recipe, substituting tofu puffs or frozen tofu for the spareribs for another vegetarian recipe.

This soup is so basic that you may add fungi (woodears and mushrooms), napa cabbage, zucchini squash, kabocha pumpkin, bamboo shoots, peas or peapods, or any combination thereof, to create more mixed vegetable soups of your own.

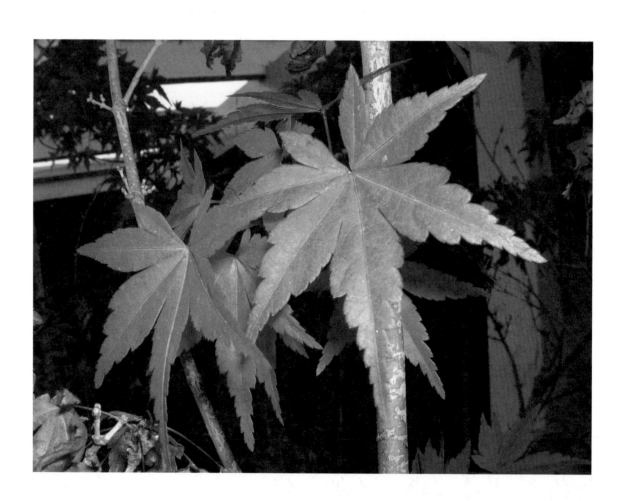

Autumn Soups

There is dryness in the air in the fall and it affects our lungs. We should maintain our good health and avoid harm by paying attention to moisture in the air we breathe, in the food we eat, and within our systems.

Pay attention to your mouth. Is it parched and bitter? Pay attention to your skin. It is dry and scaly? Pay attention to your voice. Do you have a dry cough and a scratchy throat?

In TCM terms, autumn is associated with the metal element and the pungent (or spicy-hot) taste. An appropriate amount of hot chile encourages the circulation of fluid and perspiration. Nuts, seeds, and squash harvested in the autumn season are the best lubricants for our systems. Among the medicinal herbs, the Chinese value *dendrobium nobile* as the best voice maintenance herb for opera singers.

AUTUMN SOUP RECIPES	秋季湯水
Dendrobium, American Ginseng, and Lean Pork Soup	石斛花旗參瘦肉湯
Dendrobium and American Ginseng Soup	石斛花旗參湯
American Ginseng and Partridge Soup	花旗參鷓鴣湯
Fritillary Bulb and Pear Soup	川貝燉雪梨
Chayote and Lean Pork Soup	合掌瓜瘦肉湯
Apricot Kernels, Momordica Fruit, and Pork Soup	南北杏羅漢果瘦肉湯
Gingko Nut, Bean Curd Stick, and Pork Stomach Soup	白果腐竹豬肚湯
Kabocha Pumpkin, Corn-on-the-Cob, and Sparerib Soup	南瓜粟米排骨湯
Crabmeat and Bamboo Pipe Bisque	蟹肉竹蓀羹
Chicken and Corn Bisque	雞茸粟米羹
Spinach, Oysters, and Tofu Soup	菠菜生蠔豆腐湯
Black-Eyed Pea and Chicken Feet Soup	眉豆花生煲雞腳
Oxtail, Beef Tendon, and Peanut Soup	花生牛尾牛筋湯

Dendrobium, American Ginseng, and Lean Pork Soup
石斛花旗參瘦肉湯

The "Soothing and Cooling" Orchid

The American ginseng from Wisconsin is prized as a yin tonic. Unlike the stimulating panax ginseng, American ginseng is suitable for people with high blood pressure.

The dendrobium stem clears internal heat, quenches thirst, and eliminates dryness in the mouth and throat. It is more suitable for people of the heat-type. People with cold constitution should make this soup with a few slices of fresh ginger.

The fancy, knotted dendrobium will become unfurled after boiling. Boiled dendrobium is mildly sour and salty, but, in this soup, it is balanced by the sweet flavors of pork and honey dates.

> 1 piece Mandarin orange peel (about ⅓ of a whole peel)
> 1 pound pork loin, cut into chunks
> ½ ounce knotted dendrobium
> ¼ cup sliced American ginseng, sliced (approximately ¾ ounce)
> 1 ounce poria cocos
> 1 ounce codonopsitis
> ½ ounce large, Southern apricot kernels
> 2 ounces dried wild yam
> 6 honey dates or dried figs
> 1 ounce lily bulb scales

Rinse and soak Mandarin orange peel in cold water for 30 minutes, then scrape off and discard the white pith from the inside of the peel.

Feiseui: Cook pork in boiling water for 5 minutes, then drain and rinse with cold water.

In a large pot, combine the Mandarin orange peel, pork, dendrobium, American ginseng, poria cocos, codonopsitis, apricot kernels, wild yam, and dates or figs with 2½ quarts of water. Bring to a boil over high heat and cook for 30 minutes. Reduce heat to medium-low and simmer for 1½ hours. Add lily bulb scales and cook another 30 minutes. Serve hot or at room temperature.

Serves 6.

SUGGESTIONS AND VARIATIONS:

If you use a thermal cooker, after boiling everything for 30 minutes, place the inner pot in the thermos for 6 to 8 hours.

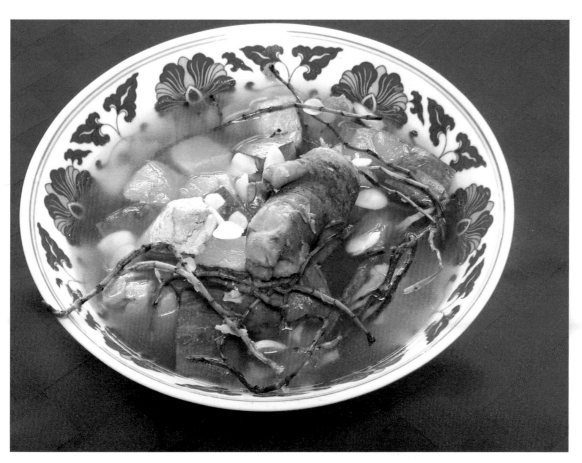

Dendrobium, American Ginseng, and Lean Pork Soup

Dendrobium and American Ginseng Soup 石斛花旗參湯

New World Energy

This "soup" is more like an herbal tea, to be taken like a beverage, for singers and for travelers whose voice may be affected by loss of sleep and jet lag.

¼ cup sliced American ginseng (approximately ¾ ounce), rinsed
½ ounce dendrobium, rinsed
2 ounces dried wild yam, rinsed
6 honey dates or dried figs
3 thin slices (about ⅛-inch thick) peeled fresh ginger (optional)

In a medium pot, combine the ginseng, dendrobium, wild yam, dates or figs, and ginger (if using) with 2½ quarts of hot water. Bring to a boil over high heat and cook for 30 minutes. Reduce heat to medium-low and simmer for 1½ hours. Strain the soup, discard solids, and serve the liquid hot or store in a thermal flask and drink throughout the day.

Serves 4 (or 1 if consumed as a tea throughout the day).

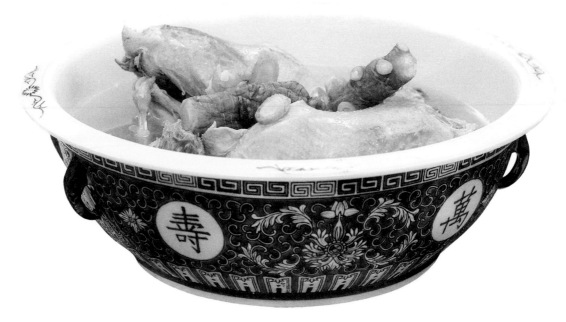

American Ginseng and Partridge Soup (opposite page)

American Ginseng and Partridge Soup 花旗參鷓鴣湯

American ginseng tonifies and moistens yin. It counteracts chronic weakness like panax ginseng, but without elevating blood pressure. American ginseng goes well with any poultry in a soup, but Chinese chefs like to pair the pricey American ginseng with delicate birds like partridges and squab.

> **2 partridges (about 1½ pounds)**
> **1½ pounds pork neck bone**
> **¼ cup sliced American ginseng, rinsed**
> **¼ cup large, Southern apricot kernels, rinsed**
> **1 teaspoon small, Northern apricot kernels (approximately**
> **⅛ ounce), rinsed**

Feiseui: Cook partridges in boiling water for 10 minutes, then drain and rinse with cold water. Cook pork neck bone in boiling water for 10 minutes, then drain and rinse with cold water.

In the inner pot of a 3½-quart thermal cooker, combine partridges, pork bone, ginseng, and apricot kernels with 2½ quarts of cold water. You may need to add more or less water to ensure that the ingredients are covered, but make sure that the water level stays at least 3 inches below the rim of the pot to avoid boiling over. Bring to a boil over high heat, then reduce heat to medium, cover, and simmer for 30 minutes. Place inner pot in the thermal cooker. Let soup slow-cook inside the thermal cooker for at least 3 hours. It won't hurt to keep it there longer.

Skim off any fat that has risen to the top. Strain out the solids, return the broth to the stovetop and reheat over medium-high heat for 5 minutes. Serve broth piping hot with the meat and other ingredients on the side.

Serves 6.

Fritillary Bulb and Pear Soup 川貝燉雪梨

To Stop Dry Coughing

This soup is reputed to soothe a scratchy throat and smooth a hoarse voice due to "dry heat" condition.

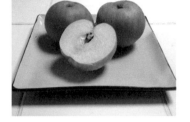

Asian pears

> **3 Asian pears (about 2¼ pounds)**
> **⅓ cup fritillary bulbs, rinsed with cold water**
> **12 small, Northern apricot kernels**
> **6 honey or brown dates**

Peel and core pears and cut into large chunks.

In a medium pot, combine pear, fritillary bulbs, apricot kernels, and dates with 2 quarts cold water. Bring to a boil over high heat, reduce heat to medium-high, and cook for 30 minutes. Reduce heat to medium and simmer for 1 hour more.

Serves 4.

SUGGESTIONS AND VARIATIONS:

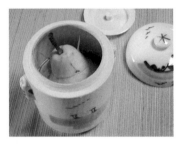

Pear in Urn for Double-Boiling

You may use different kinds of pear though Asian pear is usually preferred. Apples may be used as well.

For an individual serving, you may put the pear in a steaming urn and double-boil it with fritillary bulb powder inside.

As the pear and the date are naturally sweet, no sugar is needed for this soup. You may, however, add ¼ cup of rock crystal sugar if desired.

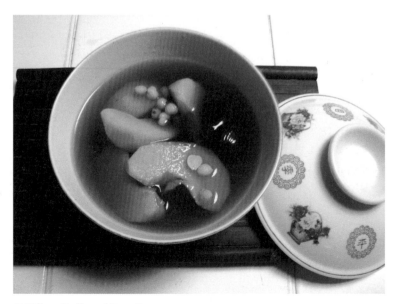

Fritillary Bulb and Pear Soup

Chayote and Lean Pork Soup 合掌瓜瘦肉湯

Good for Indian summer

Native of tropical America, the chayote is valued for its delicately sweet flavor. It belongs with summer squashes though it matures in late summer.

1 pound lean pork, cut into 2-inch cubes
6 black mushrooms
3 chayote squash (about 1¼ pounds), peeled and cut into medium chunks (1½-inch size)
1 carrot, peeled and cut into 1-inch pieces
¼ cup large, Southern apricot kernels
1 teaspoon small, Northern apricot kernels
3 honey dates, rinsed
3 thin slices (about ⅛-inch thick) peeled fresh ginger

Feiseui: Cook pork in boiling water for 5 minutes, then drain and rinse with cold water.

Rinse and soak black mushrooms in warm water for 30 minutes or until soft. Remove stem and reserve soaking liquid. Cut large ones in halves or quarters.

In a large pot, combine pork, mushrooms along with their soaking liquid, chayote, carrot, apricot kernels, dates, and ginger with 4 quarts of water. Bring to a boil over high heat and cook for 30 minutes. Reduce heat to medium and cook for 1½ hours. Salt to taste. Serve hot.

Serves 6.

SUGGESTIONS AND VARIATIONS:

The skin of the green, pear-shaped chayote must be removed. Some people have to wear rubber gloves when peeling raw chayotes because they are allergic to the slimy and sticky substance they exude. You may parboil the chayotes for a few minutes before peeling to avoid possible skin irritation.

A vegetarian version is derived by replacing pork with the Four Items, also known as the Four Flavors, which are basic for health maintenance (see recipe on pages 237–238).

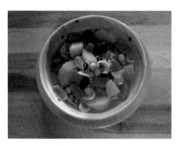

Chayote and Four Items Soup

Apricot Kernels, Momordica Fruit, and Pork Soup
南北杏羅漢果瘦肉湯

This is a traditional soup for coughs. Honey dates and momordica fruit (luo han guo) give the soup a pleasant sweetness.

4 dried scallops
1½ pounds pork tenderloin
¼ cup large, Southern apricot kernels, rinsed
1 teaspoon small, Northern apricot kernels, rinsed (approximately ⅛ ounce)
½ momordica fruit (luo han guo), rinsed
3 honey dates, rinsed
3 thin slices (about ⅛-inch thick) peeled fresh ginger

Rinse and soak dried scallops in cold water for 2 hours. Reserve the soaking liquid.

Feiseui: Cook pork tenderloin in boiling water for 10 minutes, then drain and rinse with cold water. Cut into large chunks (about 2 inches thick).

In a large pot, combine scallops along with their soaking liquid, pork, apricot kernels, momordica fruit, dates, and ginger with 4 quarts of cold water. Bring to a boil and cook over high heat for 30 minutes. Reduce heat to medium-low and simmer for 1½ hours. Salt to taste. Serve hot.

Serves 6.

Gingko Nut, Bean Curd Stick, and Pork Stomach Soup
白果腐竹豬肚湯

A Soothing Soup for the Stomach

Pork stomach, referred to in Cantonese as ju tou, is beneficial for stomachic gas. A soup made of gingko nuts and bean curd sticks is said to also help clear lung heat and ease coughing.

- 5 dried bean curd sticks
- 8 black mushrooms
- 1 pork stomach (about 2 pounds)
- 2–3 tablespoons salt, for treating pork stomach
- 3 thin slices (about ⅛-inch thick) peeled fresh ginger
- ¾ pound pork spareribs, in narrow strips
- ½ cup gingko nuts, shelled, blanched and with green centers removed (from a can)

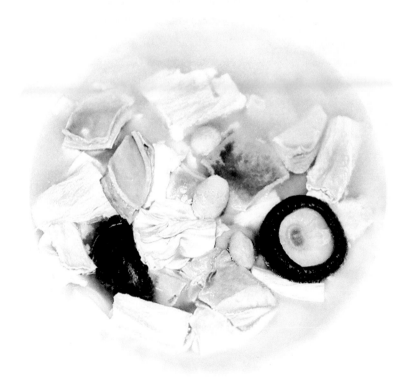

Gingko Nut, Bean Curd Stick, and Pork Stomach Soup

Soak dried bean curd sticks in warm water for 1 hour or until soft, drain, and cut into 2-inch pieces.

Soak black mushrooms in warm water for 1 hour. Reserve soaking liquid. Remove and discard mushroom stems. Use whole or cut into halves.

Turn pork stomach inside out, rub with salt, and rinse a couple of times to remove any stench and slime. Combine with ginger and place in a pot of boiling water. Cook for 10 minutes, then drain and rinse with cold water.

Cook pork spareribs in boiling water for 5 minutes, then drain, rinse with cold water, and cut into small pieces.

In a large pot, combine gingko nuts, black mushrooms and soaking liquid, pork stomach, and spareribs with 4 quarts of cold water. Bring to a boil over high heat, reduce heat to medium, and continue to cook for 2 hours.

Remove the pork stomach from the pot and set it aside to cool. Add the bean curd sticks to the pot and continue to boil over medium heat for 10 to 20 minutes more.

Cut the pork stomach into diagonal pieces about 3 inches long and 1 inch wide. Return the pieces to the pot and cook for an additional 30 minutes. Serve the soup piping-hot.

Serves 6.

SUGGESTIONS AND VARIATIONS:

For really bad stomach gas, add 2 ounces of white peppercorn.

Pickled mustard hearts may be cooked with the pork stomach, lending a sweet and sour flavor to the soup.

Kabocha Pumpkin, Corn-on-the-Cob, and Sparerib Soup
南瓜粟米排骨湯

A Nutty Treasure

The kabocha pumpkin is a gourd. Its flesh is firmer than that of the regular pumpkin we use for making pumpkin pies. Its dark green skin is edible and resembles chestnuts in taste and texture while its orange flesh is rich in potassium. The kabocha pumpkin keeps well for months after the autumn harvest.

> ¾ pound pork spareribs
> 2 ears yellow sweet corn, cut into 2-inch pieces
> 2 carrots, cut into 1-inch pieces
> ¾ pound kabocha pumpkin, seeded and cut into 1-inch chunks
>   with the skin on

Feiseui: Cook spareribs in boiling water for 10 minutes, drain, and rinse with cold water. Cut into small pieces.

In a large pot, bring 3 quarts of water to a boil. Add spareribs, corn, and carrots, and bring to a boil again. Cook over medium-high heat for 30 minutes, reduce heat to medium, and cook for 30 minutes more. Add kabocha pumpkin, and cook for another 20 minutes. Serve hot or at room temperature.

Serves 6.

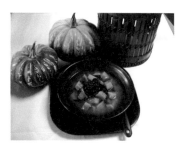

SUGGESTIONS AND VARIATIONS:

For a vegetarian version, replace the spareribs with red kidney beans or black-eyed peas. The beans need to be soaked and cooked as usual. As a shortcut, you may use canned beans. Since kabocha pumpkin does not take long to cook, this version makes for a quick and easy soup.

Kabocha Pumpkin, Corn-on-the-Cob, and Bean Soup

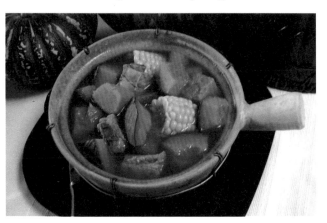

Kabocha Pumpkin, Corn-on-the-Cob, and Sparerib Soup

Crabmeat and Bamboo Pipe Bisque 蟹肉竹笙羹

Thickened soups are Autumn favorites. Their smoothness is soothing and comforting. These soups are thickened with starch, not with cream or by pureeing. The bamboo pipe fungus is a rare delicacy found in panda country.

4 ounces bamboo pipe
1 green onion, cut into 1½-inch lengths
6 slices peeled fresh ginger (about ⅛-inch thick)
1–2 pounds chicken bones
12 ounces crabmeat
½ cup Chinese broccoli stems cut crosswise into thin, round disks
2 egg whites, lightly beaten

THICKENING MIXTURE:

½ teaspoon salt
½ teaspoon sugar
½ teaspoon ground white pepper
2 tablespoons cornstarch
¼ cup water

Cook bamboo pipe, along with green onion and 3 slices of the ginger, in 2 quarts of boiling water for 10 minutes. Drain and cut off head and end of bamboo pipe and cut crosswise into ¼-inch long pieces.

Feiseui: Cook chicken bone in boiling water for 5 minutes, drain, and rinse with cold water.

In a large pot, combine chicken bone and the remaining 3 slices of ginger with 2½ quarts water and cook over medium heat for 1 hour. Discard the chicken bone and ginger, reserving the liquid. Add bamboo pipe to the hot broth and cook for 10 minutes. Add crabmeat and broccoli and bring to a boil. Salt to taste.

In a small bowl, dissolve cornstarch in ¼ cup water, add other thickening ingredients, mix well and stir into the hot soup. Remove pot from heat and add beaten egg white. Serve hot.

Serves 6.

SUGGESTIONS AND VARIATIONS:

When asparagus is in season, it may be used for the little green disks instead of Chinese broccoli. If neither Chinese broccoli nor fresh asparagus are available use a quarter cup of peas and carrots for color.

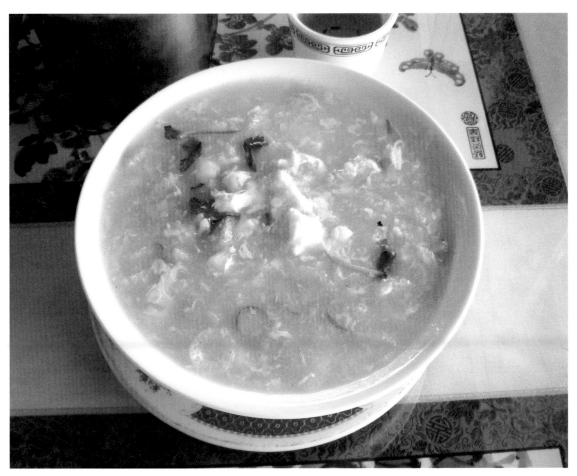

Crabmeat and Bamboo Pipe Bisque

Chicken and Corn Bisque 雞茸粟米羹

This is an all-time favorite for children and adults alike.

½ pound skinless, boneless chicken breast
1 teaspoon dry sherry
5 cups chicken broth
1 cup corn kernels (freshly shucked, if possible)
2 teaspoons ginger, minced
2 egg whites, lightly beaten but not frothy
2 tablespoons finely chopped green onion (optional)
1 tablespoon finely minced ham (optional)

THICKENING MIXTURE:

½ teaspoon salt
½ teaspoon white pepper
2 tablespoons cornstarch
½ teaspoon sugar
¼ cup water

Cut chicken into chunks and put into a food processor. Add sherry and process until meat is a smooth puree.

In a large pot, combine the chicken broth, corn, and minced ginger and bring to a boil over medium heat. Stir in chicken puree and cook until the chicken meat turns white.

In a small bowl, combine the thickening mixture ingredients, then stir into the hot soup. Remove from heat and pour in the egg white, stirring continuously. Garnish with chopped green onion and minced ham. Serve hot.

Serves 4–6.

SUGGESTIONS AND VARIATIONS:

For variety, finely chop 3 ounces of fresh button mushrooms and add along with the corn.

For a quick-and-easy version, you may use canned, creamed-style corn kernels. That is the version used in the recipe for Tai Chi Bisque (see recipe on page 251).

Spinach, Oysters, and Tofu Soup 菠菜生蠔豆腐湯

Spinach is rich in iron. Spinach should never be overcooked because, like most dark leaf vegetables, it turns dark and tastes like mud.

4 dried scallops
¾ pound pork neck bone, chopped into medium pieces
½ pound lean pork, sliced
½ teaspoon salt
½ teaspoon sugar
½ teaspoon soy sauce
1 teaspoon cornstarch
1 10-ounce jar fresh oysters, rinsed
1 teaspoon shredded peeled ginger
1 12-ounce package silken or regular tofu, cut into 1-inch cubes
1 bunch spinach (approximately 12 ounces), washed and drained

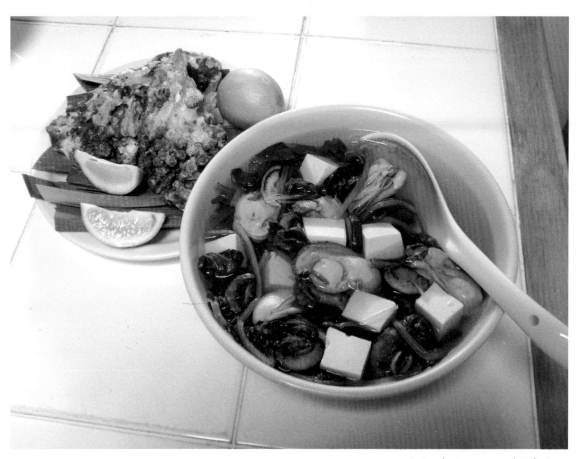

Spinach, Oysters, and Tofu Soup

Soak dried scallops in cold water for 2 hours, then shred, reserving the soaking liquid.

Feiseui: Cook pork neck bone in boiling water for 10 minutes, drain, and rinse with cold water.

In a medium bowl, combine pork, salt, sugar, soy sauce, and cornstarch. Marinate for 30 minutes.

Parboil oysters in boiling water for 2 minutes. Drain.

In a large pot, combine pork neck bone, ginger, and shredded scallops along with their soaking liquid with 4 quarts of cold water. Bring to a boil and cook over high heat for 30 minutes. Reduce heat to medium and cook for another 30 minutes.

Remove pork bone and skim off obvious fat. Add tofu and spinach. Bring to a boil, add pork, and cook, uncovered, for 10 minutes. Add oysters and boil, uncovered, for 5 more minutes. Serve piping hot.

Serves 6.

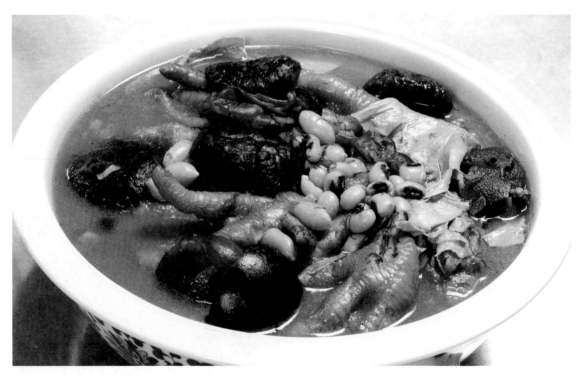

Black-Eyed Pea and Chicken Feet Soup (opposite page)

Black-Eyed Pea and Chicken Feet Soup 眉豆花生煲雞腳

A Soup that Lubricates Skin

Chicken feet and pork bone are favorite ingredients for everyday soups. They are well suited for the family budget. Besides, the Chinese people do not cook a lot of meat except on special occasions. For daily fare, whole chicken or whole pork butt is hardly used in soups. Low in protein and fat but high in gelatin, chicken feet are said to help with skin complexion and strengthen ligaments.

> ¼ cup blanched peanuts
> 12 chicken feet (approximately 1¼ pounds)
> 1 pound pork spareribs, cut into narrow strips
> ¼ cup black-eyed peas, soaked in water overnight and drained
> 4 thin slices (about ⅛-inch thick) peeled fresh ginger

Soak blanched peanuts in cold water for 30 minutes, then drain.

Clean and cut toenails off of chicken feet with a pair of scissors.

Feiseui: Cook spareribs in boiling water for 10 minutes, drain, and rinse with cold water. Cut into small pieces.

In a large pot, combine black-eyed peas, peanuts, spareribs, and chicken feet with 4 quarts of cold water. Bring to a boil over high heat. Reduce heat to medium and continue to boil with the lid elevated by a pair of bamboo chopsticks set across the rim of the pot for 2 to 3 hours. Skim off any obvious fat and serve the soup piping hot. The solids may be removed and served on the side, if desired.

Serves 6.

Oxtail, Beef Tendon, and Peanut Soup 花生牛尾牛筋湯

Tendons provide collagen for joints and ligaments. Beef tendon paired with oxtail gives a balanced form and texture as well as a delicious soup.

> **1½ pounds oxtail**
> **½ pound beef tendon**
> **¼ cup blanched peanuts**
> **3 thin slices (about ⅛-inch thick) peeled fresh ginger**
> **4 stalks celery, cut into 1-inch pieces (optional)**
> **2 carrots, roll-cut into 1½-inch pieces (optional)**

Feiseui: Cook oxtail in boiling water for 10 minutes, drain, and rinse with cold water. Cook beef tendon in boiling water for 10 minutes, drain, and rinse with cold water. Boil on high for 30 minutes. Reduce heat to medium and boil covered for 3 hours. Cool off and cut into 1½-inch sections.

Soak peanuts for 30 minutes, then drain.

In a large pot, combine oxtail, beef tendon, ginger, and peanuts with 4 quarts of water. Bring to a boil and cook for 30 minutes. Reduce to medium heat, cover, and cook for 2½ hours. Add celery and carrots and return to a boil. Reduce heat to medium and boil for an additional 30 minutes. Serve hot.

Serves 6.

SUGGESTIONS AND VARIATIONS:

Oxtail, beef tendon, and peanuts take time to cook. It is easier to cook them in a pressure cooker for 20 minutes before adding to the soup pot.

You may cook the beef tendon overnight in a thermal cooker before cutting it into big pieces and adding it to the other ingredients for another round of cooking in the thermal cooker.

Try adding a pound of fresh tomatoes cut into wedges into this soup, which will give it a Western flair.

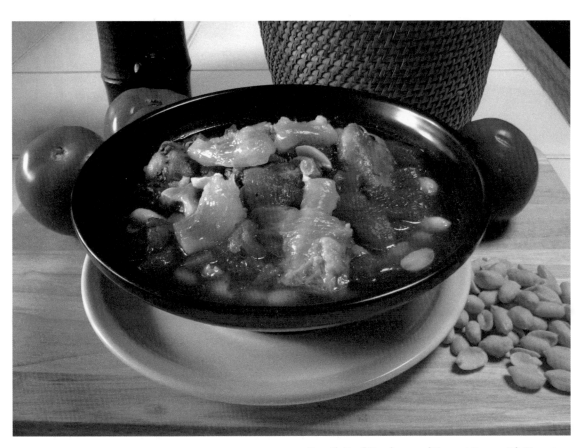

Oxtail, Beef Tendon, and Peanut Soup with Tomatoes

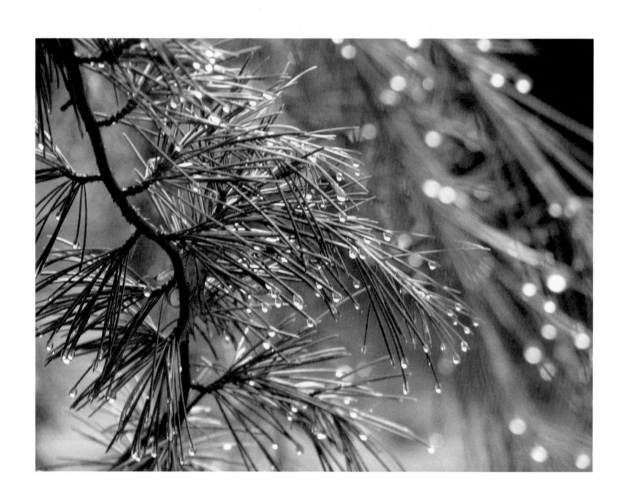

Winter Soups

Winter, the cold season, is associated with the Water element. As winter days are the shortest of the year, the yang energy in our bodies is also at its lowest point during this time. It is a time for us to follow nature's quiet mode to hold, to rest, and to conserve. It is correct to have daylight savings time and to modify our activities accordingly. Get as much sunlight as possible during the day and go to bed early.

Coldness and excessive yin during the winter months tend to obstruct yang energy, aggravating arthritis pain. Winter is the time for tonic soups to replenish and restore kidney deficiency, strengthening our immunity and curing chronic fatigue. Tonic soups help build a solid foundation for our health. In winter, we should have more root vegetables and warming foods such as fresh ginger, and chicken. The best cooking method is, of course, *louhfo* or slow cooking. A warming soup is as comforting as it is easy to digest and assimilate.

WINTER SOUP RECIPES 冬季湯水

White Ginseng and Black Chicken Soup	白參烏雞湯
Lotus Root, Octopus, and Pork Soup	蓮藕鱆魚煲豬肉
Black Mushroom and Chicken Soup	冬菇雞湯
Chestnut, Wild Yam, and Wolfberry Soup	栗子淮山杞子湯
Mom's Chinese-Style Borscht	中式羅宋湯
Black Bean and Catfish Soup	烏豆煲塘虱魚
Abalone and Chicken Soup	鮑魚雞湯
(see recipe under Exotic and Expensive Soups)	
Cordeceps and Chicken Soup	冬蟲草煲雞
(see recipe under Exotic and Expensive Soups)	
The Big Ten Tonic Soup	十全大補湯
(see recipe under Medicinal Soups)	
The Hot Pot (see recipe under Festive Soups)	打甌爐

White Ginseng and Black Chicken Soup 白參烏雞湯

Anti-Aging

White ginseng has not been processed like the red ginseng and is therefore less potent. There are two kinds of white ginseng: fresh and dried. They can be used interchangeably in soup recipes. Ginseng tonifies qi and rejuvenates older people.

> **10 dried chestnuts, blanched**
> **3 sticks Korean white ginseng**
> **10 jujube dates, pitted**
> **1 black chicken (silkie)**
> **2 tablespoons sweet rice**

Rinse dried chestnuts and soak in warm water for 3 hours, then drain.

Soak white ginseng in warm water for 3 hours, or until it is soft. Drain, cut off the head, and slice.

Rub the inside of the chicken with salt, then rinse and chop into big pieces.

Place the chicken along with the ginseng, chestnuts, dates, and rice into a lidded *dahnjung* (double-boiling urn) and fill it with enough hot water to just cover the ingredients. Put the urn, covered, in a steamer and fill the outside pot with water, being careful not to let the water level come up to more than two-thirds the height of the urn. Steam for 5½ hours. Serve hot.

Serves 4.

SUGGESTIONS AND VARIATIONS:

Instead of using the dahn method, put ingredients into 3 quarts of boiling water in a ceramic pot, cook over high heat for 30 minutes, then reduce heat to medium and simmer covered for 2½ hours.

If dried chestnuts are unavailable, use fresh ones. Boil whole chestnuts in shell for 30 minutes. Then remove shell and skin inside.

Lotus Root, Octopus, and Pork Soup 蓮藕鱆魚煲豬肉

Drive Away the Chill

This soup will warm the body inside and out. Its sweet aroma drives the chill away and brightens up a gray day.

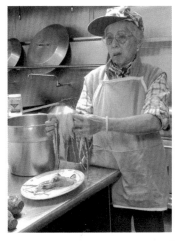

Mrs. Sun Kwong Preparing Dried Octopus in Jene Wah's Kitchen

1 dried octopus (approximately 2½ ounces)
1 pound pork loin
1 pound lotus root
4 red jujube dates, pitted
2 thin slices (about ⅛-inch thick) peeled fresh ginger

Rinse dried octopus and soak in hot water for 2 hours, then cut into bit-sized pieces, straining and reserving the soaking liquid.

Feiseui: Cook pork loin in boiling water for 5 to 10 minutes, drain, and rinse with cold water. Cut into 1½-inch chunks.

Remove lotus root joints, peel, and cut into big chunks by first cutting into 2-inch cross sections and then quartering them vertically.

In the inner pot of a 3½-quart thermal cooker, combine the octopus along with its soaking liquid, pork, lotus root, jujube dates, and ginger with 2½ quarts of water. Bring to a boil and cook over medium heat for 30 minutes. Place pot inside the thermal cooker and let the soup cook slowly for 6 to 8 hours. Serve hot.

Serves 4.

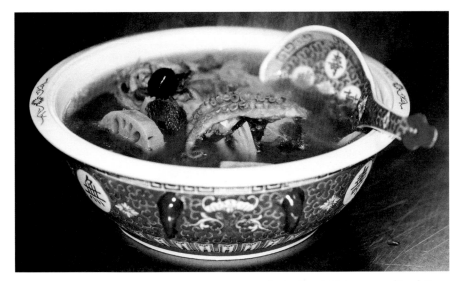

Lotus Root, Octopus, and Pork Soup

Black Mushroom and Chicken Soup 冬菇雞湯

The black mushroom or shiitake mushroom is said to be good for lowering high blood pressure and cholesterol. Its stem and mycelium are said to be good for liver health, so boil the stems in the soup after separating them from the succulent caps. Remove before serving.

> 4 dried scallops
> 10 black mushrooms
> 6 cups chicken broth
> 1 skinless, boneless chicken breast, sliced
> ¼ teaspoon salt
> ¼ teaspoon sugar
> ¼ teaspoon soy sauce
> 1 teaspoon vegetable oil
> 1 teaspoon cornstarch
> 2 ounces bamboo shoots, sliced (optional)
> 2 carrots, peeled and roll-cut into 1½-inch pieces (optional)
> 2 thin slices (about ⅙-inch thick) peeled fresh ginger

Rinse and soak dried scallops in warm water for 2 hours. Save the soaking liquid.

Rinse and soak black mushrooms, then remove their stems, reserving the soaking liquid. The stems may be thrown into the soup pot. Use mushrooms whole or cut mushroom caps into halves or quarters.

In a medium bowl, combine chicken breast with salt, sugar, soy sauce, vegetable oil, and cornstarch. Marinate for 30 minutes.

Cook soaked scallops and mushrooms in the chicken broth and liquid from soaking scallops and mushroom for an hour. Add bamboo shoot, carrots (if using), and chicken slices. Bring to a boil over high heat. Lower heat to medium and simmer for another 10 minutes. Serve piping hot.

Serves 4.

SUGGESTIONS AND VARIATIONS:

Instead of skinless and boneless chicken breast meat, you may use a silkie or Cornish game hen. You may cut chicken into larger pieces.

A number of winter greens like bok choy, napa cabbage, and *yàuh choi* (rape) or turnip green may be added when you put in the other vegetables. Be sure not to cover the pot, lest the greens will turn brown. For extra color, add 2 teaspoons of goji berries.

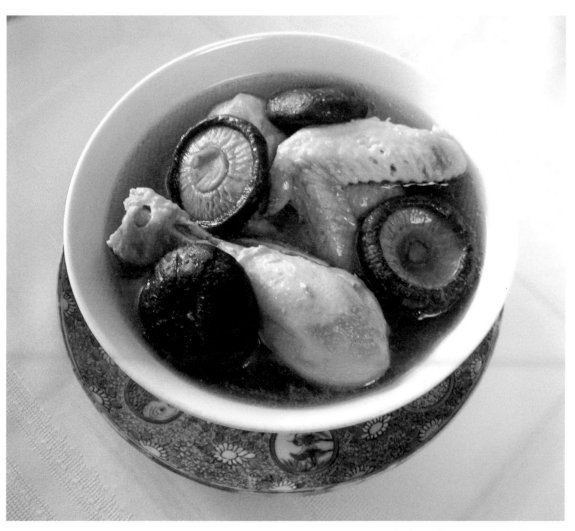

Black Mushroom and Chicken Soup

Chestnut, Wild Yam, and Wolfberry Soup 栗子淮山杞子湯

Combating a Cold with Soup

Both chestnuts and Chinese wild yams strengthen the spleen and boost the body's immunity. This soup helps build up resistance to colds caused by sudden temperature and weather changes. It also helps people with bronchitis in their recovery.

> **12 dried chestnuts**
> **7 slices dried Chinese wild yam**
> **1 pound lean pork**
> **¼ cup Chinese wolfberries**

Soak the chestnuts in warm water for 30 minutes, then drain and remove skin.

Rinse wild yam, then drain.

Feiseui: Cook pork in boiling water for 10 minutes, drain, and rinse with cold water.

In the inner pot of a thermal cooker, combine chestnuts, wild yam, pork, and wolfberries and cover with cold water (about 2½ quarts). Bring to a boil over high heat. Reduce heat to medium and cook for another 15 minutes.

Place the inner pot in the thermal cooker and slow-cook the soup for 6 to 8 hours. Place the inner pot on stovetop and bring to a boil again. Serve piping hot.

Serves 6.

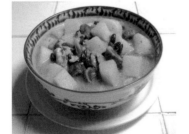

Chestnut, Wild Yam, and Wolfberry Soup

SUGGESTIONS AND VARIATIONS:

Substitute a pound of fresh wild yam for the dried Chinese wild yam. The fresh wild yam is known as nakaimo or yamaimo in Japanese. It looks somewhat like a daikon and may exceed 2 feet in length. It is sold in sections in the Asian grocery store. Trim both ends of each yam section, peel, and cut into large pieces crosswise (about 1 inch thick). Minimize contact with fingers as the cut edge is slimy and some people are allergic to the raw yam.

Mom's Chinese-Style Borscht 中式羅宋湯

My mother probably learned to make borscht from the White Russians in Shanghai. She did not use red beets because she did not like the bloody color of the soup. Instead, she used fresh tomatoes.

2½ pounds beef shank, Chinese or American cut

2 teaspoons vegetable oil

2 yellow onions, halved and sliced crosswise

4 carrots, peeled and sliced

2 potatoes, peeled and sliced

½ head of cabbage, cut into large pieces

2 golden beets, sliced (optional)

2 large tomatoes, cut into wedges

4 ounces mushrooms, sliced

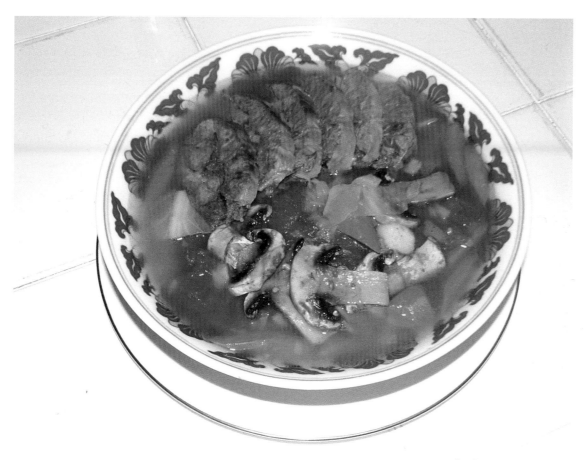

Mom's Chinese-Style Borscht

Feiseui (only necessary if you are using the American crosscut beef shank): Cook beef shank in 2 quarts of boiling water for 10 minutes, drain, and rinse with cold water.

In a frying pan, heat the vegetable oil and sauté the onions until soft.

In a 3½-quart inner pot of a thermal cooker, combine the beef, sautéed onions, carrots, potatoes, tomatoes, mushrooms, cabbage, and beets (if using), cover with 2½ quarts water, and bring to a boil.

Place the inner pot in the thermos and leave the soup there to slowly cook for 4 to 6 hours.

Remove beef shank from the pot, let cool, and thinly slice. Put the inner pot with the soup on the stove again and cook for another 30 minutes over medium heat. Salt to taste. Ladle the vegetables and broth into a soup bowl or tureen and garnish with the sliced beef. Serve immediately.

Serves 6–8.

Suggestions and Variations:

As fresh tomatoes are more expensive during winter months, use canned tomatoes. The essential nutrient lycopene keeps well with cooking and heat processing, but do watch out for sodium content.

If you are cooking in a regular pot, after the initial preparation and boiling, cover with a lid elevated by a pair of bamboo chopsticks laid across the rim, simmer on medium-low heat for 2 to 3 hours, adding more boiling water if needed.

Black Bean and Catfish Soup 烏豆煲塘虱魚

Black beans and catfish are both yin tonics, making for a perfect wintry soup. As black beans are hard to cook and to digest, a special technique is employed.

- 1 catfish (approximately 1 pound)
- 1 cup black beans
- 8 jujube dates, pitted (optional)
- 1 piece dried Mandarin orange peel (about ⅓ of a whole peel)
- 2 teaspoons vegetable oil
- 6 thin slices (about ⅙-inch thick) peeled fresh ginger
- 2 tablespoons cooking wine
- 1 tablespoon sesame oil

Clean the catfish and remove the black lining inside the belly.

Stir-fry the black beans in a dry pan over medium heat until the shells crack open, and then rinse with cold water.

Soak Mandarin orange peel for 30 minutes, drain, then scrape off and discard the white pith inside of the peel. Cut the peel into thin strips.

In a skillet, heat the vegetable oil, then add 2 slices of the ginger and the catfish. When both sides of the fish are browned, add the cooking wine and 1 cup of water. Retain the liquid.

In a large pot, combine the fish, black beans, Mandarin orange peel, jujube dates (if using), and the rest of the ginger with 4 quarts of water and bring to a boil. Raise the lid of the pot with a pair of a bamboo chopsticks laid across the rim. Reduce heat to medium-low and simmer for 2½ hours. Drizzle with sesame oil and serve piping hot.

Serves 4–6.

SUGGESTIONS AND VARIATIONS:

You may use catfish fillet instead of a whole catfish.

12
Healthful Soups for All Seasons

Year-Round Soups

Advances in refrigeration and preservation technology have greatly stretched the shelf life of fresh produce. We can get winter vegetables in summer, and vice versa. Any time of the year, we can make the Tai Chi Bisque (see recipe on page 251) with frozen corn and chopped spinach.

Canning has enabled us to get food from all over the world. For example, we can get canned lychee fruit, longan fruit, baby corn, bamboo shoots, and straw mushrooms from China, and canned abalone from Mexico. Chinese restaurants in the U.S. use canned water chestnuts and the Japanese love canned white asparagus. When I grew up in Hong Kong, canned peaches and fruit cocktails from California were special treats. But no matter how exotic they sound, canned foods are poor substitutes where taste and texture are concerned.

With dried herbs, pickles, grains, nuts, and legumes available year-round, we have even more choices across seasons. Such choices should then be guided by health reasons, regardless of the time of the year. For example, if you want to shed a few pounds, fibrous vegetables like bamboo shoots and great burdock root (牛蒡, *gobo* in Japanese) may help. If you want smooth skin and a radiant complexion, gelatinous food like hasmar, white woodear, swallow's nest, or chicken feet should be included in your diet. If you want to cleanse the system of heavy metal and radiation, take sea vegetables, such as purple laver and kelp. Make a *donggwai* soup with chicken for hot flashes. I can go on and on because there are hundreds of Chinese medicinal teas and soups for myriad ailments, documented and passed down through generations.

There are also soups for general health maintenance. For example, Ching Bo Leung is loaded with antioxidants while The Big Ten Soup features an assortment of tonic herbs to boost vitality. Often, the soup ingredients are pre-packaged and available in Chinese grocery and herb stores so that we do not need to measure out the herbs each time we make these popular soups.

Maybe we don't even need a health condition to enjoy a pot of soup. As the Reverend Aaron Zerah has so aptly put it in *Chicken Soup for the Soul at Work,* "Mom always made her chicken soup at the right time. Rarely did she make it for someone already sick; yet she knew instinctively when you needed some as preventive medicine. Somehow she also knew when hard times were coming. When a slew of salesmen would arrive, all demanding payment, there was a soul-soothing pot of chicken soup. Let the refrigerator break down, the taxman call, the employees leave without notice! We had chicken soup with fresh dill and we would be okay!" No wonder I have always felt that the Great Wall should be linked to the Wailing Wall ever since I had a roommate in college with the name Rappaport. There is no denying Mom's wisdom about chicken soup in all cultures.

Year-Round Soup Recipes	保健養生湯
Sugar Cane, Rhizome of Woolly Grass, Arrowroot, Water Chestnut, and Carrot Soup	竹蔗茅根粉葛馬蹄紅蘿蔔湯
Water Chestnut, Cilantro, and Carrot Soup	馬蹄芫茜紅蘿蔔水
Papaya and Fishtail Soup	木瓜魚尾湯
Four Tonics Fortified with Eucommia	四物杜仲湯
Danggui Chicken Soup	當歸雞湯
Danggui Duck Soup	當歸鴨湯
Fish Trim with Mustard Green and Tofu Soup	一魚兩吃芥菜豆腐湯
Chrysanthemum, Lycii Leaves, Lycii Berry, and Pork Liver Soup (see recipe under Spring Soups)	菊花豬肝枸杞湯
Cereus Blossom and Lean Pork Soup (see recipe under Spring Soups)	霸王花煲豬肉
Ching Bo Leung Soup (see recipe under Summer Soups)	清補涼
Soybean Sprouts and Kelp Soup (see recipe under Summer Soups)	黃豆芽菜海帶湯
Dendrobium, American Ginseng, and Lean Pork Soup (see recipe under Autumn Soups)	石斛花旗參瘦肉湯
Oxtail, Beef Tendon, and Peanut Soup (see recipe under Autumn Soups)	花生牛尾牛筋湯
Mushroom Chicken Soup (see recipe under Winter Soups)	冬菇雞湯

Sugarcane, Rhizome of Woolly Grass, Arrowroot, Water Chestnut, and Carrot Soup 竹蔗茅根粉葛馬蹄紅蘿蔔湯

This soup is antipyretic. It clears heat and replenishes body fluid. It also helps soothe red eyes caused by fatigue or heat conditions.

1 pound pork loin, cut into chunks
1 pound arrowroot, peeled and cut into large pieces
½ pound carrots, peeled and cut into 2-inch pieces
½ pound water chestnuts, top shoot removed, scrub clean
2 ounces rhizome of woolly grass, rinsed
4 honey dates
1 pound sugarcane, each piece halved lengthwise

Feiseui: Cook pork in 2 quarts of boiling water for 10 minutes, drain, and rinse with cold water.

In a large pot, combine pork, arrowroot, carrots, water chestnuts, rhizome of woolly grass, dates, and sugarcane with 4 quarts of boiling water and cook for 1 hour over high heat. Reduce heat to medium and simmer for 1½ hours.

Serves 6.

SUGGESTIONS AND VARIATIONS:

A vegetarian soup can be derived from the above recipe by simply omitting the pork.

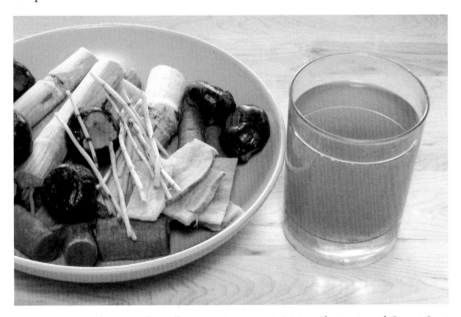

Sugarcane, Rhizome of Woolly Grass, Arrowroot, Water Chestnut, and Carrot Soup

This soup is a more specialized variation of the preceding recipe, commonly served to children suffering from small pox or measles. The herbs allow the affliction to be released through the skin or exterior rather than suppressed and trapped inside.

> ½ pound carrots, peeled and cut into 2-inch pieces
> ½ pound water chestnuts, top shoot removed, scrubbed clean
> 1 bunch cilantro, cut into 4 pieces

In a large pot, combine the carrots and water chestnuts with 2½ quarts of water and bring to a boil over high heat. Reduce heat to medium and simmer for 1½ hours. Add cilantro and continue to cook for 30 minutes more. Strain and serve the broth hot or at room temperature.

Serves 4.

SUGGESTIONS AND VARIATIONS:

You may serve the broth as a beverage throughout the day. The vegetables, especially the cooked water chestnuts, may be eaten as a snack. The peel comes off easily when you bite into it. If you dislike having to spit out the skin, peel the water chestnuts before serving or even cooking. I would not recommend using canned water chestnuts.

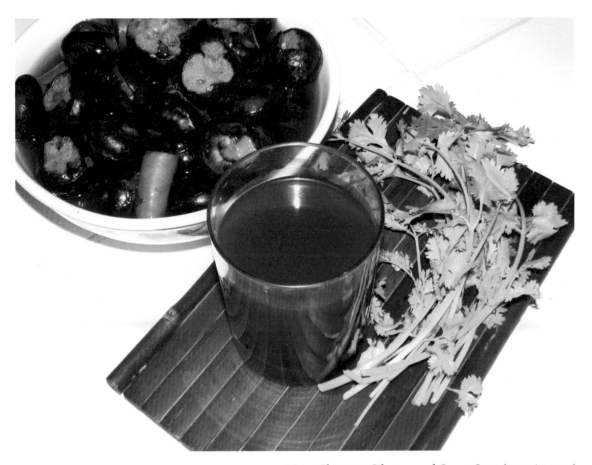

Water Chestnut, Cilantro, and Carrot Soup (opposite page)

Papaya Fish Tail Soup 木瓜魚尾湯

Good Nutrition for Nursing Mothers

Protein in fish is easy to digest. This soup is a pick-me-up for the entire family, not just for the nursing mother and her baby.

    1 papaya (approximately 1¼ pounds), medium ripe
    ½ cup blanched peanuts
    ½ ounce Mandarin orange peel (about ⅓ of a whole peel)
    2 teaspoons vegetable oil
    7 thin slices (about ⅛-inch thick) peeled fresh ginger
    1 fish tail (approximately 1 pound), cleaned
    2 tablespoons cooking wine
    4 honey dates, rinsed

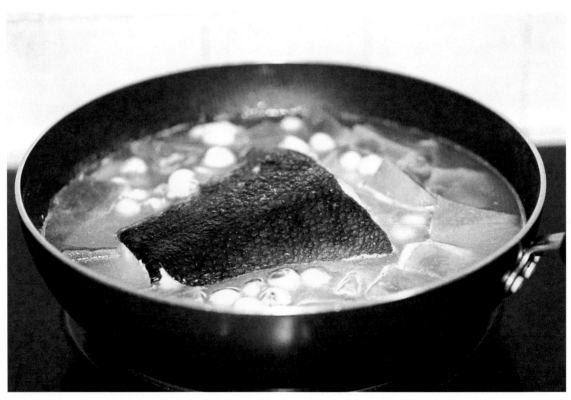

Papaya Fish Tail Soup

Peel the papaya. Remove seeds and pulp and cut into chunks.

Boil peanuts, in the inner pot of a thermal cooker with 1 quart of water for 30 minutes. Place the inner pot in the thermal cooker and let cook for 3 to 5 hours, until the peanuts are soft.

Soak orange peel in cold water for 30 minutes. Scrape off and discard the white pith on the inside of the peel.

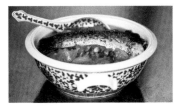

Papaya Fish Tail Soup

In a nonstick pan, heat the vegetable oil over medium-high heat. Add 4 slices of the ginger and the fish. Pan-fry both sides of the fish until they turn golden brown. Add cooking wine and 2 cups of water. Cook for 2 minutes. Set aside.

In a large pot, combine peanuts, dates, orange peel, and the remaining 3 slices of ginger with 2½ quarts of cold water. Cook over high heat for 30 minutes. Add papaya and bring to a boil. Reduce heat to medium and cook for 30 minutes more. Add fish tail and liquid and simmer for 15 minutes. Season to taste with salt and serve hot.

Serves 4.

Four Tonics Fortified with Eucommia 四物杜仲湯

The four tonics are good for tonifying blood. They come pre-packaged. Eucommia tonifies the liver and kidneys. This soup helps to lower high blood pressure and reduce severe pain during a woman's menstrual period. This is a vegetarian version.

> ½ ounce angelica sinensis
> ¼ ounce lovage root (cnidium)
> ½ ounce white peony root
> ½ ounce foxglove root (rehmannia)
> ½ ounce eucommia bark
> 4 ounces vegetarian or mock sausage, rinsed and cut into ½-inch pieces
> 5 jujube dates, pitted

Place the angelica senensis, cnidium, peony root, foxglove root, and eucommia bark in a mesh bag or wrap them in cheesecloth and tie with string.

Place the bag of herbs along with the vegetarian sausage and dates in a clay pot with 2 quarts of water. Bring to a boil over high heat and cook for 30 minutes. Reduce heat to medium and simmer, covered, for another 30 minutes. Remove the bag. Serve hot.

Serves 4.

SUGGESTIONS AND VARIATIONS:

Four Tonics Soup may be cooked with ½ pound of pork spareribs that have been parboiled and rinsed, if desired.

Danggui Chicken Soup 當歸雞湯

Blood Tonic and Hormone Regulator

Danggui (angelica sinensis) has a unique aroma and taste. A soup made with danggui is a blood tonic.

4 boneless, skinless chicken thighs
10 red jujube dates, pitted and rinsed
2 chunks danggui roots
½ ounce fresh ginger root, thinly sliced

Feiseui: Cook chicken in 1 quart of boiling water for 5 minutes, drain, and rinse with cold water.

In a large pot, combine dates, danggui roots, chicken, and ginger with 2 quarts of water. Bring to a boil over high heat. Reduce heat to medium-low and simmer covered for 2½ hours. Serve hot.

Serves 4.

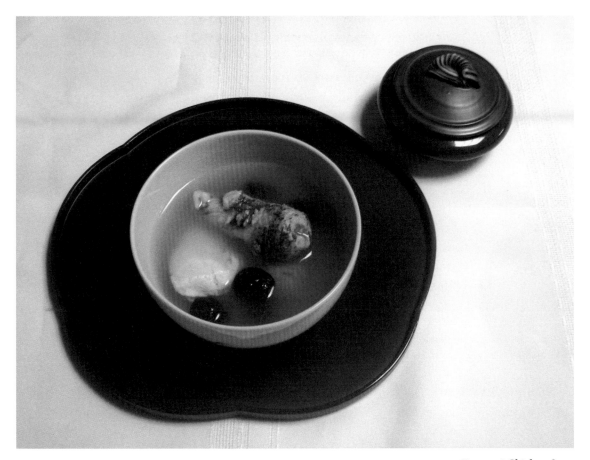

Danggui Chicken Soup

Danggui Duck Soup 當歸鴨湯

Fabulous Flavor from Taiwan

Angelica sinensis, commonly known as danggui, has been used widely in herbal formulas for women with proven results for centuries. Danggui helps with pre-menstrual and post-partum cramps, as well as hot flashes. Its success has led to the misconception that danggui is to be used only by women. This is simply not true. It should be understood that danggui is not a female hormone. It only helps regulate our sex hormone.

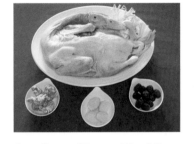

Ingredients of Danggui Duck Soup

Danggui contains bitter elements that complement the flavor of poultry well. Men and women alike in Taiwan enjoy this soup, though Cantonese men would laughingly decline to have a bowl of danggui duck soup. I have included this recipe because I have come to appreciate it very much through my husband's family.

> 8 red jujube dates, pitted, rinsed
> ½ duck (approximately 1½ pounds), skin and fat removed
> 1 ounce fresh ginger, thinly sliced
> ½ ounce danggui root slices, rinsed
> ½ ounce astragalus root slices, rinsed
> ½ ounce codonoposis root, rinsed
> ½ ounce cnidium *(chuanxiong),* rinsed
> 3 tablespoons Chinese wolfberries
> 2 tablespoons cooking wine

Cook duck in boiling water with sliced ginger for 10 minutes, drain, and rinse with cold water. Chop into medium-sized pieces.

In a large pot, combine dates, duck, danggui, astragalus, codonoposis, and cnidium with 4 quarts of water. Bring to a boil over high heat. Reduce heat to medium-low and simmer for 2½ hours. Add wolfberries and continue to boil for 30 minutes more. Add wine, cook 1 more minute, then skim off obvious fat and serve the soup piping-hot.

Serves 6.

SUGGESTIONS AND VARIATIONS:

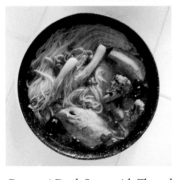

Danggui Duck Soup with Thread Noodles

In Taiwan, Danggui Duck Soup is often served with thin noodles, similar to angel's hair pasta.

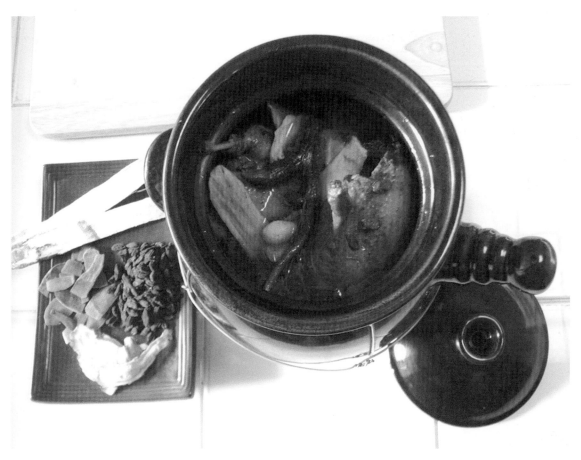

Danggui Duck Soup with Ginseng

Fish Trim with Mustard Green and Tofu Soup
一魚兩吃芥菜豆腐湯

One Fish, Two Delicious Ways to Eat

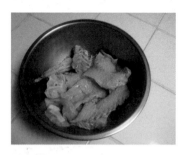

Fish Trim

When one gets a sizeable fish weighing 3 pounds or more, it is common practice to cut it into steaks or fillets. In the West the head and the bones are usually discarded. Asians, on the other hand, salvage the trims to make soup. To the fish stock is added tofu and mustard green.

> 1 whole sturgeon or grouper (about 3 pounds)
> 1 pound mustard green, cut into 2-inch sections
> 1 16-ounce package of regular tofu, cut into domino pieces or
>   1-inch cubes
> 6 thin slices (about ⅛-inch thick) peeled fresh ginger
> 1 12-ounce can of straw mushrooms, drained
> 4 tablespoons vegetable oil
> 2 tablespoons cooking wine

Fillet the fish, leaving the head, the collar, the bones, and other trim. Total weight is about one pound. Cut the back bone into 3-inch sections and chop the head into large chunks.

In a deep, non-stick frying pan, heat vegetable oil and brown the fish head and trim pieces with ginger on medium-high heat, turning to brown both sides. Add cooking wine and 1 quart of water. Bring to a boil.

Add mustard green (stems fist) and tofu. Add more water to cover the ingredients, return to a boil. Reduce heat to medium and simmer uncovered for at least 45 minutes. Add leafy sections of mustard green. Cook until leaves wilt, adding more hot water as needed. Salt to taste.

Strain and serve the broth, with the solids served as a side dish.

Serves 6.

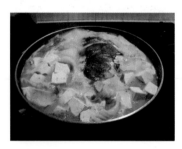

Fish Trim with Mustard Green and Tofu Soup

Suggestions And Variations:

Fish stock tends to be milky white in color. You may further enhance the color by stirring in 1 cup of non-fat milk or soybean milk.

Festive Soups

The Chinese celebrate by the lunar calendar. The most notable celebratory days are New Year's Day, Everyone's Birthday (on the seventh day of the first moon), the first full moon, Memorial Day (the third day of the third moon), Dragon Boat Festival (the fifth day of the fifth moon), Festival of Celestial Love (the seventh day of the seventh moon), Mid-Autumn Festival (the fifteenth day of the eighth moon), Double-Yang Festival (the ninth day of the ninth moon), the Winter Solstice, and New Year's Eve. Overlapping with the solar calendar, the lunar calendar also recognizes the Spring Equinox, Summer Solstice, Autumn Equinox, and Winter Solstice. Family reunions on Chinese New Year's Eve precede fifteen days of New Year's celebrations, culminating with the first full moon. Sweet dumpling soups are served then as well as on the eighth full moon, reputedly the brightest of the year. A comforting savory dumpling soup is served on the Winter Solstice to drive away the chills and the blues.

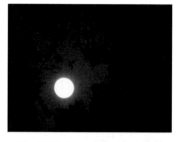

The Full Moon in Mid-Autumn

Chinese Buddhists also celebrate the dates of Buddha's birth and *nirvana*, and the birthday of Guanyin, the Goddess of Mercy.

In China, birthday celebrations are the privilege of the elderly. Everyone else acknowledges their coming into this world on Everyone's Birthday (*yàhn yát* 人日), which falls on the seventh day of the first moon. On that day, braised long-life noodles are served with a steaming pot of rice soup. Nothing fancy. Children do not have birthday parties. In the old days, all that a birthday boy or birthday girl would get was a bowl of long-life noodle soup and a hard-boiled egg, with perhaps some lucky money in a small red envelope, *laihsih* 利是.

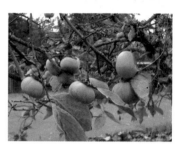

Persimmons in Late Autumn

Grown-ups start celebrating birthdays when they reach sixty. Then, it is a big event every ten years. While patriarchs are given big parties when they become sixty, seventy, eighty, and so on, matriarchs celebrate at sixty-one, seventy-one, eighty-one, and so on. These event call for gatherings of family and friends far and near, gifts, wining and dining, and banquets with expensive soup ingredients like shark's fin, fish maw, abalone, sea cucumber, and swallow's nest.

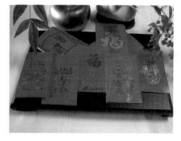

Laihsih—Red Envelopes for Lucky Money

A wedding is of course an event for celebration. The price for each banquet table is pretty much based on the grade of shark's fin used for the first course. No self-respecting Chinese would dare to skimp on the shark's fin lest they lose face and social status. This creates market demand, which results in the crude and cruel harvesting practice of shark's fin by commercial fishing fleets. A report by the National Geographic Society led to a worldwide outcry and boycott, but shark's fin soups continue to be served up at Chinese wedding banquets, probably because the image of sharks as dangerous predators themselves and the fact that sharks are not endangered do not inspire humane protective efforts.

During the wedding ceremony, a sweet tea is offered to the bride consisting of red jujube dates (*hohng jou* 紅棗), lotus seeds (*lihn ji* 蓮子), and a hard-boiled egg with the good wish of *jou-sang-gwai-ji* 早生貴子, meaning "get a baby boy soon."

The birth of a grandchild, especially of a grandson, is also cause for celebration. Chinese grandparents throw a Red Egg and Ginger party when a baby is one month old. Besides getting red hard-boiled eggs and pickled ginger, guests are treated to pig's feet cooked in black vinegar and a chicken soup spiked with port or whisky, partaking in tonic food normally served to the new mother.

FESTIVE SOUPS: CELEBRATIONS THROUGHOUT THE YEAR · 佳節喜慶湯

Crabmeat, Yellow Chives, and Long-Life Noodle Soup	蟹肉韭黃伊麵(長壽麵)
Abalone, Shark's Fin, and Chicken Bisque	鮑魚雞絲魚翅羹
The Wedding Tea = Red Jujube, Lotus Seed, and Egg Tea	新抱茶
Eight Treasure Diced Melon Soup	八寶瓜粒湯
Enoki, Shiitake, Bamboo Pipe, and Tofu Bisque (see recipe under Vegetarian Soups Recipes)	金針菇竹笙豆腐羹
Red Bean Paste Dumpling Soup with Sweet Osmanthus	桂花紅豆湯圓
Winter Solstice Savory Dumpling Soup	冬至鹹湯圓
The Hot Pot	打甂爐
New Year Soup	新年湯
Chicken Wine Soup	雞酒

Crabmeat, Yellow Chives, and Long-Life Noodle Soup
蟹肉韭黃伊麵 (長壽麵)

This is a noodle soup for birthday parties. The long-life noodle is a single strand of noodle coiled into the shape of a cake and lightly deep-fried. It symbolizes longevity.

2 ounces lean pork, shredded
1 teaspoon oyster sauce
½ teaspoon sugar
1 teaspoon cornstarch
6 stalks tender greens (such as Chinese broccoli or rape)
1 tablespoon vegetable oil
1 slab dried long-life noodle
2 dried black mushrooms
½ pound cooked crabmeat
2 quarts chicken broth
4 ounces yellow chives, cut into 1-inch pieces

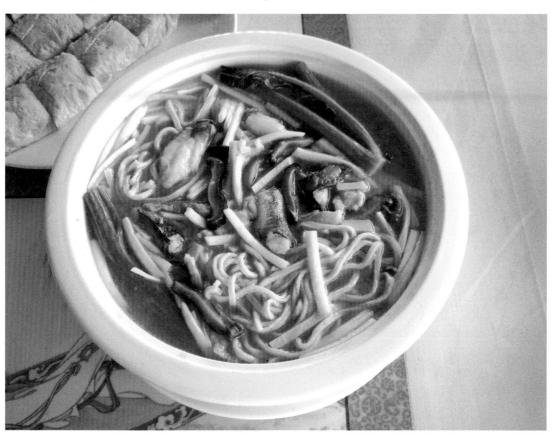

Crabmeat, Yellow Chives, and Long-Life Noodle Soup

Rinse and soak dried black mushrooms in hot water for 30 minutes, until soft, then drain. Cut off and discard stems and shred mushrooms.

In a medium bowl, combine pork with oyster sauce, sugar, cornstarch, and 1 tablespoon of water and set aside to marinate for 30 minutes.

Place greens in a pot of boiling water with 1 teaspoon of the vegetable oil. Blanch (5 to 10 minutes) until tender. Set aside.

Cook dried noodle in 3 quarts of boiling water for 3 minutes or until it softens. Drain and rinse thoroughly with cold water. Set aside.

In a frying pan, heat the vegetable oil, add mushrooms and pork, and stir-fry for about 2 minutes, until pork is cooked through.

In a medium pot, combine chicken broth with 1 quart of water and bring to a boil. Add the chives and cook for 1 minute more, then remove the chives and set aside.

Place noodle in a big bowl and top with pork, mushrooms, crabmeat, and chives. Pour broth over and serve immediately, garnished with blanched greens.

Serves 6.

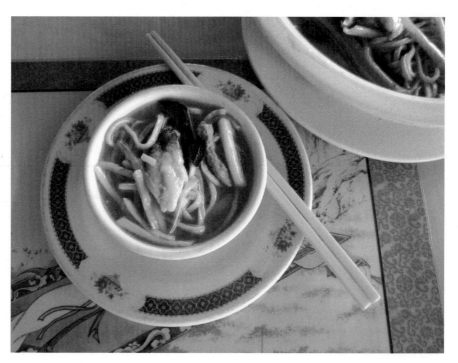

Crabmeat, Yellow Chives, and Long-Life Noodle Soup in Individual Serving Bowl

Abalone, Shark's Fin, and Chicken Bisque 鮑魚雞絲魚翅羹

8 ounces shark's fin, dried

7 thin slices (about ⅛-inch thick) peeled fresh ginger

4 green onions, divided

1 whole chicken (approximately 2 pounds), skin and fat removed

¾ pound lean pork

1 12-ounce can abalone, sliced

2 slices ham (preferably Jinhua or Virginia ham), shredded

2 ounces mung bean sprouts, both ends pinched off

3 tablespoons red vinegar

2 tablespoons Chinese mustard

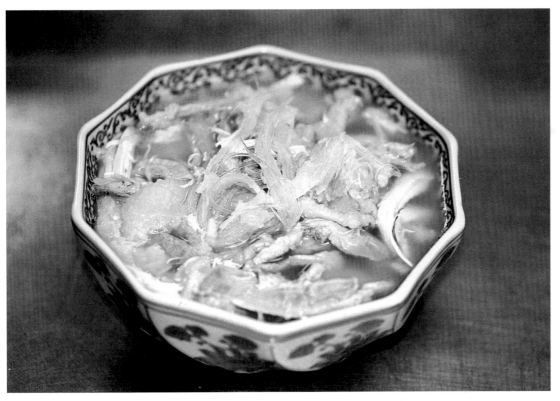

Shark's Fin and Chicken Soup

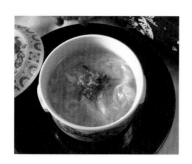

Shark's Fin and Chicken Soup with Shreds of Ham as Garnish

In a large pot, bring 2 quarts of water to a boil and add the shark's fin, 2 slices of the ginger, and 2 of the green onions. Remove from heat, cover, and let sit overnight. When the shark's fin is soft, drain, and rinse with cold water. Set aside.

Feiseui: Cook chicken in 2 quarts of boiling water for 10 minutes, drain, and rinse with cold water. Cook pork in 2 quarts of boiling water for 10 minutes, drain, and rinse with cold water.

Fill the inner pot of a thermal cooker with 2½ quarts of boiling water. Add chicken, pork, and the remaining ginger slices. Cook over high heat for 30 minutes.

Place the inner pot in the thermal cooker and let soup slow-cook inside for at least 3 hours. Remove chicken and pork and set aside. Skim any visible fat off the top of the soup.

Bone the chicken and shred the meat.

Add shark's fin, chicken, pork, abalone, and its juice (from the can) to the soup. Bring to a boil and simmer over medium-low heat for 30 minutes.

If so desired, combine cornstarch and water and gradually add the mixture to the hot soup a little at a time until it reaches the desired thickness.

Serve in individual bowls and garnish with shreds of ham, with side dishes of raw mung bean sprouts, red vinegar, and Chinese mustard as condiments.

Serves 6.

Suggestions and Variations:

When crab is in season in the fall, substitute crabmeat (along with crab roe) for the abalone. In that case, finely chop the ham and sprinkle it over the soup just before serving.

Dried scallops may also be used to substitute for the abalone. Soak the scallops in warm water for 2 hours, reserve the soaking liquid to add to the soup, and shred the scallops.

Instead of going through the trouble of reconstituting shark's fin, you may buy frozen reconstituted ones in large Asian markets.

The Wedding Tea = Red Jujube, Lotus Seed, and Egg Tea 新抱茶

This sweet offering to the wedding party, especially to the bride and groom, is attractive, delicious, and well meaning. While the egg is a symbol of fertility, the other ingredients sound like jóu-sàng-gwai-jí 早生貴子, a wedding wish for the couple to soon beget a baby boy who will grow up to be both rich and prominent in society.

8 eggs
16 red jujube dates
4 ounces lotus seeds, blanched
16 longan fruits
1 cup rock crystal sugar or ¼ teaspoon stevia powder

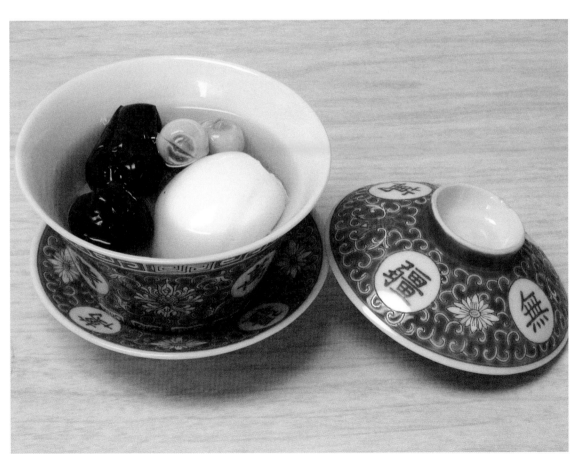

The Wedding Tea

Place eggs in a pot and cover with cold water. Bring to a boil and simmer on low heat for an additional 7 to 10 minutes. Drain and rinse eggs with cold water. When the eggs are cool, remove the shells and the membrane.

Soak lotus seeds in warm water for 1 hour. Drain and remove the green embryo in the center.

Boil red jujube dates, lotus seeds, and longan meat in 2½ quarts of water for 1 hour. Add rock crystal sugar or stevia powder and stir to dissolve.

Place one hard-boiled egg in each serving bowl or cup. Divide lotus seeds, jujube dates, and longan fruit among the tea bowls or tea cups (at least 2 pieces of each for every bowl of tea). Pour the hot liquid over the top.

Serves 8.

Suggestions and Variations:

You should remove the pit from the jujube date so the bride does not need to spit it out during the wedding ceremony. However, you must do it delicately so the dates look intact. You may also buy pitted jujube dates and select the best ones.

Eight Treasure Diced Melon Soup 八寶瓜粒湯

The winter melon is a huge squash, weighing anywhere from 25 to 40 pounds when it matures in early winter. If stored properly, in a cool and dark place off the ground, winter melons can keep through the next summer.

The winter melon can be cut into big chunks and cooked with the rind on. On special occasions, the melon is diced and cooked with small morsels including black mushrooms, bamboo shoots, chicken meat and giblets, shrimp, white woodears, peas and carrots, and abalone tidbits.

> **6 dried black mushrooms**
> **1 white woodear**
> **2 skinless, boneless chicken breasts, trimmed of fat and diced**
> **½ teaspoon soy sauce**
> **½ teaspoon vegetable oil**
> **½ teaspoon cornstarch**
> **6 chicken gizzards**
> **5 cups top stock (see recipe in chapter 5)**
> **6 ounces fresh white button mushrooms, coarsely chopped**
> **2 bamboo shoots, diced**
> **1 cup frozen peas and carrots, thawed**
> **2 pounds winter melon or fuzzy melon, peeled, seeds and pulp**
>   **removed, and diced**
> **½ pound shrimp, peeled, deveined, and coarsely chopped**

Rinse and soak dried mushroom in hot water for 30 minutes, or until soft. Reserve soaking liquid. Cut off and discard stems and finely dice mushrooms.

Soak white woodear in cold water for 1 hour, drain, remove hard stem and separate into florets.

In a bowl, combine chicken, soy sauce, vegetable oil, and cornstarch. Marinate for 30 minutes.

Parboil chicken gizzards in hot water for 10 minutes. Rinse in cold water and cut into ¼-inch dice.

In a large pot, combine the soup stock with 5 cups of water (2½ quarts total) and bring to a boil. Add the chopped gizzards along with both the dried and fresh mushrooms, woodear, chicken, bamboo shoots, peas and carrots, winter melon, and shrimp and boil for 30 minutes over high heat. Reduce heat to medium, cover, and simmer for 1½ hours. Serve hot.

Serves 6.

Suggestions and Variations:

More elaborate versions include crabmeat, roast duck meat, finely diced Smithfield or Virginia ham(⅛-inch pieces), bamboo pipe (¼-inch pieces), and even loose shark's fin needles.

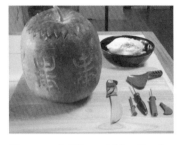

Homemade Winter Melon Bowl

To make a Dung Gwa Jung, or Winter Melon Bowl, get a small winter melon (about 10 pounds, and less than 8 inches in diameter). Cut off the top and save as a lid for the tureen. Scoop out seeds and pulp. Rinse clean. Draw a design on the surface of the melon and, using tools for carving pumpkins on Halloween, carve the outside to reveal the pale inner rind. Steam the melon in a pot of boiling water for 1 hour without any soup inside, then add top stock and ingredients, return to the steamer and double-boil covered for another 1½ hours. Most families do not have steamers that big and that tall, so this presentation is best left for restaurant chefs (see page 290).

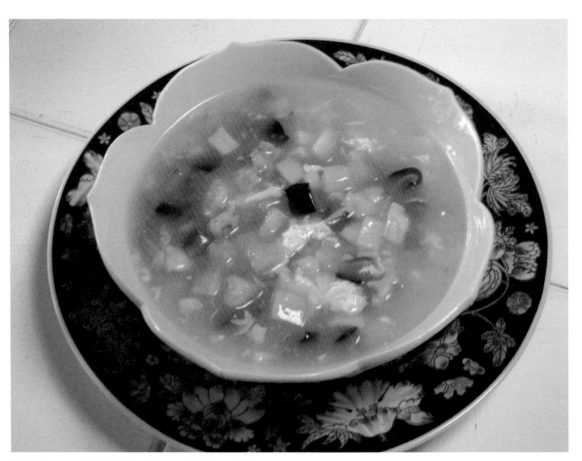

Eight Treasure Diced Melon Soup with Fuzzy Melon

Red Bean Paste Dumpling Soup with Sweet Osmanthus
桂花紅豆湯圓

Fragrance at Mid-Autumn Moon

This is a sweet soup served at the Mid-Autumn Moon Festival along with moon cakes and pomelos. The sweet osmanthus flowers bloom during this season and have enjoyed a legendary and poetic association with the moon.

> 1 cup glutinous rice powder
> ¼ cup boiling water
> 2 tablespoons cold water
> ½ cup sweetened red bean paste (24 teaspoons), canned or in package

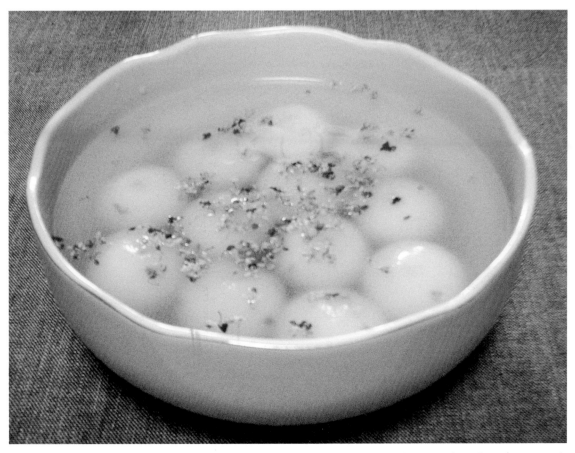

Red Bean Paste Dumpling Soup with Osmanthus Flowers as Garnish

Mix glutinous rice powder with boiling water and cold water. Knead into a smooth dough. Shape the dough into a roll about 2 inches in diameter. Cut into 20 pieces. Roll each piece of dough into a ball, then flatten it into a round patty, about 3 inches in diameter.

Place one portion (about 1 teaspoon) of the bean paste in the center of each patty of dough, gather the edges of the dough around the filling, pinch to seal, and roll gently into a ball. Repeat until of the filling and dough are used up. Yields 20 dumplings.

Bring 1½ quarts of water to a boil, add the dumplings, and let cook for 5 to 10 minutes over medium heat, until the dumplings rise to the surface. Add 1 cup of cold water and continue to cook until the dumplings rise again.

Ladle dumplings and soup into serving bowls. Sprinkle sweet osmanthus flowers on top and stir gently. Serve hot or at room temperature.

Serves 4–5.

SUGGESTIONS AND VARIATIONS:

You may make dumplings with ground sesame seed filling instead of the store-bought red bean paste (see recipe on pages 339–340).

Shanghai people like to add fermented sweet rice to the soup along with the dumplings.

Winter Solstice Savory Dumpling Soup *(xián tāng yuán, haàhm tòng yún)* 冬至鹹湯圓

To Start Winter Right

Summer and winter solstices, as well as the spring and autumn equinoxes, are the only times of the year when the solar and the lunar calendars agree. To herald in winter on December 22, dumplings are made. Characteristically, the Cantonese celebrate this solstitial event with a soup of plain dumpling balls cooked with winter vegetables and meat.

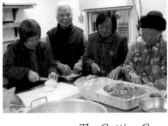

The Cutting Crew

> 4 ounces lean pork, sliced
> 2 teaspoons oyster sauce
> 1 teaspoon sugar
> 2 teaspoons cornstarch
> 2 tablespoons water
> 4 dried black mushrooms
> ¼ cup dried shrimp
> 1 ounce black woodears (optional)
> 2 cups shredded napa cabbage
> 2 cups shredded daikon
> 2 Chinese broccoli stems (optional), thick skin removed and cut
>   into thin coin-shape discs
> 60 plain dumplings (see recipe on page 205)

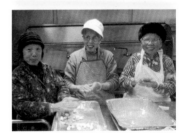

Making Dumplings

In a bowl, combine pork oyster sauce, sugar, cornstarch, and water. Marinate for 30 minutes.

Rinse and soak dried black mushrooms, dried shrimp, and black woodears (if using) separately in cold water for 30 minutes each. Reserve the soaking liquid from the mushrooms and shrimp. Cut mushrooms and woodears in long strips or shreds.

In a large pot, bring 2 quarts of water to a boil. Add cabbage, daikon, mushrooms, woodears, pork, shrimp, and the mushroom and shrimp soaking liquids. Return to a boil, then reduce heat to low and simmer for 45 minutes.

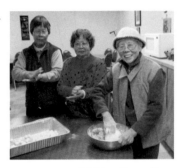

Making Dumplings

In a separate pot, add the dumplings to boiling water. When they float to the top, pour in 1 cup of cold water and wait for it to boil again. Repeat one more time. Drain dumplings and rinse thoroughly in cold, running water. Add the dumplings to the soup pot.

Cook the broccoli (if using) in 1 cup of boiling water for 5 minutes. Drain. Serve the soup hot, garnished with the broccoli disks, if using.

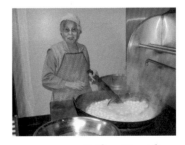

Boiling Dumplings

Serves 5–6.

If a vegetarian version is desired, substitute pressed tofu or tofu puffs cut into strips for the pork.

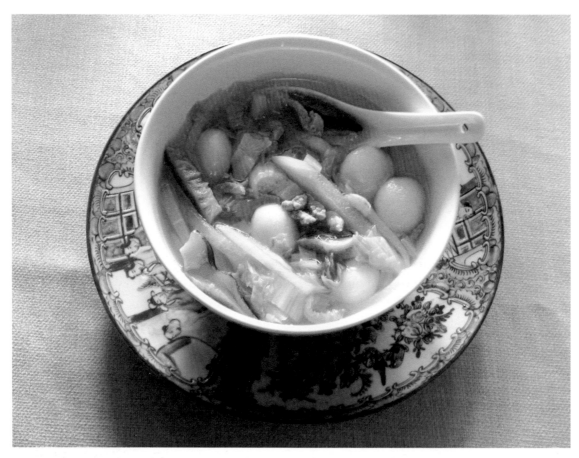

Winter Solstice Savory Dumpling Soup

Plain Dumplings 無餡湯圓

Plain dumplings are made of glutinous rice powder. These little dough balls may be added to a sweet bean soup (see page 344) or to a savory soup with meat and vegetables (see page 203).

1 cup glutinous rice powder
¼ cup boiling water
2 tablespoons cold water

In a bowl, combine the glutinous rice powder with both boiling water and cold water and mix well. Knead mixture into a smooth dough. Shape the dough into a roll about 2 inches in diameter and cut into four pieces. Shape each piece into a thin roll, and cut into pieces, about ½-inch wide. Roll each piece of dough into a small ball. Sprinkle the balls with dry rice powder and roll them gently.

Makes about 30 dumplings.

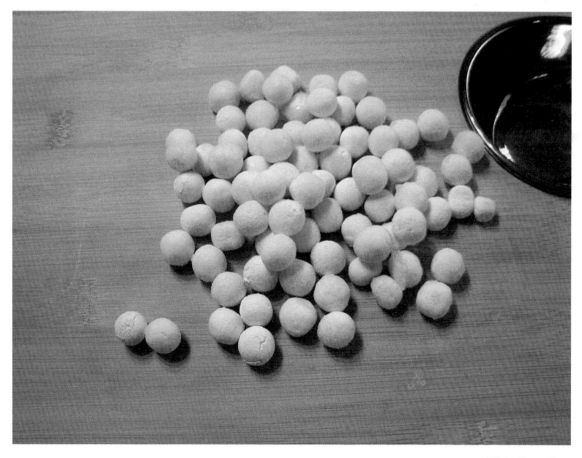

Plain Dumplings

The Hot Pot (*Dá-bìn-lòuh*) 打邊爐

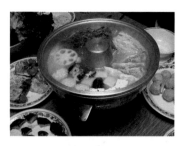

The Hot Pot

In the cold winter months when the wind cuts like a sharp knife, even Southerners enjoy the Mongolian hot pot. A portable stove is placed in the middle of the table with a pot of hot water or clear broth on top. Fresh ingredients, raw or parboiled, are prepared ahead of time and placed on platters. There are sliced meat, fish fillets, seafood, vegetables, and noodles. Food items are dropped into the hot soup, where they cook very quickly. Once ready, they are taken out immediately and dipped into a sauce, individually prepared in one's own bowl to one's own taste. Family members sit around the pot chatting as they cook and eat.

In the old days, people cooked and ate with the same pair of chopsticks, but now people are more hygiene-minded. However, even when people are given extra pairs of chopsticks to cook with, they still get mixed up, so I provide everyone with personal ladles.

The hot pot way of eating is warm and cozy. Throughout the country, it is practiced on cold winter nights and on Chinese New Year's Eve when all family members gather under one roof. Hence, the hot pot has become synonymous with annual family reunions in China. For a vegetarian version of hot pot, see the recipe on pages 254–256 under Vegetarian Soups.

The Chinese are not the only ones who cook on the table and eat around the hot pot. The French *fondue* (called "cheese hot pot" in Hong Kong), the Japanese *shabushabu,* and the Korean *sinsonlo* 神仙爐 are all based on the same idea. I learned from an Indian cookbook that Indians also eat hot pot style, with curry flavor of course.

Ingredients for *da-bin-louh* include the following:

The Soup Base

Nowadays, few people would start the hot pot with plain hot water. A clear broth is preferred. A vegetable stock can be made from napa cabbage, white turnip (daikon), mushrooms, and/or soybean sprouts. Chicken and meat trimmings, including gizzards and bones, can also go into the stockpot. Some Cantonese put in a "thousand-year" egg to balance the yin and yang.

Meatballs

Since the food is cooked at the table, it must be in small pieces that will cook quickly. For the hot pot, meatballs, shrimp balls, fish balls, and/or squid balls are a must. Besides, they look pretty, both on the platter and in the soup.

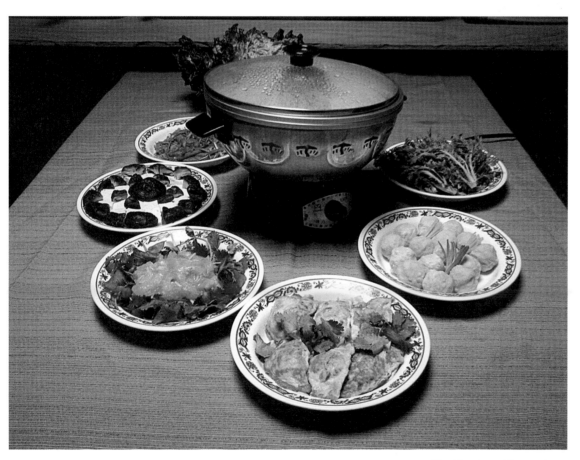

The Hot Pot and Ingredients

Mini Omelets

In my family, we have always had mini omelets filled with ground pork or fish paste mixed with other finely chopped ingredients. I did not realize until recently that the mini omelet is not a Cantonese tradition. I got it from my mother's side, from Shanghai cuisine.

Sliced Meat and Fish

Chicken, pork, beef, and mutton can all be thinly sliced and quickly cooked in the hot pot. The meat is then dipped into your own bowl of individualized sauce before eating. Thin slicing is made easy by placing the meat in the freezer for 20 minutes before cutting with a very sharp knife.

The fish preferred for quick cooking in the hot pot, as well as in juk, is the grass carp. While the grass carp of the Pearl River Delta is not readily available in the U.S., fresh cod, sole, or black bass may be used. Thinly slice the fish fillet and season with ground white pepper, slivers of fresh ginger, and green onion.

Some people prepare slices of pork liver and crisscross-cut pork kidney for the hot pot, but, unless treated properly, the scum from cooking liver will make the soup murky while the kidney has a stench that overpowers the other ingredients. Therefore, I rarely use these items for da-bin-lou. Rinsing the liver slices and kidneys under cold tap water may help to wash off the liver's slime and remove the kidney's stench.

Seafood

The most frequently used seafood for the hot pot is shrimp. Remove the head and shell, devein, and use whole, halved, butterflied, or skewered. No matter what, shrimp always looks presentable.

Live clams are also used and are considered to bring good fortune, since the cooked clams open up like old-fashioned Chinese silver nuggets.

Vegetables

Quick-cooking green vegetables—such as leaf lettuce, spinach, and snow pea leaves and tendrils—are commonly used. Garland chrysanthemum, when available, is a welcomed bonus. The leafy parts of napa cabbage and bok choy may also be used, but their stems need to be parboiled, just as white turnip (daikon) slices, carrot slices, and bamboo shoots need to be cooked ahead of time.

Mushrooms, either fresh or dried and reconstituted, can be used. Bear in mind that all kinds of fungi should be cooked longer and consumed in smaller quantity because they are hard to digest.

Tofu and Tofu Puffs

Due to the blandness of tofu and tofu puffs, add them to the pot halfway through the cooking to absorb the flavor from the soup. As tofu may fall apart with stirring, cut it into big, thick pieces. Tofu puffs may be cut in half, straight or diagonally.

Noodles

The hot pot is normally not accompanied by rice. Put in mung bean noodles, udon, or pasta shells toward the end because they are more filling. Cook some rice for those who must have rice to call it a meal.

Sauce

Quick-cooked meat and vegetables taste good, but most people like to dip them in a sauce for flavoring. Offer satay sauce, soy sauce, sesame oil, and even chile sauce that can all be mixed together according to individual taste. A raw egg used to be added to the sauce for cooling down the food taken straight from the pot, but this custom has been dropped due to the threat of avian flu.

New Year's Eve Da-Bin-Lou 年卅晚打甌爐

From the above list, you may create your own combination according to the preferences of your family members and the availability of certain ingredients. The following is just an example.

24 mini omelets (see recipe on pages 212–214)
1 boneless, skinless chicken breast, sliced
8 ounces pork, thinly sliced
8 ounces beef, thinly sliced
8 ounces fillet of sole, sliced
8 ounces shrimp, peeled, deveined, and butterflied
8 ounces squid, crisscross-cut
1 12-ounce package tofu, cut into 1-inch cubes
8 ounces leaf lettuce
8 ounces spinach
1 pound daikon, peeled and cut into 2 x 1-inch pieces
1 pound napa cabbage, trimmed and cut into 3 x ½-inch pieces
2 ounces mung bean vermicelli

CONDIMENTS:

8 raw eggs (optional)
Soy sauce
Satay sauce
Chile sauce
Red chiles, thinly sliced
Chopped green onion
Chopped cilantro
Sesame oil

Boil white stem of the napa cabbage and daikon separately for 30 minutes, drain, reserving the cooking liquid, and pile on separate plates. Combine the cooking liquid from the napa cabbage and daikon and add hot water to yield 5 quarts of clear vegetarian stock. Bring to a boil. Bring the hot pot to the table and fill it with the boiling stock.

Arrange the plates around the hot pot and set the table. Make sure each person has a soup bowl, a pair of chopsticks, and a ladle to cook with. When everyone is seated, and after greetings, start by making a personal dipping sauce using the dipping sauce ingredients in any combination that appeals to you. A beaten raw egg may be added for cooling off the quickly cooked food.

As the soup gets boiled down, more hot stock or hot water can be added to the pot. Each person picks up the morsel he or she intends to eat (with the extra pair of chopsticks) from the plates and puts it into the pot. When the leaf vegetable withers or the meat changes color, pick it up with a ladle.

Toward the end of the meal, when all seem to have had their fill of meat and vegetables, cook the noodles and mix with the remaining sauce. Enjoy the hot soup last, now rich with flavors from all the ingredients.

Serves 8.

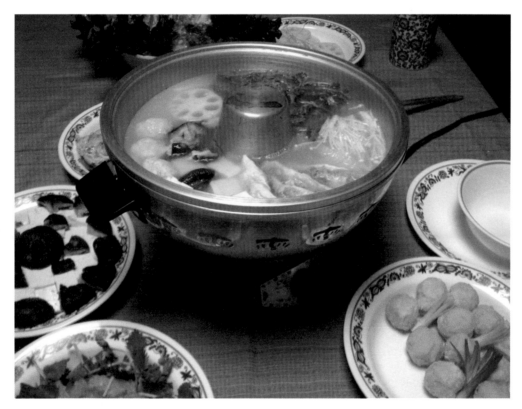

Da-Bin-Lou

Mini Omelets Filled with Ground Meat 蛋餃

These Mini Omelets, to be included on the platter of items to be cooked in the hot pot, are filled with ground pork. You may substitute ground chicken or ground turkey, if desired. The meat may not be thoroughly cooked when the omelets are formed, so cook the meat omelets for at least 5 more minutes in the hot pot.

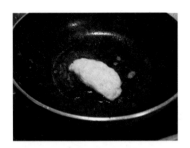

A Mini Omelet in the Making

6 ounces ground pork
3 water chestnuts
2 ounces raw shrimp, peeled, deveined, and minced
1 teaspoon finely chopped ginger
1 teaspoon finely chopped green onions or finely chopped cilantro
½ teaspoon salt
½ teaspoon rice wine
½ teaspoon sugar
¼ teaspoon black pepper
1 teaspoon cornstarch
8 eggs, beaten
½ cup vegetable oil

In a medium bowl, combine pork, water chestnuts, shrimp, ginger, green onions or cilantro, salt, rice wine, sugar, pepper, and cornstarch. Mix well.

Heat a flat, nonstick skillet over medium-high heat. When hot, reduce heat to medium and add 1 teaspoon of vegetable oil. Pour in 2 tablespoons of beaten egg. As the egg spreads to form a thin layer about 2½ inches in diameter, add 1 teaspoon of the pork mixture to the center. Fold one half of the egg over to form a pocket with the filling inside. Quickly flip the omelet over, cook for 1 minute, then flip it over again, cooking until both sides are golden. Remove from pan and place on serving platter. Repeat this method until the filling is used up. If you run out of eggs before you run out of filling, beat one or two more.

Makes 24 mini omelets.

SUGGESTIONS AND VARIATIONS:

If you want the pork in your filling to be fully cooked before the omelets are added to the stock, stir-fry it for 5 to 8 minutes before mixing it in with the other filling ingredients.

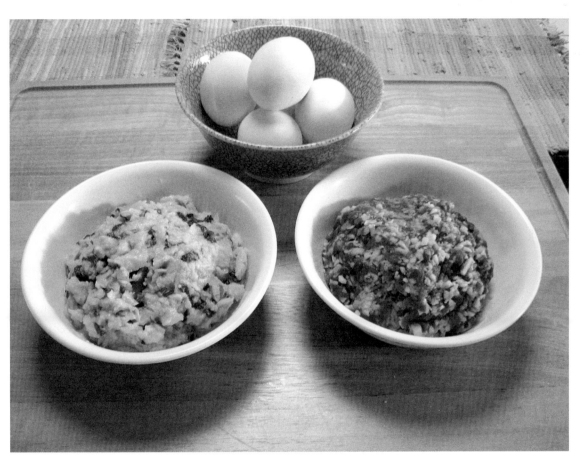

Ingredients for Mini Omelets—Fish Paste (left) and Ground Pork (right)

Fish Paste Omelets 魚肉蛋餃

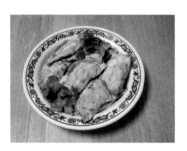

A Plateful of Mini Omelets

3 dried black mushrooms
½ cup plus 1 teaspoon vegetable oil
8 ounces fish paste
5 shallots, finely chopped
⅓ cup finely chopped carrot
1 teaspoon finely chopped ginger
1 teaspoon finely chopped green onion
1 teaspoon finely chopped cilantro
8 eggs, beaten

Rinse and soak dried black mushrooms in hot water for 30 minutes, until soft, then drain, reserving the soaking liquid, and mince.

In a medium skillet, heat 1 teaspoon of vegetable oil over medium-high heat. Add minced shallots, carrots, and mushrooms and stir-fry until shallot is soft, about 3 minutes. Add cooking wine and 2 tablespoons of the mushroom's soaking liquid. Stir well and remove from heat. Let cool, then mix in ginger, green onion, and cilantro. Add to the fish paste and mix well.

Heat a flat, nonstick skillet over medium-high heat. When hot, reduce heat to medium and add 1 teaspoon of vegetable oil. Pour in 2 tablespoons of beaten egg. As the egg spreads to form a thin layer about 2½ inches in diameter, add 1 teaspoon of the fish paste mixture to the center. Fold one half of the egg over to form a pocket with the filling inside. Quickly flip the omelet over, cook for 1 minute, then flip it over again, cooking until both sides are golden yellow. Remove from pan and place on serving platter. Repeat this method until the filling is used up. If you run out of eggs before you run out of filling, beat one or two more.

Makes 24 mini omelets.

New Year Soup 新年湯

1 frozen reconstituted fish maw (approximately 6 ounces), thawed

2 frozen reconstituted sea cucumbers (approximately 1 pound), thawed

2 frozen conch (approximately 4 ounces), thawed

8 thin slices (about ⅛-inch thick) peeled fresh ginger

1 frozen fresh abalone (approximately ½ pound), thawed

6 dried scallops

10 dried black mushrooms

⅛ ounce black moss

6 dried oysters

4 ounces dried bean curd sticks

2 teaspoons vegetable oil

2 carrots, peeled and sliced on the diagonal

1 pound lotus root, peeled, joints removed, cut in half lengthwise, and thickly sliced

4 honey dates

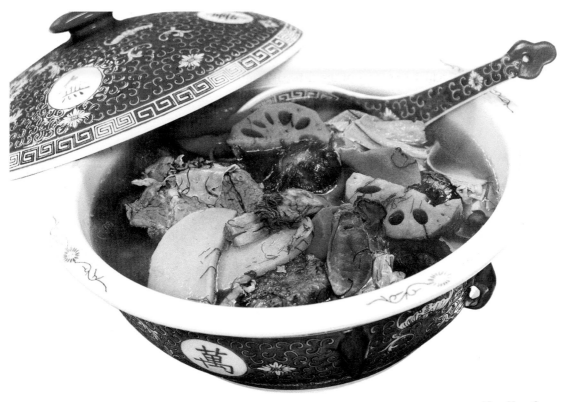

New Year Soup

Cover the fish maw with boiling water and soak overnight. Drain and rinse with cold water.

Clean and remove the intestine from the sea cucumber. Cook in 1 quart of boiling water with 4 slices of the ginger for 5 minutes. Drain and rinse with cold water.

Cut each conch in half from the stomach and remove the intestines. Treat it the same way as with the sea cucumber. Cook in 1 quart of boiling water with the remaining 4 slices of the ginger for 5 minutes. Drain and rinse with cold water.

Scrub the edge of the abalone with a brush, clean with salt, and rinse twice. Pound with a wooden mallet, then cook in a pot of boiling water together with the sea cucumbers for 30 minutes.

Soak dried scallops in warm water for an hour. Reserve the liquid.

Rinse and soak dried black mushrooms in hot water for 30 minutes, until soft. Reserve the liquid and cut off and discard stems.

Soak black moss in cold water and vegetable oil for 1 hour, drain, rinse thoroughly, and pat dry.

Rinse and soak dried oysters in warm water for 30 minutes.

Soak dried bean curd sticks in warm water for 30 minutes. Drain and cut into 2-inch pieces.

In a large pot, combine bean curd sticks, scallops, mushrooms, lotus root, honey dates, and dried oysters with 5 quarts of cold water. Cook over high heat for 30 minutes. Add abalone and conch, bring to a boil, reduce heat to medium, and cook for 1½ hours. Add sea cucumbers and fish maw and continue to cook for 30 minutes.

Take the sea cucumbers and fish maw out and cut them into 1 inch wide pieces. Set aside.

Pull out and slice the abalone and conch and set aside.

Add carrots and black moss to the soup and cook for another 45 minutes.

Return the sea cucumbers, fish maw, abalone, and conch to the soup pot and bring to a boil. Salt to taste. Serve the soup hot in a fancy soup tureen.

Serves 8–10.

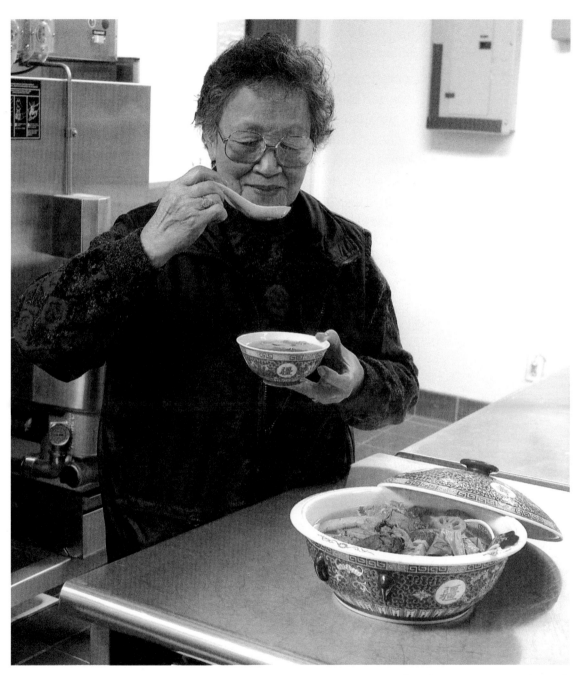

Mrs. Lee Wai Ying Tam Sampling the New Year Soup She Made

Chicken Wine Soup 雞酒

This is an all-time blood tonic that improves blood circulation. It is a popular tonic soup to offer to women after childbirth. This soup is also offered to guests at a Ginger-and-Red-Egg party, thrown when a baby turns one month old.

> 10 black mushrooms
> ½ pound blanched peanuts
> 10 red jujube dates
> 1 ounce tigerlily buds
> 4 ounces black woodears
> 1½ pounds pork neck bone
> ½ cup sliced ginger
> 1 whole chicken (about 2 pounds), skin and fat removed, cut into pieces
> ½ cup rice wine

Rinse and soak black mushrooms in warm water until soft (about 2 hours), drain, remove and discard stems, and cut into halves.

Rinse peanuts.

Soak red jujube dates in warm water for 30 minutes, drain and remove pits.

Soak tigerlily buds in warm water for 30 minutes. Remove and discard hard ends and tie into a knot in the middle.

Soak black woodears in warm water for 30 minutes, drain, rinse well, and remove and discard hard stem.

Feiseui: In a large pot, cook chicken and pork neck bone in 3 quarts of boiling water for 15 minutes. Discard fat and foamy residue and rinse chicken and bones.

Add mushrooms, peanuts, dates, ginger, and bones to 5 quarts of water, bring to a boil, and cook for 2 hours. Remove the bones. Add chicken, woodears, and tigerlily buds and return to a boil. Continue to boil for 10 minutes. Add rice wine, reduce heat to medium, and continue to simmer for at least another 30 minutes. Serve piping hot.

Serves 6.

SUGGESTIONS AND VARIATIONS:

Do not overcook woodears and lily buds or they will turn slimy and sour.

Depending on individual taste, you may prefer to substitute hard liquor for the rice wine. Cantonese like to use port, whisky, or brandy as well as rice wine.

Quick and Easy Soups

For the Chinese, soups are daily fare. Light soups are served with meals and as light meals themselves (see chapter 16). These soups are quick and easy to make, consisting usually of clear broth (or just hot water) with some tender greens, small pieces of vegetables, and thin slices of meat. The soup may be consumed throughout the meal like a beverage. When noodles or dumplings such as wonton are added to a simple soup like that, the soup becomes a meal in itself.

Traditionally, as noted by Martin Yan in his *Chinese Cooking for Dummies*, "The typical Chinese soup is a far cry from a thick chowder or a cream bisque." Some Chinese-American restaurants have adapted to the western idea of thick and smooth soups by serving up cream of potato soup, cream of corn soup, cream of tomato soup, and so on, using cornstarch as a thickener instead of cream. The Tai Chi Bisque is a vegetarian invention that uses the combination of cream of mushroom and cream of corn soups. You can create your own yin-yang combination with two *gang* or thickened soups.

You can find quick and easy soups year-round. The recipes in this section simply recapture daily soups I have enjoyed and have learned to make. As this dummy of a cook has learned, all Cantonese soups are simple and easy to make in the first place. They only get complicated with added ingredients.

These soups may look simple, but the warm liquid provides a great pick-me-up for people constantly on the go. Soups rehydrate the body without the excessive amount of refined sugar and salt in soft drinks. Soups contain water-soluble fibers, minerals, and vitamins. And there are so many interesting flavors.

I use only water to start my Quick and Easy Soups, but you may use chicken or beef stock as starter. If you have learned to make top stock, just get it out of the freezer and use that.

QUICK AND EASY SOUP RECIPES	快捷湯水
Watercress and Fish Fillet Soup	西洋菜魚片湯
Soybean Sprout and Sparerib Soup	大豆芽菜黃芽白排骨湯
Four Items Plus Chayote Soup	四味合掌瓜湯
Spinach and Tofu Soup	菠菜豆腐肉片湯
Loofah and Mung Bean Vermicelli Soup	絲瓜粉絲湯
Asparagus, Shiitake Mushroom, and Sliced Chicken Soup	蘆筍冬菇滾雞片
Hot and Sour Soup	酸辣湯
West Lake Beef Bisque	西湖牛肉羹
Simplified Chicken and Corn Bisque	簡易雞茸粟米湯

Watercress and Fish Fillet Soup 西洋菜魚片湯

This is not a louhfo (slow-cooking) soup. The watercress stays green and crisp, with strong cleansing properties to dissolve phlegm, clear lung heat, and clear facial blemishes.

> ¾ pound grouper fillet, thinly sliced (about ³⁄₁₆ inch thick)
> ½ teaspoon salt
> ½ teaspoon ground pepper
> ½ teaspoon sugar
> 1 teaspoon vegetable oil
> 1 teaspoon cornstarch
> 2 bunches watercress (approximately 12 ounces), cut into 2-inch
>   pieces
> 1 carrot, peeled and sliced
> 4 honey dates, rinsed
> 3 thin slices (about ⅛-inch thick) peeled fresh ginger, finely
>   julienned (less than ¹⁄₁₆ inch wide)

In a bowl, combine grouper with salt, pepper, sugar, cornstarch, and vegetable oil. Mix to coat fish evenly. Marinate for 20 minutes.

In a large pot, combine watercress, carrots, and honey dates with 2½ quarts of water and bring to a boil over high heat. Reduce heat to medium and cook for 30 minutes. Add grouper fillet and ginger and cook for 3 minutes more. Remove from heat and serve hot.

Serves 6.

SUGGESTIONS AND VARIATIONS:

You may use frozen, ready-made fish balls in place of fish fillet.

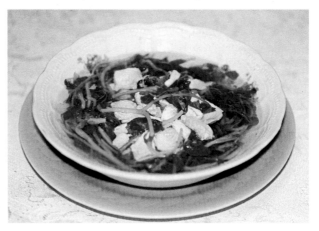

Watercress and Fish Fillet Soup

Soybean Sprout and Sparerib Soup　大豆芽菜黃芽白排骨湯

Thinly sliced meat cooks in minutes, but soybeans and spareribs need to be cooked longer. The thermal cooker is the simplest and greenest way to do the cooking.

½ pound soybean sprouts, washed, drained, and with the stringy
　　ends removed
1¼ pounds pork spareribs, cut into narrow strips
1 pound napa cabbage, cut into 1-inch sections
4 ounces fresh mushrooms, sliced (optional)
2 carrots, peeled and sliced on the diagonal (optional)
3 thin slices (about ⅛-inch thick) peeled fresh ginger

Feiseui: Cook spareribs in 2 quarts of boiling water for 10 minutes, drain, and rinse with cold water. Cut into small pieces.

　In the inner pot of a thermal cooker, combine spareribs, soybean sprouts, cabbage, ginger, carrots, and mushrooms (if using) with 2½ quarts of water. Bring to a boil over high heat and cook for 15 minutes. Remove the inner pot from the heat and place it into the thermal cooker. Let cook in the thermal cooker for 3 hours or until you are ready to serve dinner.

Serves 6.

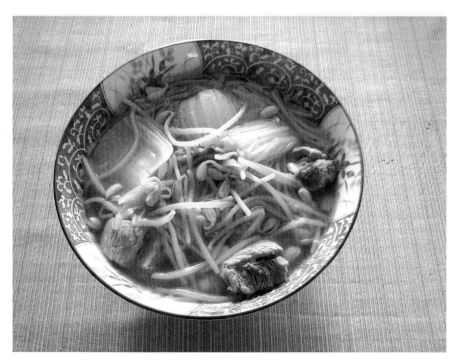

Soybean Sprout and Sparerib Soup

Four Items Plus Chayote Soup 四味合掌瓜湯

This is a variation of Lai King Chan's vegetarian Four Items Plus Winter Melon Soup (see page 237), the four main ingredients being lotus seeds, lily bulb scales, foxnuts, and pearl barley. These are all rich in antioxidants and are recommended for frequent consumption.

> 4 dried scallops
> 1½ ounces lotus seeds
> 1 pound pork tenderloin, cut into 2-inch chunks
> 1 ounce lily bulb scales, rinsed
> 1 ounce foxnuts, rinsed
> 2 ounces pearl barley, rinsed
> 3 chayote squash (approximately 1¼ pounds), peeled and cut into
>   2-inch chunks
> 2 carrots, peeled and cut into 1-inch pieces
> 3 honey dates, rinsed
> 3 thin slices (about ⅛-inch thick) peeled fresh ginger

Rinse and soak dried scallop in warm water for 2 hours. Strain and retain soaking liquid.

Rinse and soak the lotus seeds in warm water for 1 hour, drain, and remove the green centers if there are any.

Feiseui: Cook pork tenderloin in 2 quarts of boiling water for 10 minutes, drain, and rinse with cold water.

In the inner pot of the thermal cooker, combine scallops, lotus seeds, orange peel, pork, lily bulb scales, foxnuts, barley, chayote squash, carrots, dates, and ginger with 2½ quarts of water and bring to a boil over high heat. Cook for 30 minutes with the lid on. Place inner pot inside the thermal cooker and let slow-cook for 3 hours or more, until you are ready to serve. Salt to taste.

Serves 6.

SUGGESTIONS AND VARIATIONS:

You may add many things to the basic four items, such as American Ginseng and fresh wild yam. Adding dried wild yam, Solomon's Seal, and longan meat actually turns the mix into Ching Bo Leung.

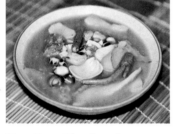

Four Items Plus American Ginseng Soup

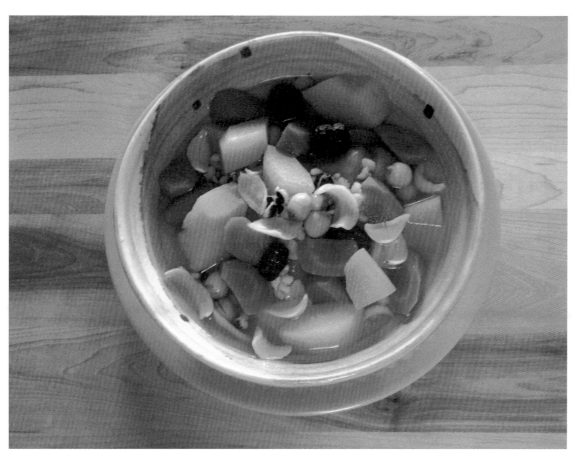

Four Items Plus Chayote Soup

Spinach and Tofu Soup 菠菜豆腐肉片湯

Quick and Colorful

¾ pound pork tenderloin, sliced
¼ pound peeled shrimp, deveined and halved lengthwise
½ teaspoon salt
½ teaspoon sugar
½ teaspoon vegetable oil
1 teaspoon cornstarch
3 thin slices (about ⅛-inch thick) peeled fresh ginger
1 pound spinach, washed and cut into 3-inch pieces
1 6-ounce package regular tofu, rinsed and cut into 1-inch cubes
    or domino-sized pieces

In a bowl, combine pork, shrimp, salt, sugar, cornstarch, and vegetable oil. Marinate for 20 minutes.

In a large pot, combine ginger and 2½ quarts of water and bring to a boil. Add spinach and tofu and return to a boil. Add marinated pork and shrimp. Cook for 10 minutes more, until shrimp turns pink and pork turns white. Serve hot or at room temperature.

Serves 6.

SUGGESTIONS AND VARIATIONS:

Any leafy vegetable—such as amaranth, water spinach, spring chrysanthemum, baby bok choy, tender rape, or watercress—may be substituted for the spinach. You may even substitute with snow peas.

Skinless, boneless chicken breast or fish fillet may be used in place of pork.

Loofah and Mung Bean Vermicelli Soup 絲瓜粉絲湯

1 pound loofah squash
1 bunch mung bean threads (½ ounce)
¾ pound chicken breast, sliced
¼ teaspoon salt
¼ teaspoon sugar
¼ teaspoon vegetable oil
½ teaspoon cornstarch
6 fresh shiitake mushrooms, sliced
6 tofu puffs, cut diagonally
¼ pound bamboo shoots, sliced (optional)
2 carrots, peeled and sliced (optional)

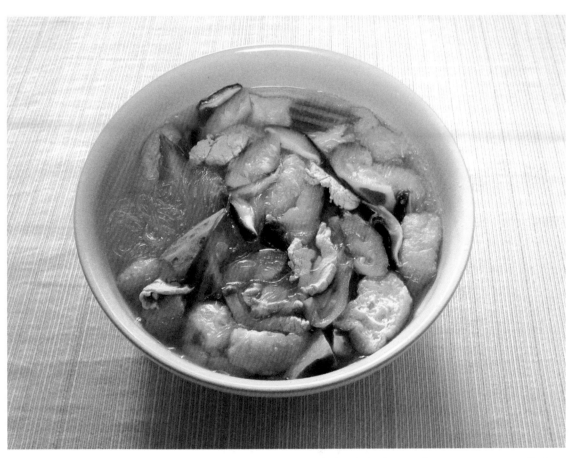

Loofah Squash, Tofu Puff, Sliced Chicken, and Mung Bean Vermicelli Soup

Remove the rib part of the loofah squash and roll-cut into 1-inch lengths.

Soak mung bean threads in cold water for 15 minutes. Cut into 6-inch pieces.

In a bowl, combine chicken with salt, sugar, vegetable oil, and cornstarch, stirring to coat evenly. Marinate for 30 minutes.

In a large pot, combine squash, mushrooms, tofu puffs, bamboo shoots, and carrots (if using), with 2½ quarts of water and cook over high heat for 30 minutes. Add chicken and continue to cook on medium for 10 more minutes. Add mung bean threads and cook for 3 more minutes. Serve hot or at room temperature..

Serves 6.

SUGGESTIONS AND VARIATIONS:

Instead of loofah squash, any summer squash will do. Fuzzy melon, zucchini, and winter melon are excellent candidates for this recipe.

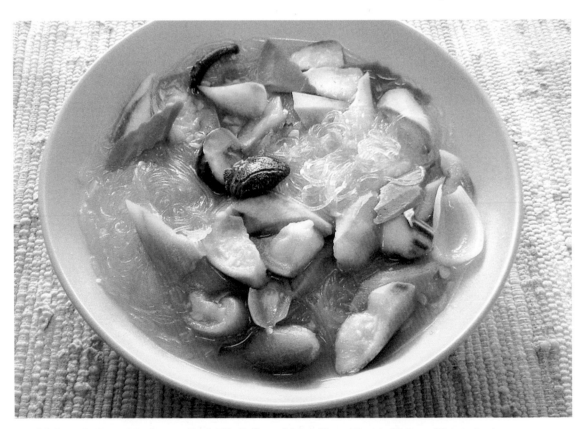

Loofah Squash, Straw Mushroom, Fresh Lily Bulb, and Mung Bean Vermicelli Soup (Vegetarian)

Asparagus, Shiitake Mushroom, and Sliced Chicken Soup
蘆筍冬菇滾雞片

1 pound asparagus, trimmed and sliced on the diagonal
¾ pound boneless, skinless chicken breast, sliced
¼ teaspoon salt
¼ teaspoon sugar
¼ teaspoon vegetable oil
½ teaspoon cornstarch
¼ pound fresh shiitake mushrooms, with stems removed and cut
    into strips
5 cups chicken stock

In a bowl, combine chicken with salt, sugar, cornstarch, and vegetable oil, stirring to coat evenly. Marinate for 30 minutes.

In a large pot, combine chicken broth with 5 cups of water and bring to a boil over high heat. Add mushrooms and asparagus and return to a boil. Reduce heat to medium and cook uncovered for 5 more minutes. Add chicken and cook about 15 minutes until the meat turns white. Serve hot or at room temperature.

Serves 6.

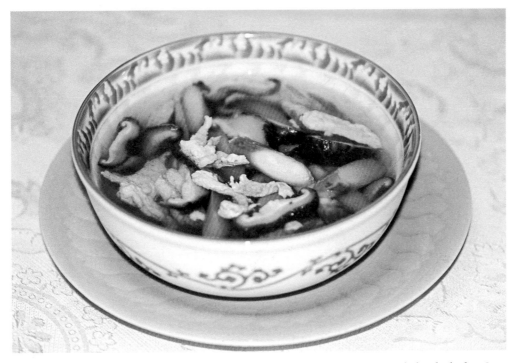

Asparagus, Shiitake Mushroom, and Sliced Chicken Soup

Hot and Sour Soup 酸辣湯

Hot and Sour Soup was not originally a Cantonese soup. It was brought to Hong Kong in the 1950s by Sichuan people and by people who had been in Sichuan during the eight-year Sino-Japanese War, which ended with the end of WWII. Later on, it was brought to the United States by those who passed through Hong Kong in the 1960s. Hot and Sour Soup so captured the American palate that even Cantonese restaurants began serving it before long.

I was totally amazed when I found Hot and Sour Soup included in a cookbook for Cantonese cuisine published in Guangzhou (Canton), of all places, but it legitimizes somewhat my inclusion of this recipe here.

1 skinless, boneless chicken breast (approximately 8 ounces), cut into ¼ inch wide strips

¼ teaspoon salt

1 teaspoon cornstarch

¼ teaspoon sugar

1 teaspoon soy sauce

1 ounce dried black woodears

5 dried black mushrooms

1 green onion (optional)

5 cups chicken stock or top stock

2 tablespoons cooking wine

2 thin slices (about ⅙-inch thick) peeled fresh ginger, finely minced

1 tablespoon chile sauce or paste

2 tablespoon red vinegar (*jit chou* 浙醋)

1 carrot, peeled and shredded

2 canned bamboo shoots, julienned

1 cup julienned baked or firm tofu (6–8 ounces)

4 ounces shrimp, peeled, deveined, and cut into ½-inch pieces (optional)

1 egg, lightly beaten

1 dash ground white pepper

THICKENING MIXTURE:

½ teaspoon salt

½ teaspoon sugar

2 teaspoons cornstarch

¼ cup water

In a bowl, combine chicken with salt, cornstarch, sugar, and soy sauce, stirring to coat evenly. Marinate for 30 minutes.

Soak woodears in warm water for 30 minutes. Drain, rinse, and cut off and discard hard ends, then shred woodears finely.

Rinse and soak dried black mushrooms in hot water for 30 minutes or until the caps are soft. Cut off and discard stems. Cut mushroom caps into a fine julienne (less than ¼-inch wide).

Clean and remove both ends of the green onion (if using). Make several vertical cuts and then cut crosswise into 2-inch pieces, resulting in fine shreds. Set aside for garnishing the finished soup.

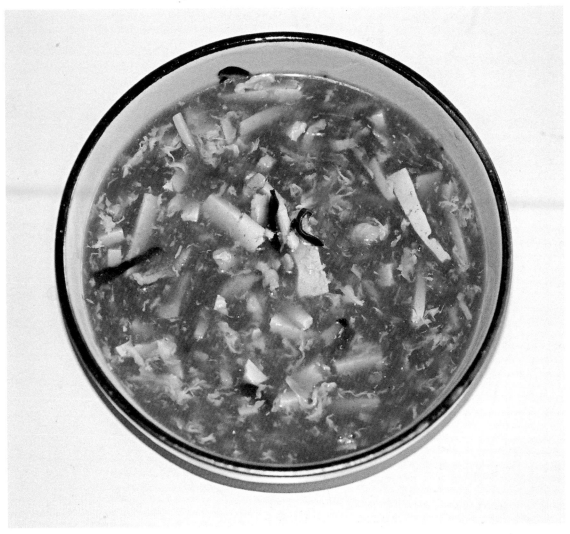

Hot and Sour Soup

In a large pot, combine soup stock, cooking wine, ginger, chile sauce, and vinegar with 1½ quarts of water and bring to a boil. Add carrots, bamboo shoots, mushrooms, woodears, and tofu and return to a boil. Add chicken and shrimp and cook until they turn opaque. Remove from heat, stir in egg and ground white pepper.

In a small bowl, combine thickening mixture ingredients and gradually stir into hot soup, adding a little at a time until soup reaches desired thickness. Serve hot, garnished with the shredded green onion.

Serves 6.

Suggestions and Variations:

Shredded pork may be substituted for the chicken.

For a vegetarian hot and sour soup, omit the chicken and shrimp, add enoki mushrooms, and double the amount of tofu.

Some like it hot. You may increase the amount of chile sauce while maintaining a ratio of 1 part chile sauce to 2 parts vinegar.

West Lake Beef Bisque 西湖牛肉羹

Tonifying the Spleen and Stomach

Beef is considered neutral, not as warming as chicken nor as cooling as pork. It is therefore the ideal meat for tonifying the middle burner or the center, often recommended for people with conditions of deficiency or vacuity.

½ pound lean ground beef
1 teaspoon salt
1 teaspoon sugar
1 teaspoon vegetable oil
1 teaspoon cornstarch
2 ounces frozen peas and carrots, thawed
5 cups top stock, chicken stock, or beef stock
1 8-ounce package silken tofu, cut into 1-inch cubes
2 egg whites, lightly beaten
2 sprigs cilantro (optional), finely chopped

THICKENING MIXTURE:

½ teaspoon salt
½ teaspoon sugar
2 tablespoons cornstarch
¼ cup water

Mix lean ground beef with salt, sugar, vegetable oil, and cornstarch. Marinate for 30 minutes.

Cook peas and carrots in boiling water for 2 minutes, then drain.

Combine soup stock with 5 cups of water (2½ quarts total) and bring to a boil. Add tofu, peas and carrots, and ground beef and return to a boil. Stir in egg white, and remove from heat. In a small bowl, combine thickening mixture ingredients and gradually stir into hot soup, adding a little at a time until soup reaches desired thickness. Garnish with cilantro, if using.

Serves 6.

Simplified Chicken and Corn Bisque 簡易雞茸粟米羹

A Family Favorite Made Easy

5 cups chicken stock
1 skinless, boneless chicken breast, finely minced
1 15-ounce can "cream style" corn
2 egg whites, lightly beaten but not frothy

THICKENING MIXTURE (OPTIONAL):

½ teaspoon salt
½ teaspoon sugar
2 tablespoons cornstarch
¼ cup water

In a 2-quart pot, bring 2 cups of water and chicken stock to a boil and stir in the chicken and corn. Return to a boil, remove from heat, and stir in the egg whites. If a thicker consistency is desired, stir in some thickening mixture.

Serves 4.

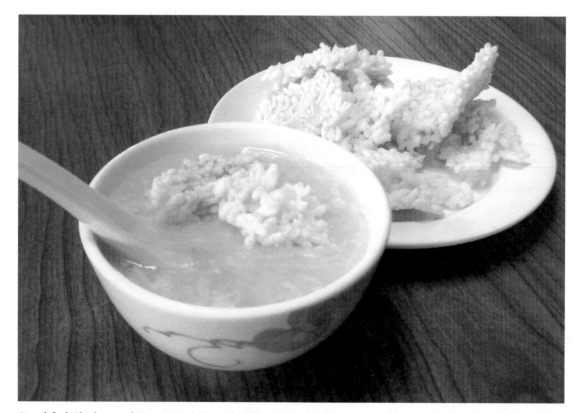

Simplified Chicken and Corn Bisque Served with Crispy Rice

13
Vegetarian Soups

~~~~~~~~~

If you sought out this chapter first, I do not need to talk too much about the health benefits of plant-based food. Go directly to the recipes and enjoy. If, on the other hand, you have simply landed here after having read other parts of this book, it is to our mutual benefit that you read on.

Please understand that I am not a purist. Though I have cooked vegetarian food for my husband, who eschews meat, for many years, I also have also cooked meat for my children and myself. Depending on who is coming to dinner, I can always alter a meat dish into a vegetarian dish and vice versa. On New Year's Eve, I have two hot pots going, one designated as "vegetarian only." In this section, you will encounter soup recipes that are meatless alternatives to meat recipes listed elsewhere in the book. I want to make the point that it is possible to make soups without using meat, poultry, fish, or eggs, or even seasonings from the allium family (onions, garlic, shallots, chives, etc.) for members of certain Buddhist sects who believe that these are stimulants of desire.

Surprisingly, it was the Chinese Buddhists who first developed imitation meat products to allow the faithful to enjoy the food they loved without killing animals. In Taiwan, Hong Kong, and Mainland China, fancy vegetarian restaurants are known to feature a banquet menu complete with imitation shark's fin, chicken, beef, fish, prawn, abalone, and ham. If you really miss eating meat, this is an easy way to go, whether it is for religious or health reasons. These ingenious copies of animal products are derived from plant proteins from soybeans and wheat. You are spared the saturated fat, cholesterol, growth hormones, and antibiotics found in most commercially raised meat and poultry (including eggs). Do watch out, however, for additives such as monosodium glutamate (MSG) and chemicals used to re-create the taste and texture of meat. I usually like to avoid using any processed imitation meat in packages or in cans, unless the labels clearly indicate the absence of these additives. You may also want to keep your eye out for excessive amounts of added salt and sugar, which may contribute to a host of health problems. For protein, I prefer to use plain tofu or tofu puffs, plain gluten, or legumes instead of imitation meat.

The American Cancer Society has recommended 36 cancer-preventing vegetables such as broccoli, kale, and tomato, and fruits such as apple and cantaloupe that help rid our bodies of toxins and build up our immunity. In this section, I have included several Asian vegetables commonly used for cleansing the system. Among them are sea vegetables, known as seaweeds in the West, and fungi, as well as leafy vegetables, root vegetables, legumes, and grains.

Until their recent Westernization, the Cantonese did not drink ice-cold water, fruit juice, or soda. Instead, soup had always been their mealtime beverage. A vegetable soup provides fluid, vegetable fiber, vitamins, and minerals, absolutely cholesterol-free.

VEGETARIAN SOUP RECIPES	素菜湯類
Fruit Trio Soup	三果湯
Four Items Plus Winter Melon Soup	四味冬瓜湯
Vegetarian Ching Bo Leung Soup	清補涼湯(加胡蘿蔔)
Mung Beans, Kelp, Lotus Seeds, and Lily Bulb Soup	海帶綠豆蓮子百合湯
Two-Tone Bok Choy and Louhfo Tofu Soup	金銀菜老火豆腐湯
Napa Cabbage, Tofu Puffs, and Mung Bean Thread Soup	黃芽白豆腐泡粉絲湯
Soybean Sprouts, Kelp, and Frozen Tofu Soup	大豆芽海帶老豆腐湯
Watercress and Honey Date Soup	西洋菜蜜棗湯
Mixed Vegetable Bisque	什錦素菜羹
Vegetarian Borscht	素羅宋湯
Enoki, Shiitake, Bamboo Pipe, and Tofu Bisque	金針菇竹笙豆腐羹
Tai Chi Bisque	太極羹
Vegetarian Hot Pot	素火鍋
Fermented Black Bean and Tofu Soup (see recipe under Spring Soups)	薑蔥淡豆豉豆腐湯
Water Chestnut, Cilantro, and Carrot Soup (see recipe under Year-Round Soups)	馬蹄芫茜紅蘿蔔水

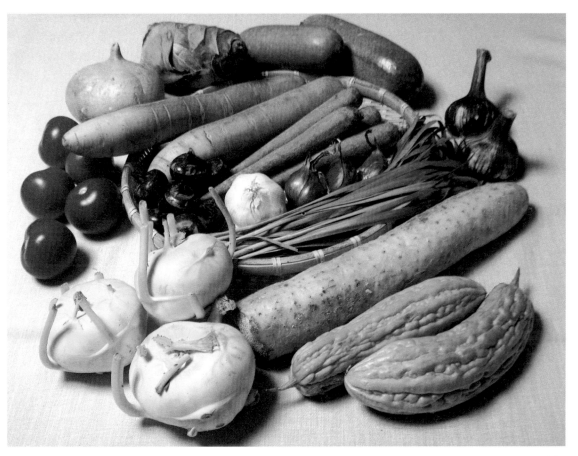

Vegetables

Fruit Trio Soup 三果湯

Appetizing and Fruity

The dried pale-yellow figs available in Chinese grocery stores are smaller and less flavorful than European varieties such as black mission and golden Calimyrna. Red apples and green apples are both used in soups. Though both green and ripe papayas can be used in soups, ripe ones are preferred in vegetarian soups.

Fruits are usually cooked in soups to balance their "cold" nature according to TCM theory and folk belief. As fruits are naturally sweet, no added sugar is needed, but vegetarian or fruit soups may be sweetened and served as between-meals snacks or as dessert at the end of a meal.

> **3 large red Delicious apples (approximately 1½ pounds), cored and cut into chunks**
> **6–8 dried Chinese figs**
> **1 large papaya (approximately 1 pound), peeled, seeded, and cut into chunks**

In a large pot, combine apples and figs with 2½ quarts of cold water and bring to a boil over high heat. Reduce heat to medium and simmer for 1½ hours. Add papaya and cook 30 minutes more. Serve hot or at room temperature.

Serves 6.

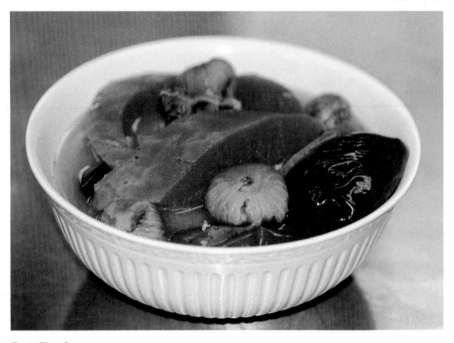

Fruit Trio Soup

Four Items Plus Winter Melon Soup 四味冬瓜湯

Strict vegetarian Lai King Chan provided this recipe. Many devout Buddhists, regarding members of the allium family to be stimulating and aphrodisiac, shun onions and chives in their cooking. Ginger, which is not a member of the allium family, may be used to balance the "coolness" of fruits and vegetables. The "four items"—lotus seeds, lily bulbs, foxnuts, and pearl barley—also translated as the "four flavors"—are noted antioxidants. They are good for general health maintenance.

¼ cup lotus seeds (1½ ounces)

1 piece Mandarin orange peel (about ⅓ of a whole peel)

3 tablespoons foxnuts (1 ounce), rinsed

1 cup raw pearl barley (2 ounces), rinsed

3 honey dates, rinsed

2 pounds winter melon, scrubbed, seeded, and cut into 2-inch
    cubes with rind on

3 carrots, peeled and roll-cut into 2-inch pieces (optional)

3 thin slices (about ⅛-inch thick) peeled fresh ginger

4 ounces fresh mushrooms, sliced (optional)

¼ cup lily bulb scales (1 ounce), rinsed

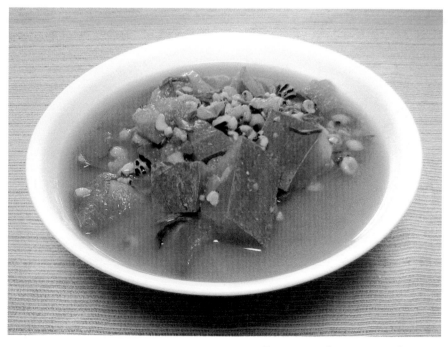

Four Items Plus Winter Melon Soup

Rinse and soak lotus seeds in warm water for 1 hour, drain, and remove any green centers.

Soak Mandarin orange peel, drain, and scrape off and discard the white pith on the inside of the peel.

In a large pot, combine lotus seeds, orange peel, foxnuts, barley, and dates with 2½ quarts of water and bring to a boil over high heat. Continue to cook for 30 minutes. Add winter melon, carrots, and ginger, return to a boil, then reduce to medium and simmer for 1½ hours. Add fresh mushrooms and lily bulb scales and cook for an additional 30 minutes. Serve hot.

Serves 6.

Suggestions and Variations:

Winter melon may be substituted with chayote, fuzzy melon or zucchini squash to create more variations (see page 155).

Fresh porcini, button, or shiitake mushrooms may be used for this soup, but not dried black mushrooms, as their strong flavor may overpower the other ingredients.

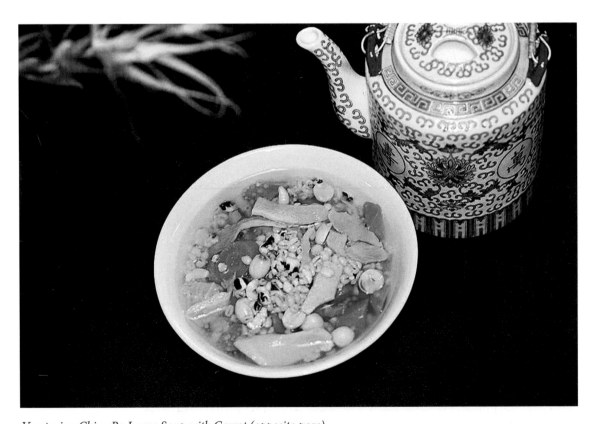

Vegetarian Ching Bo Leung Soup with Carrot (opposite page)

Vegetarian Ching Bo Leung Soup 清補涼湯 （加胡蘿蔔）

Ching Bo Leung is loaded with antioxidants. In this vegetarian version carrot is used to give the bland ingredients a flavor lift.

Instead of buying the prepackaged Ching Bo Leung, you may assemble the ingredients yourself from your own pantry, as they are all very common Chinese food items.

> 1¼ cups raw pearl barley (2½ ounces)
> ¼ cup lotus seeds (1½ ounces)
> 6 pieces dried wild yam (½ ounce)
> ½ cup Solomon's seal (½ ounce)
> 1½ tablespoons foxnuts (½ ounce)
> 2 tablespoons lily bulb scales (½ ounce)
> 2 ounces bamboo pith (optional)
> 2 tablespoons dragon-eye or longan fruit (¼ ounce)
> 4 honey dates, rinsed
> 2 thin slices (about ⅛-inch thick) peeled fresh ginger
> 3 carrots, peeled and roll-cut into 1- to 2-inch pieces

Rinse and soak the barley in cold water for 30 minutes or more.

Rinse and soak lotus seeds in cold water for 1 hour, drain, and remove any green centers.

Rinse and soak wild yam in cold water for 30 minutes or more. Drain.

Rinse and soak Solomon's seal in cold water for 30 minutes. Drain.

Rinse and soak foxnuts in cold water for 30 minutes or more. Drain.

Rinse and soak lily bulb scales in cold water for 30 minutes. Drain.

Rinse and soak bamboo pith (if using) in cold water for 1 hour. Drain.

Cook bamboo pith and ginger in 2 quarts of boiling water for 2 minutes. Drain. Remove and discard the ends of the bamboo pith and cut it into 2-inch pieces.

In a large pot, combine carrot, barley, lotus seeds, wild yam, Solomon's seal, foxnuts, dragon-eye fruit, and dates with 2½ quarts of water and bring to a boil over high heat. Cook for 30 minutes. Reduce heat to medium and cook for 1 more hour. Add lily bulbs and bamboo pith, and cook for an additional 30 minutes. Serve hot or at room temperature.

Serves 6.

Suggestions and Variations:

One may sweeten the vegetarian Ching Bo Leung with ¼ cup of sugar (or a dash of stevia powder) to make it into a snack or dessert soup. My Vietnamese friends refrigerate the sweet Ching Bo Leung and serve it cold in the summer.

Mung Beans, Kelp, Lotus Seeds, and Lily Bulb Soup
海帶綠豆蓮子百合湯

Cooling and Cleansing

Mung beans are cooling by nature and are anti-pyretic. Kelp, like other sea vegetables, helps cleanse the body of pollutants, especially heavy metal and radiation. This soup also helps with acne.

> 3 ounces kelp
> ½ cup mung beans (4 ounces)
> ¼ cup lotus seeds (1½ ounces)
> ¼ cup lily bulb scales (1 ounce)
> ¾ pound fuzzy melon, peeled and cut into 2- x 1- x ¼-inch pieces
> 3 thin slices (about ⅛-inch thick) peeled fresh ginger
> 4 ounces canned straw mushrooms
> 2 carrots, peeled and cut into ½-inch pieces
> 4 honey dates, rinsed
> 1 tablespoon vegetable oil

Rinse and soak kelp in cold water overnight until soft, drain, and cut into 1-inch lengths. Reserve 2 cups of soaking liquid.

Rinse and soak mung beans overnight. Discard liquid.

Rinse and soak lotus seeds in cold water for 1 hour, drain, and remove any green centers.

Rinse and soak lily bulb scales in cold water for 30 minutes. Drain and set aside.

Slow-cook mung beans and lotus seeds in a thermal cooker for 8 hours or overnight.

Heat vegetable oil in a frying pan or wok, add fuzzy melon, and cook until lightly browned. Add ginger and 2 cups of water and cook, covered, over high heat for 5 minutes.

In a large pot, combine kelp, kelp soaking liquid, mung beans, lotus seeds, lily bulb scales, mushrooms, carrots, dates, browned fuzzy melon along with the ginger and cooking liquid with 2½ quarts of water, bring to a boil over high heat, and cook for 30 minutes. Reduce heat to medium and cook for 45 minutes more uncovered.

Serves 8.

SUGGESTIONS AND VARIATIONS:

The standard recipe for treating zits calls for only kelp, mung beans, and rue. You may add a few sprigs of fresh rue to this soup to help with acne.

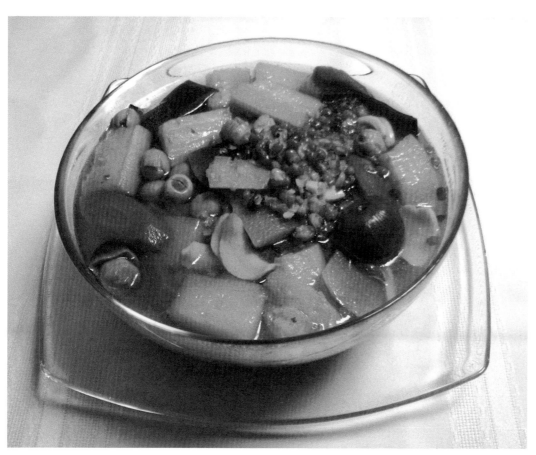

Kelp and Mung Bean Soup

Two-Tone Bok Choy and Louhfo Tofu Soup 金銀菜老火豆腐湯

A soup that has been boiled for a long while (at least 1 hour) is referred to as louhfo meaning "aged by fire." Louhfo tofu becomes spongy and honeycomb-like, and readily absorbs the flavor of other ingredients, making it delicious.

> 4 ounces dried bok choy
> 4 dried black mushrooms
> 3 thin slices (about ⅛-inch thick) peeled fresh ginger
> 4 honey dates, rinsed
> ¼ cup large, Southern apricot kernels (2 ounces), rinsed
> 1 teaspoon small, Northern apricot kernels (½ ounce), rinsed
> 1 14-ounce package regular tofu, cut into 1-inch cubes
> 2 carrots, peeled and cut into 1-inch pieces
> ¾ pound fresh bok choy, cut into 2-inch pieces

Soak dried bok choy overnight, rinse thoroughly and cut into 2-inch pieces.

Rinse and soak dried black mushrooms in hot water for 30 minutes, until soft, strain and reserve the soaking liquid, cut off and discard stems, and cut mushrooms into strips.

In a large pot, combine mushrooms along with their soaking liquid, ginger, dates, both types of apricot kernels, tofu, carrots, and dried bok choy with 2½ quarts of water and bring to a boil over high heat. Reduce heat to medium, cover with lid elevated by a pair of bamboo chopsticks set across the rim of the pot, and continue to cook for 1½ hours. Add fresh bok choy and boil for an additional 30 minutes. Salt to taste. Serve hot.

Serves 6.

Napa Cabbage, Tofu Puffs, and Mung Bean Thread Soup
黃芽白豆腐泡粉絲湯

Chinese cooks consider napa cabbage and carrots to be the sweetest-tasting vegetables.

2 ounces mung bean threads
¾ pound napa cabbage, cut into (¼- to ½-inch wide strips
2 ounces *ja choi* (preserved turnip), rinsed and cut into ⅙-inch slices
4 ounces canned straw mushrooms, rinsed and halved
4 ounces canned bamboo shoots, sliced
2 carrots, peeled and sliced on the diagonal into ¼-inch thick slices
12 tofu puffs, halved
2 ounces snow peas, ends trimmed off and strings removed

Soak mung bean threads in cold water for 30 minutes, drain, and cut into 4-inch pieces. Set aside.

In a large pot, bring 2½ quarts of water to a boil in high heat. Add napa cabbage, *ja choi* mushrooms, bamboo shoots, and carrots, cook for 30 minutes over high heat, reduce heat to medium, cover with a lid elevated by a pair of bamboo chopsticks set across the rim of the pot, and cook for 30 minutes. Add tofu puffs and snow peas and cook, uncovered, for 10 minutes more. Add mung bean threads last and cook for an additional 10 minutes. Salt to taste. Serve hot.

Serves 6.

SUGGESTIONS AND VARIATIONS:

In the summer when loofah squash and fresh lily bulbs are available, use them instead of napa cabbage and ja choi.

Soybean Sprouts, Kelp, and Frozen Tofu Soup
大豆芽海帶老豆腐湯

This soup is rich in soybean protein, essential fatty acids (EFA), and isoflavones.

Thawed frozen tofu is very spongy, but firm with a meat-like texture. Its sponginess is different from that of louhfo tofu.

> 1 16-ounce package tofu, frozen
> 4 ounces kelp
> 2 ounces frozen peas, thawed
> ½ pound soybean sprouts, ends pinched off and discarded
> 2 carrots, peeled and roll-cut into 1- to 2-inch pieces
> ¼ pound bamboo shoots, sliced
> 3 thin slices (about ⅛-inch thick) peeled fresh ginger
> ¼ pound fresh mushrooms, sliced

Remove the tofu from the freezer and defrost overnight. Squeeze to remove excess water, and cut into 1-inch cubes.

Soak kelp overnight until soft, drain, and cut into 1-inch pieces.

Cook peas in boiling water for 2 minutes, then drain.

In a large pot, bring 2 quarts of water to a boil over high heat. Add soybean sprouts, kelp, tofu, carrots, bamboo shoots, and ginger and cook, uncovered, over high heat for 30 minutes. Reduce heat to medium, continue to cook, covered with the lid elevated by a pair of bamboo chopsticks set across the rim of the pot, for 1½ hours. Add mushrooms and peas, and cook for 15 minutes more. Serve hot.

Serves 6.

Watercress and Honey Date Soup 西洋菜蜜棗湯

This is a soothing soup for the lungs in windy or dry season.

¼ cup lily bulb scales (1 ounce)

6 dried black mushrooms

3 carrots, peeled and roll-cut into 1- to 2-inch pieces

¼ cup large, Southern apricot kernels (2 ounces), rinsed

1 teaspoon small, Northern apricot kernels (½ ounce), rinsed

6 honey dates, rinsed

1 18-ounce package regular or firm tofu (optional)

2 bunches watercress (approximately 12 ounces), cut into 3-inch
   pieces

Rinse lily bulb scales and soak in cold water for 30 minutes. Drain.

Rinse and soak dried black mushroom in hot water for 30 minutes, or until soft, drain, reserving the soaking liquid, remove and discard stems, and cut mushrooms in halves or quarters.

In a large pot, combine mushrooms along with their soaking liquid, carrots, both types of apricot kernels, and dates with 2½ quarts of water and bring to a boil over high heat. Cook for 30 minutes. Add tofu (if using), lily bulb scales, and watercress and return to a boil. Reduce heat to medium and continue to cook, covered with the lid elevated by a pair of bamboo chopsticks set across the rim of the pot, for 30 minutes. Serve hot or at room temperature.

Serves 6.

Mixed Vegetable Bisque 什錦素菜羹

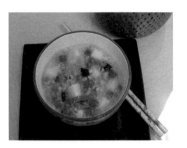

Mixed Vegetable Bisque

This is a colorful Soup. This recipe calls for winter melon and pearl barley, all-time Chinese vegetarian favorites, because the squash resembles white jade while the barley resembles pearls.

2 ounces raw pearl barley
4 ounces frozen green peas and diced carrots, thawed
4 dried black mushrooms or fresh shiitake mushrooms, finely diced
½ ounce dried orange peel (1/3 of a whole peel) (optional)
1 teaspoon peeled fresh ginger, minced
1¼ pounds winter melon, peeled, seeded, and diced
2 egg whites, lightly beaten (optional)

THICKENING MIXTURE:

1 teaspoon salt
1 teaspoon sugar
2 tablespoons cornstarch
¼ cup water

Rinse and soak barley in warm water for 30 minutes. Drain.

Cook frozen peas and carrots in boiling water for 2 minutes. Drain.

If using dried mushrooms, rinse and soak in hot water for 30 minutes, or until soft, strain and reserve the soaking liquid, remove and discard stems, and finely dice the mushroom caps.

Soak dried orange peel in cold water for 30 minutes, drain, and scrape off and discard the white pith from the inside of the peel. Mince finely.

In a large pot, combine melon, barley, mushrooms along with their soaking liquid, orange peel, and ginger with 2½ quarts of water and cook over high heat for 30 minutes. Reduce heat to medium, cover with a lid elevated by a pair of bamboo chopsticks set across the rim of the pot, and continue to cook for 1 hour. Add peas and carrots and cook for 10 minutes more.

In a small bowl, beat the egg whites by hand (with a fork or a pair of chopsticks) until they have an even consistency but are not frothy.

In another small bowl, combine the thickening mixture ingredients and stir slowly into the hot soup, adding a little at a time until desired thickness is achieved. Remove from heat and stir in the beaten egg white. Serve hot.

Serves 6.

Diced winter melon can be replaced by diced white turnip or daikon, which also resemble white jade. Diced fuzzy melon will do, as well. The stem portion of napa cabbage, either shredded or diced, also assumes a jade-like translucence upon cooking. The sweetness of napa cabbage has made it my favorite ingredient in a mixed vegetable soup.

Leafy green vegetables like spinach turn dark and acrid after cooking for more than an hour and are therefore not recommended in a mixed vegetable soup.

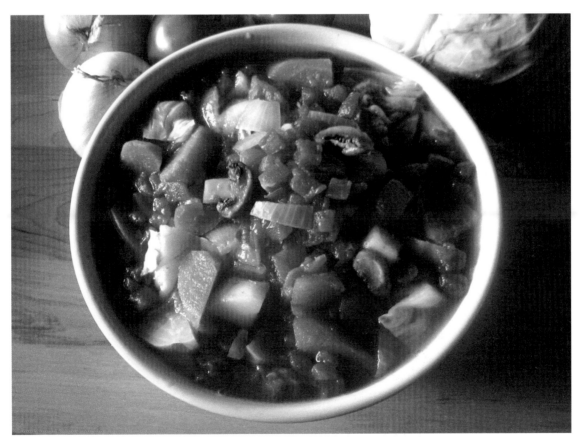

Vegetarian Borscht (next page)

Vegetarian Borscht 素羅宋湯

This is adapted from Mom's Chinese-Style Borscht (see recipe on pages 175–176 under Winter Soups).

> 2 tablespoons vegetable oil
> 1 medium yellow onion, sliced
> ½ pound cabbage, cut into 1- x 2-inch pieces
> 2 russet potatoes, peeled and cut into 1-inch cubes
> 1 golden beet, peeled, halved, and sliced crosswise
> 4 ounces fresh mushrooms, halved
> 2 medium tomatoes, peeled, seeded, and cut into wedges
> 2 carrots, peeled and roll-cut in 1- to 2-inch pieces
> 3 thin slices (about ⅛-inch thick) peeled fresh ginger

In a frying pan, heat the vegetable oil over high heat. Add onion and sauté until soft and translucent, about 5 minutes.

In a large pot, combine the sautéed onion, cabbage, potatoes, beet, mushrooms, tomatoes, carrots, and ginger with 2½ quarts of water, bring to a boil over high heat, and cook for 30 minutes. Reduce heat to medium, cover with a lid elevated by a pair of bamboo chopsticks set across the rim of the pot, and cook for 1½ hours more. Serve hot.

Serves 6.

SUGGESTIONS AND VARIATIONS:

If you prefer to use a thermal cooker, after the onions are sautéed, boil all of the ingredients together for 20 minutes, then place the inner pot in the thermos for at least 3 hours.

If desired, you may finely dice or slice all of the ingredients of the vegetarian borscht and thicken the soup into a gang. Then you get a bisque out of the vegetarian borscht.

You may choose to puree the tomatoes, or use a small (4-ounce) can of tomato sauce. Then you get a vegetable borscht with a western touch.

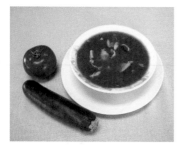

Vegetable Borscht with Tomato Puree

Enoki, Shiitake, Bamboo Pipe, and Tofu Bisque
金針菇竹笙豆腐羹

A Fungi Delight

Chinese vegetarians delight in using fungi in their cuisine. This is a creation of Mr. Lai Wong of the Golden Palace Restaurant in Stockton. No ingredients from the allium family, such as green onions or chives, are used in order to strictly observe the Buddhist vegetarian code.

   1 white woodear
   2 bamboo pipe fungus
   2 thin slices (about ⅛-inch thick) peeled fresh ginger
   1 bunch enoki or *gamjam* (golden needle) mushrooms (about 4
      ounces), trimmed and cut into 1-inch pieces
   5 fresh shiitake mushrooms cut into strips
   1 16-ounce package soft or silken tofu, cut into 1-inch cubes
   1 egg white, lightly beaten but not frothy

THICKENING MIXTURE:

   1 teaspoon salt
   1 teaspoon sugar
   2 tablespoons cornstarch
   ¼ cup water

Soak white woodear in cold water for 1 hour until it turns snowy white and expands in size. Drain, cut off the hard ends, and separate the florets.

Soak bamboo pipe in cold water for 2 hours until it expands and turns white. Cut off the ends. Cut into ¼-inch cross-sections.

Cook bamboo pipes, along with the ginger, in boiling water for 5 minutes, drain, and discard ginger.

In a large pot, combine enoki mushrooms, shiitake mushrooms, woodear, and bamboo pipes with 2½ quarts of cold water and bring to a boil. Lower heat to medium and continue to cook for 30 minutes. Add tofu and boil for 5 more minutes.

In a small bowl, stir together thickening mixture ingredients and stir into the hot soup. Remove pot from heat. Pour in beaten egg white as you continue to stir. Salt to taste and serve hot. Garnish with minced carrot.

Serves 6.

To create a more colorful soup, add peas and/or thinly sliced Chinese broccoli stems or asparagus along with the tofu.

This soup may be used inside a carved *dung gwa jung* (Winter Melon Bowl) for a vegetarian feast.

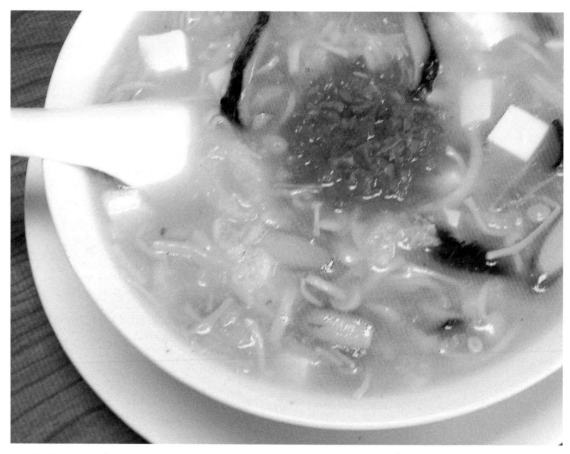

Enoki, Shiitake, Bamboo Pipe, and Tofu Bisque

Tai Chi Bisque 太極羹

This recipe sports two thickened soups presented in the same bowl in the shape of the yin-yang symbol.

Cream of Mushroom Soup with Chopped Spinach

1 8-ounce package frozen, chopped spinach, thawed
1 10.75-ounce can Campbell's Cream of Mushroom Soup
    (Reduced Salt)

In a 2-quart pot, bring 2 cups of water to a boil. Stir in the cream of mushroom soup and chopped spinach. Remove from heat as soon as the soup is smooth and warm.

Cream of Corn Soup with Egg White

2 egg whites
1 10-ounce can cream-style corn

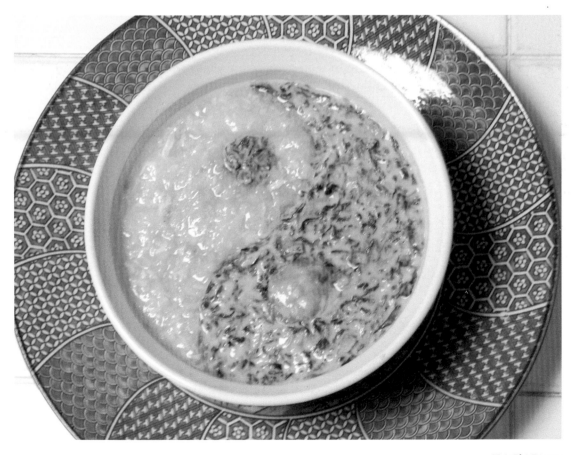

Tai Chi Bisque

THICKENING MIXTURE:

½ teaspoon salt
½ teaspoon sugar
1 tablespoon cornstarch
2 tablespoons water

Beat the egg whites lightly by hand (with a fork or a pair of chopsticks) until they are an even consistency, but not frothy.

In a 2-quart pot, bring 2 cups of water to a boil and stir in the corn. If a thicker consistency is desired, slowly stir in thickening mixture, as with a *gang* or bisque. Remove from heat and stir in the egg white.

PRESENTATION OF THE TAI CHI BISQUE

First you'll need a template for shaping the two soups into the yin-yang symbol. Cut a strip from a disposable aluminum baking pan. The width should be at least as deep as your bowl, and the length, at least 1.6 times the diameter of the bowl. If you plan to use a flat-bottomed bowl, you may cut a straight edge. If you are using a regular soup bowl, you'll have to trim the aluminum to follow the curvature of the bowl.

Wrap the strip of aluminum foil around two tumblers, the diameter of which is about half of that of the soup bowl, in a reverse S-shape, as shown in the diagram. Secure the ends with scotch tape and let it set for an hour or so.

When you are ready to serve the soup, place the template into the bowl (you'll need a second pair of hands to hold the template in place while you pour the soups into the bowl).

Be sure the template is centered and the ends are touching the bowl, leaving no gaps.

Pour in one soup, preferably the thicker one, on one side of the aluminum barrier. Usually a bisque thickens more when it comes down to room temperature. Adjust the template delicately to make sure the corners are sharp and the yin-yang sides are even.

Pour in the next soup. Delicately adjust the template once more.

Carefully remove the aluminum template by lifting it vertically up without disturbing the yin-yang pattern.

Complete the design by using a teaspoon to add a drop of the yin soup to the yang side, and a drop of the yang soup on the yin side. It is important to place the drops half way between the center and the edge of the bowl as shown in the picture.

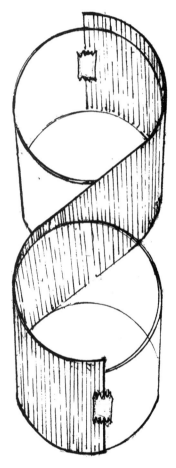

Template for Making Tai Chi Bisque

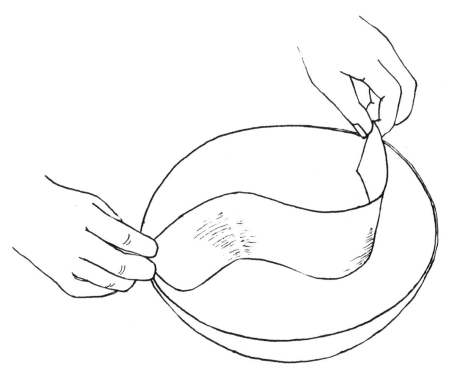

Holding the template in place

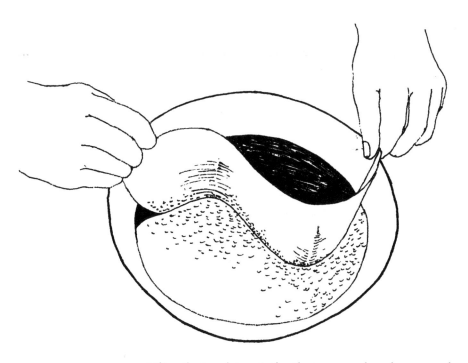

Lifting the template out after the two soups have been poured

Vegetarian Hot Pot 素火鍋

Here is a recipe that would charm a gathering of vegetarians. Emphasis should be placed on varying the color and texture of the food. Asian stores offer a wide variety of mock meat and seafood made of bean curd, koniyaku powder, and wheat gluten. While I am generally of the opinion that to a vegetarian, fake meat is somewhat pointless, I must admit that imitation shrimp, fish ball, chicken, and abalone do add interesting form and texture to a vegetarian hot pot.

1 pound daikon turnip, peeled and cut into 2- x 1-inch pieces
1 pound napa cabbage
10 fresh mushrooms, sliced
10 dried black mushrooms
4 arrowhead roots, sliced (optional)
2 bamboo shoots, sliced
4 carrots, sliced
1 pound lotus root, peeled and cut into ½-inch rounds
8 ounces taro root, peeled and diced
8 ounces fresh wild yam, peeled and cut into ½-inch rounds
8 ounces leaf lettuce
8 ounces spinach
8 ounces snow pea tendrils or pea pods
8 ounces edible chrysanthemum greens
24 vegetarian mini omelets (see recipe on page 257)
1 6-ounce package regular tofu, cut into 1-inch cubes
6 tofu puffs, halved
1 ounce kelp
2 ounces mung bean vermicelli
Mock abalone, sea cucumber, pork kidney, and chitterling, sliced

CONDIMENTS:

8 raw eggs (optional)
Soy sauce
Sesame seed oil
Vegetarian satay sauce (without the dried shrimp)
Chile sauce
Thinly sliced red chiles (optional)

Parboil the daikon, cabbage, carrots, and lotus root separately for 30 minutes each. Remove the vegetables and drain them, reserving the liquid (the different liquids may be combined after parboiling), and arrange the vegetables on serving plates.

Rinse and soak dried black mushrooms in hot water for 30 minutes, until soft, reserve the liquid (may be combined with the liquid used to parboil the daikon, cabbage, carrots, and lotus root), and remove and discard the mushroom stems.

Soak kelp in cold water for 3 hours, drain, and cut into 1½-inch lengths.

Soak mung bean vermicelli in cold water for 10 minutes or until softened and cut into 4-inch lengths.

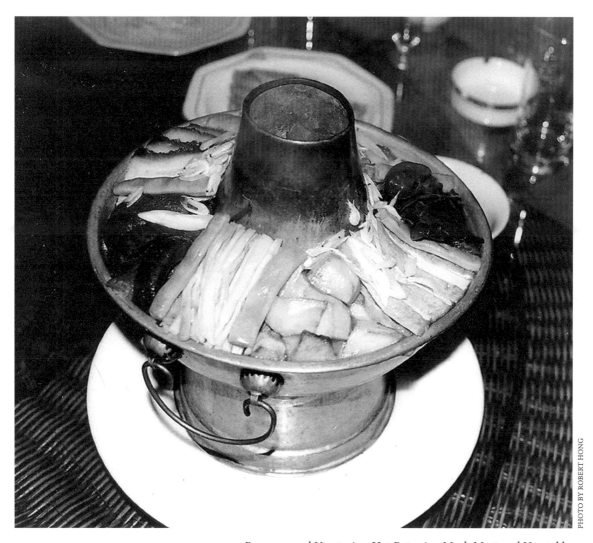

PHOTO BY ROBERT HONG

Pre-arranged Vegetarian Hot Pot using Mock Meat and Vegetables

Clean all the green vegetables, drain, pat dry, and place in separate serving bowls or colanders.

Arrange mini-omelets on a plate and garnish with sprigs of cilantro, if desired.

Fill the hot pot with boiling water and the liquid used to parboil the vegetables. Put hot pot in the center of the dining table, surrounded by dishes of food.

Set the table with individual soup bowls, spoons, chopsticks, and condiments.

Gather the people around the table to do their own cooking and eating and add merriment and laughter.

Serves 8.

SUGGESTIONS AND VARIATIONS:

A space-saving way of serving Hot Pot is to pre-arrange everything inside the hot pot before cooking at the table (see picture on previous page). Hot water can be added as food and broth are being consumed.

Pre-arrangement is common with Korean Hot Pot where most of the ingredients are pre-cooked or parboiled.

Vegetarian Mini Omelets 素蛋餃

½ ounces black woodears
½ ounce white woodears
½ cup plus 1 tablespoon vegetable oil
1 medium onion, finely chopped (optional)
2 carrots, finely chopped
2 ounces bamboo shoots, finely chopped
4 ounces baked tofu, finely chopped
4 ounces fresh mushrooms, finely chopped
1 teaspoon finely chopped green onion or cilantro (optional)
½ teaspoon rice wine
½ teaspoon salt
½ teaspoon sugar
¼ teaspoon black pepper
8 eggs, beaten

Soak the black and white woodears, then drain, rinse, remove and discard the hard stems, and finely chop.

Heat 1 tablespoon of vegetable oil in a large skillet over medium-high heat. Reduce heat to medium, and add onion (if using), carrots, and bamboo shoots. Stir-fry until onion is soft, about 5 minutes. Add chopped woodears, tofu, mushrooms, and green onion or cilantro (if using) and continue to stir-fry for 2 more minutes. Stir in rice wine, salt, sugar, and pepper and remove from heat. Set aside to cool.

Heat a flat, nonstick skillet over medium-high heat. When hot, reduce heat to medium and add 1 teaspoon of vegetable oil. Pour in 2 tablespoons of beaten egg. As the egg spreads to form a thin layer about 2½ inches in diameter, add 1 teaspoon of the tofu and vegetable mixture to the center. Fold one half of the egg over to form a pocket with the filling inside. Quickly flip the omelet over, cook for 1 minute, and then flip it over again, cooking until both sides are golden. Remove from pan and place on serving platter. Repeat this method until the filling is used up. If you run out of eggs before you run out of filling, beat one or two more.

Makes 24 mini omelets.

14
Medicinal Soups

~~~~~~~~~~

The goal of traditional Chinese nutrition, more narrowly defined as "food therapy," is twofold: to heal and to prevent illness. By correcting the conditions of a disease, food as well as medicine restores health.

Based on their synergistic actions, herb formulas can be grouped into four broad categories:

1. 補 Tonifying: to supplement deficiency of qi, blood, yang, and yin
2. 瀉 Eliminating: to expel or disperse excessive wind, heat, cold, dryness, dampness, and fire, thus clearing the system
3. 調 Harmonizing: to regulate the function, direction, and tendency (for example, of qi and blood) in harmony with the internal and external environment
4. 衛 Fortifying: to strengthen the root and the center, to build up defense and immunity

It is not unusual for a formula (and medicinal soup) to offer multiple benefits.

While the taste, color, aroma of some ingredients of medicinal soups may take a little getting used to, the health benefits are undeniable.

MEDICINAL SOUP RECIPES	藥膳湯
Six-Herb Regulating Soup	六味地黃湯
Notoginseng and Chicken Soup	田七雞湯
Panax Ginseng and Chicken Soup	人參雞湯
Seahorse Soup	海馬湯
Eucommia Bark and Alpinia Oxyphylia Tea	杜仲益智仁湯
Smilax Glabra, Rehmannia, and Sparerib Soup	土茯苓大生地排骨湯
The Medicinal Herb Soup	藥材湯
Sha Shen, Solomon's Seal, and Dried Fig Soup	沙參玉竹無花果湯
Selfheal, Mulberry Leaf, and Chrysanthemum Tea	夏桑菊(下火茶)
The Big Ten Tonic Soup	十全大補湯

Cross-Reference

The following list cross-references more than a dozen soups from other categories that may also be considered "medicinal" because medicinal herbs are involved.

Cordeceps and Chicken Soup (Version 1) (see Exotic and Expensive Soup Recipes)	冬蟲草煲雞湯
Fritillary Bulb and Partridge Soup (see Exotic and Expensive Soup Recipes)	川貝燉鷓鴣
Sea Cucumber, Dried Scallop, and Selfheal Soup (see Exotic and Expensive Soup Recipes)	海參干貝夏枯草湯
Chrysanthemum, Lycii Leaves, Lycii Berry, and Pork Liver Soup (see Spring Soup Recipes)	菊花杞子枸杞豬肝湯
Ligusticum and Angelica Dahurica with Fish Head Soup (see Spring Soup Recipes)	川芎白芷燉魚頭
Dendrobium, American Ginseng, and Lean Pork Soup (see Autumn Soup Recipes)	石斛花旗參湯
White Ginseng and Black Chicken Soup (see Winter Soup Recipes)	白參烏雞湯
Four Tonics Fortified with Eucommia Soup (see Year-Round Soup Recipes)	四物杜仲湯
Danggui Chicken Soup (see Year-Round Soup Recipes)	當歸雞湯
Sugar Cane, Rhizome of Woolly Grass, Arrowroot, Water Chestnut, and Carrot Soup (see Year-Round Soup Recipes)	竹蔗茅根粉葛馬蹄紅蘿蔔湯
Chicken Wine Soup (see Festive Soup Recipes)	雞酒
Dispel Dampness Juk (see Rice Soup Recipes)	去濕粥
Cistanche and Lamb Rice Soup (see Rice Soup Recipes)	肉蓯蓉羊肉粥

Six-Herb Regulating Soup 六味地黃湯

All the herbs in this soup are neutral in nature, thus tonifying spleen and stomach. Drinking this soup regularly will help to improve both your physical and mental health.

¾ ounce cornus or Cornelian cherry fruit
½ ounce alisma
¾ ounce treated rehmannia
¾ ounce poria cocus
½ ounce white peony root
¾ ounce wild yam

Rinse herbs with cold water and pat dry.

Place herbs into a ceramic pot with 4 cups of water and bring to a boil over high heat. Reduce heat to low and simmer for 30 minutes or until mixture is reduced to 2 cups. Strain, reserving the herbs, and serve the soup as a beverage, two or three times a day.

Boil the herbs once more in 4 cups of water to make an additional 2 cups. Drink this second batch twice a day.

Serves 2.

SUGGESTIONS AND VARIATIONS:

Basic top stock made from pork and chicken bones may be used in place of some of the water if meat flavor is desired.

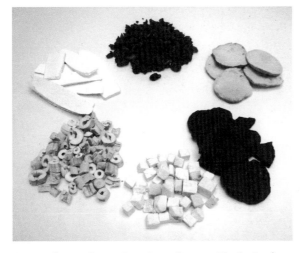

Six-Herb Regulating Soup Ingredients—Clockwise from top: cornus, alisma, rehmannia, poria cocus, white peony root, and wild yam

Notoginseng and Chicken Soup 田七雞湯

This soup is effective as a blood tonic and for lowering cholesterol. Drinking this soup regularly helps boost the immune system; however, it is not recommended for women who are pregnant or menstruating.

> 1 ounce notoginseng root slices
> 6 dried black mushrooms
> ½ chicken, skin and fat removed, chopped into large pieces
> 12 jujube dates, pitted
> 6 slices fresh ginger, ⅛-inch thick

Feiseui: Cook pork in 1 quart of boiling water for 5 minutes, drain, and rinse with cold water.

Rinse jujube dates.

In a large pot, combine chicken, mushroom, dates, notoginseng, and ginger with 2 quarts of water. Cook over medium-high for 30 minutes. Reduce heat to medium-low and simmer for 1½ hours, covered.

Serves 2.

SUGGESTIONS AND VARIATIONS:

Yunnan people invented a steaming pot called qiguo specifically for making notoginseng and chicken soup, their regional specialty. See picture of Yunnan Notoginseng Soup made in a qiguo by Dr. and Mrs. George Wang on next page.

We may substitute chicken with 8 ounces of pork. Also, the rock-hard notoginseng is readily available in powder form.

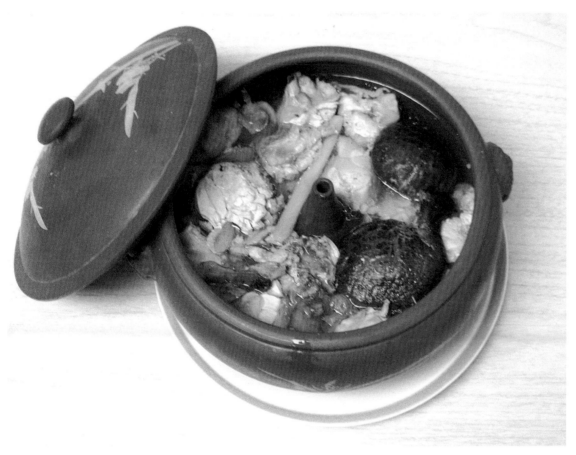

Notoginseng and Chicken Soup in a Qiguo

Panax Ginseng and Chicken Soup 人參雞湯

Energizer Supreme for Stamina and Rejuvenation

This soup is good for older people and people convalescing from surgery or illness, but it is not suitable for younger people with lots of yang energy as the potent panax ginseng may cause them vertigo. Even for those with the right constitution, do not use more than the small quantity of ginseng called for in the recipe.

> 1 whole chicken (approximately 2 pounds), skin and fat removed
> and cut into large pieces
> 10 slices Korean red ginseng (approximately 0.05 ounce)
> 3 slices ginger, 1/16-inch thick
> 2 green onions
> 1/4 cup cooking wine or dry sherry

Feiseui: Cook chicken in 2½ quarts of boiling water for 10 minutes, drain, and rinse with cold water.

In a large pot, combine chicken, ginseng, ginger, green onions and wine with 2½ quarts of boiling water and cook over high heat for 30 minutes. Reduce heat to medium-low and simmer covered for 3 to 6 hours. Serve hot.

Serves 6.

SUGGESTIONS AND VARIATIONS:

For those with dryness and heat conditions, it is best not to use chicken. Duck, domestic pigeon, partridge and quail are good substitutes due to their moistening qualities.

Ginseng alone can be made into a vegetarian beverage, called Ginseng Solo Soup 獨參湯. In this case, use 3 pieces (approximately 1½ ounces total) of Korean white ginseng or the Chinese *sehk chyúh sàm* 石柱參. Remove the top of the ginseng, slice it, and boil it in 3 quarts of water for 3 hours. As these types of ginseng are less potent, or yang, than the Korean red ginseng, they are better for those with high blood pressure.

Seahorse Soup 海馬湯

Seahorse is classified as a yang tonic. According to Doreen Leung's book, drinking this soup three or four times per week for a total of twenty servings will help lower your cholesterol.

2 cups top stock
¼ ounce seahorse, rinsed

In a medium pot, bring the broth to a boil over medium-high heat and add the seahorse. Reduce heat to medium and continue to boil until liquid is reduced to 1 cup, about 35 to 40 minutes. Serve hot.

Serves 1.

SUGGESTIONS AND VARIATIONS:

For a better tasting soup, add 1 ounce of lotus seeds, 4 ounces of lean pork or spareribs, wild yam, jujube dates, and a small piece of Mandarin orange peel along with the seahorses. By adding ¼ ounce of pipe fish, known as "sea dragon" 海龍 in Chinese, we get a soup with a fancy name: Sea Dragon and Seahorse Soup.

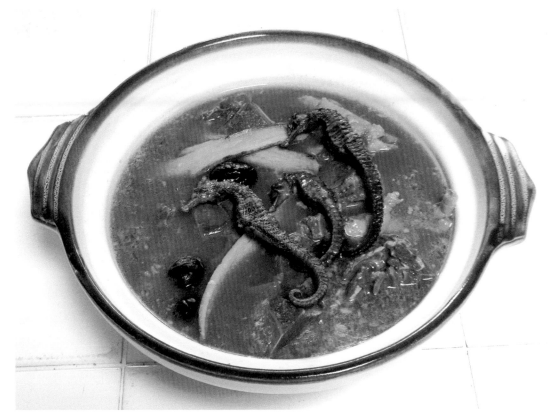

Seahorse Soup with Wild Yam, Wolfberries, and Spareribs

Eucommia Bark and Alpinia Oxyphylia Tea 杜仲益智仁湯

Tonify Blood and Nourish the Brain

> ½ ounce eucommia bark, rinsed
> ½ ounce alpinia oxyphylia, rinsed
> ½ ounce hawthorne, rinsed
> 4 honey dates
> 2 tablespoons crushed rock crystal sugar (or a pinch of stevia powder)

In a large pot, bring 2 quarts of water to a boil and add eucommia bark, alpinia oxyphylia, hawthorne, and dates. Cook over medium-high heat for 30 minutes. Reduce heat to medium-low and simmer uncovered for another 30 minutes. Add crystal sugar (or stevia) and boil until sugar dissolves. Strain and serve the tea hot.

Serves 4.

SUGGESTIONS AND VARIATIONS:

Since Chinese food therapy taps into the power of association, animal brain and walnut kernels are used with Alpinia Oxyphylia to improve brain power in many known recipes, both savory and sweet.

Smilax Glabra, Rehmannia, and Sparerib Soup 土茯苓大生地排骨湯

To combat heat and fatigue, red eye and hoarseness of voice

Normally, only pork is used with these cooling herbs. Chicken is deemed too hot and dry in nature.

   1½ pounds pork spareribs, cut in strips
   1 ounce smilax glabra (7 thick slices)
   ½ untreated rehmannia (6 slices)
   1 piece Mandarin orange peel (about 1/3 of a whole)

Feiseui: Cook spareribs in separate pots of boiling water for about 10 minutes until foamy residues and fat rise to the surface. Drain and rinse with cold water. Cut in between bones into small pieces.

   In a large pot boil 2½ quarts of water and add spareribs, smilax glabra, rehmannia, and orange peel. Bring to a boil. Reduce to medium and simmer for 3 hours. Serve hot.

Serves 6.

The Medicinal Herb Soup 藥材湯

Tonify Qi and Boost Immunity

This all-time tonic soup consists of four tonic herbs: wàhn lìhng (poria cocos) baahk seuht (Atractylodes), bāk kèih (astragalus) and fòhng dóng (codonositis). It is so popular that every Po-Po can rattle off the eight syllables wahn-lihng-baahk-seuht-bak-keih-fohng-dong 雲苓白朮北芪防黨 in one breath. This tonic soup is simply referred to as yeuhk chòih tong 藥材湯 (the medicinal herb soup).

> 1 whole black-bone chicken or juk si gai (silkie), whole or chopped into large pieces
> ½ pound pork sparerib
> 6 poria cocos or tuckahoe roll (about ½ ounce)
> 6 atractylodes slices (about ½ ounce)
> 3 slices astragalus root (about 1 ounce)
> 3 pieces codonopsitis root (about 1 ounce), cut into 2-inch sections
> 3 honey dates
> ½ cup rice wine or red wine

Feiseui: Cook chicken and spareribs separately in boiling water for 10 minutes, drain, and rinse with cold water.

Rinse the herbs.

In a large pot, bring 3 quarts of water to a boil. Add chicken, tuckahoe roll, atractylodes, astralagus root, codonopsitis root, and dates and return to a boil. Reduce heat to medium-low and simmer covered for 3 hours. Remove astragalus, atractylodes, and tuckahoe. Add wine, salt to taste, and serve hot.

Serves 6.

SUGGESTIONS AND VARIATIONS:

For a variation that will strengthen the lower limbs, add achyranthes bidentata and eucommia bark and simmer for an extra 2 hours. According to Wai Kuen Szeto, this soup also tonifies qi and dispels wind.

Do not add black mushrooms to this soup as they will overwhelm the taste.

Sha Shen, Solomon's Seal, and Dried Fig Soup
沙參玉竹無花果瘦肉湯

A Soup for Beautiful Complexion

The root of Solomon's seal is known to be a lubricating herb, moistening the mouth and quenching thirst. It can help improve dry skin and liver spots. Adenophora root is sweet and slightly bitter. It is good for dry throat and dry mucous membranes.

1½ pound pounds lean pork, cut into chunks
½ ounce adenophora tetraphylia, rinsed
½ ounce Solomon's seal
6 dried figs, rinsed and halved
1 whole piece dried Mandarin orange peel

Cook pork in 2 quarts of boiling water for about 10 minutes until foamy residues and fat rise to the top. Drain and rinse the meat with cold water.

In a large pot, boil 2½ quarts of water and add pork, adenophora tetraphylia, Solomon's seal, figs, and ginger. Cook over medium-high heat for 30 minutes. Reduce heat to medium-low and simmer for 2½ hours. Salt to taste. Serve hot.

Serves 4.

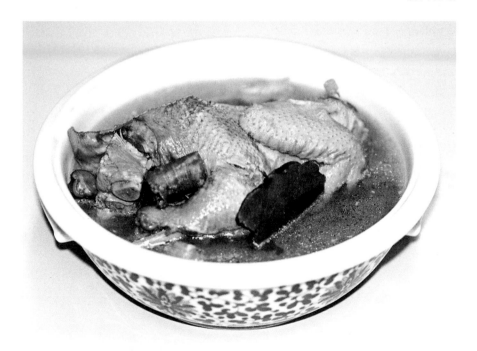

The Medicinal Herb Soup with Smilax Glabra and Old Chicken (opposite page)

Selfheal, Mulberry Leaf, and Chrysanthemum Tea
夏桑菊(下火茶)

The Eyebright Tea

This sweet soup helps tonify liver and lungs, and reduce excess heat inside the body. This soup exemplifies medicinal teas used to counter external attacks by the six evils. Both mulberry leaf and chrysanthemum are capable of dispersing wind and clearing heat, treating wind-heat patterns with fever and headache, as well as helping the liver and symptoms of red, painful, dry eyes or excessive tearing manifesting wind heat, or with such symptoms as spots in front of the eyes and blurriness manifesting liver yin deficiency.

Selfheal or prunella is also great for calming ascending liver fire and brightening the eyes. Recently selfheal is used to treat hypertension accompanied by ascending liver yang with good results.

> 1 ounce selfheal, rinsed several times with cold water until clean of
> dust and debris
> 1 ounce mulberry leaf, rinsed
> ½ ounce white chrysanthemum, rinsed
> 1 tablespoon honey

In a large pot, combine selfheal, mulberry leaf, and chrysanthemum with 2 quarts of water. Bring to a boil over high heat and cook for 10 minutes. Reduce heat to medium-low and simmer covered for 30 minutes. Strain. Add honey and serve hot.

Serves 4.

SUGGESTIONS AND VARIATIONS:

You may add lean pork and a pinch of salt (instead of honey) to make this into a savory soup.

The Big Ten Tonic Soup 十全大補湯

Just like traditional herbal formulas, there are established soup recipes for dietary purposes to clear excesses and tonify the body. Some assortments are pre-packaged and available in grocery stores. This assortment of ten tonic herbs should be decocted first before the liquid is cooked in a soup with rice, legumes, poultry, meat, and/or root vegetables.

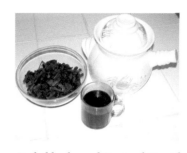

Boiled herbs and Strained Liquid

This herbal decoction does not taste bad but because of the rehmannia, everything in the soup, including the chicken, will turn black. The soup is rather tasty.

2 boneless, skinless chicken breasts (approximately 12 ounces)

1 package of assorted herbs called *sahp chyuhn daaih bo tong* **十全大補湯 (total weight: 5.3 ounces) containing: angelica sinensis當歸, astragalus 黃芪, atractylodes 白朮, cinnamon bark 桂皮, codonopsitis 黨參, glycyrrhiza/licorice 炙甘草, ligusticum/lovage root 川芎, poria cocos 茯苓, treated rehmannia/foxglove root 熟地, and white peony root 白芍**

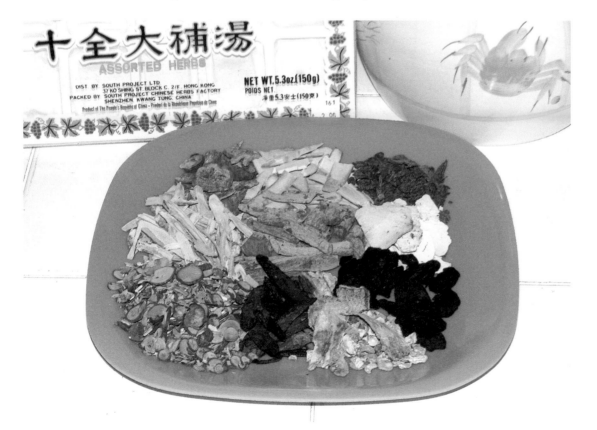

An Assortment of the Ten Tonic Herbs

Feiseui: Cook chicken breast in boiling water for 5 minutes, drain, and rinse with cold water. Cut into large pieces.

Decoct all herbs from the package in 1 quart of water in a clay pot. After bringing it to a boil, simmer for 1 hour. Strain and save the liquid, discarding the solids.

Place all the herb liquid and chicken pieces in a clay pot and add another quart of hot water. Bring to a boil and simmer over low heat for 30 minutes. Serve hot or at room temperature.

Serves 4.

SUGGESTIONS AND VARIATIONS:

If you do not like drinking a black soup, there are The Big Ten Tonic Pills 十全大補丸 available in Chinese herb shops. However, you'll miss out on a true epicurean experience. For a better presentation, add goji berries and diced fresh wild yam (nakaimo), cooked separately from the other ingredients, as a garnish to the soup.

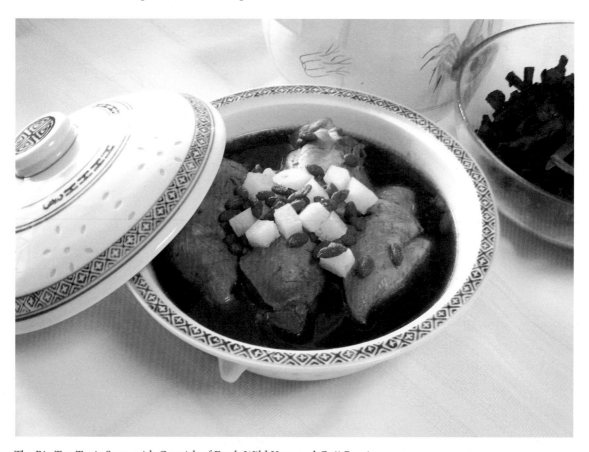

The Big Ten Tonic Soup with Garnish of Fresh Wild Yam and Goji Berries

15
Exotic and Expensive Soups

All my soup contributors are of the opinion that we would be doing a disservice to Cantonese cuisine if I chose to leave out recipes of the exotic and expensive soups. In fact, their first response to my call for recipes was to give their best, in terms of cost and perceived health benefits. These are the soups they prepare when grown children come home to visit, for special occasions like Thanksgiving, and for their own health maintenance, contradicting my assumption that they might stop making soup for just one person. I have much to learn from them. Not being selfish, they put cooking in the right perspective: Care, for oneself and one's family. It is the alpha and omega of louhfo tong. I can sense their pride and devotion in sharing their best. I am beginning to understand why Mrs. Yuk Hung Hong chose to work in the cannery to earn the extra money to make ginseng and chicken soup weekly for her frugal husband who would otherwise forbid such extravagance. Thanks to his wife's ginseng soup, Mr. Hong lived to be ninety-four years old.

To give you a rough idea of cost, I have included the going rates of many of the expensive ingredients used in this book in Part Three. Please understand that prices fluctuate and go up with time and differ from place to place.

Some of the most expensive ingredients happen to be colorless, odorless, and flavorless. These include the swallow's nest, hasmar, sea cucumber, shark's fin, fish maw, deer tendon, and velvet deer antler. Others are mild in odor and flavor, such as cordeceps, ginseng, American ginseng, dendrobium, and fritillary bulbs. For flavor, whole chicken, ham, and pork, as well as pricey seafood like abalone, dried scallops, crabmeat, and shrimp are called for.

EXOTIC AND EXPENSIVE SOUP RECIPES	名貴湯
Abalone, Sea Cucumber, Shark's Fin, and Fish Maw Soup	鮑參翅肚湯
Abalone and Chicken Soup (Version 1)	鮑魚雞湯(一)
Abalone and Chicken Soup (Version 2)	鮑魚雞湯(二)
Cordeceps and Chicken Soup (Version 1)	冬蟲草煲雞湯
Cordeceps and Chicken Soup (Version 2)	冬蟲草燉雞湯
Swallow's Nest and Chicken Soup	燕窩湯
Fritillary Bulb and Partridge Soup	川貝燉鷓鴣

Sea Cucumber, Dried Scallop,　　　　　海參干貝夏枯草湯
　　and Selfheal Soup
Crabmeat, Yellow Chive,　　　　　　　蟹肉韭黃瑤柱羹
　　and Dried Scallop Bisque
Hasmar Soup or Bisque　　　　　　　　雪蛤膏
Winter Melon Bowl　　　　　　　　　冬瓜盅
Turtle Soup　　　　　　　　　　　　水魚湯
Abalone, Shark's Fin, and Chicken　　　鮑魚雞絲魚翅羹
　　Bisque (see Festive Soup Recipes)
New Year Soup　　　　　　　　　　　新年湯
　　(see Festive Soup Recipes)

Abalone, Sea Cucumber, Shark's Fin, and Fish Maw Soup
鮑參翅肚湯

This extravagant soup brings together the four most expensive seafood items in one pot. It is prototypical of other elaborate soups like Mrs. Wai Ying Tam's New Year Soup and rich stews like *fo tiao qiang* 佛跳牆, so called because it is so enticing that "Buddha jumps over the wall" to get it.

- 4 small sea cucumbers (the size of your middle finger)
- 1½-inch thick slice fresh ginger, crushed
- 2 green onions
- 1 tablespoon cooking wine
- 1 fresh-frozen abalone, thawed
- 6 small dried shark's fins (2 ounces)
- 4 ounces fish maw, dried
- 1 pound lean pork
- 6 dried scallops
- 6 jujube dates

Place sea cucumbers in a pot of boiling water, turn off the heat, cover, and let sit overnight. Drain and discard soaking liquid. Cook sea cucumbers in boiling water along with the ginger, green onion, and wine for 15 minutes. Drain. Slit open the sea cucumber lengthwise and remove the inside. Rinse with cold water, cut each sea cucumber into 3 pieces, and set aside.

Scrub the abalone with salt and rinse twice with cold water. Pound the abalone with a wooden mallet. Slice sideways to get abalone steak pieces about ¼-inch thick. Set aside. Soak abalone in a fresh pot of boiling water overnight. Drain. Set aside.

Put shark's fin in a pot of boiling water, turn off the heat, cover, and let sit overnight. Drain, discarding the liquid, and repeat the overnight soaking process using fresh water. Drain and set aside.

Place fish maw in a pot of boiling water, turn off the heat, cover, and let sit overnight. Drain and cut into 1-inch wide pieces. Set aside.

Feiseui: Cook pork in boiling water for 10 minutes, drain, rinse with cold water, and cut into big chunks.

In the inner pot of a thermal cooker, combine abalone, shark's fin, pork, scallops, and dates with 2½ quarts of boiling water. Cook over high heat for 30 minutes. Place the inner pot inside the thermal cooker and let soup slow-cook for at least 5 hours. If time allows, leave it there for 8 hours or overnight.

Move the inner pot back to the stovetop and add sea cucumbers and fish maw. Bring to a boil again. Reduce heat and cook over medium heat for 30 minutes. Salt to taste. Serve hot.

Serves 6.

Suggestions and Variations:

It is less time consuming to use reconstituted sea cucumbers and reconstituted shark's fin, which can be bought frozen in big Asian markets. You may use canned abalone if fresh abalone is not available. Dried abalone is a lot of work, but once reconstituted, it tastes even better than fresh.

To balance the "cold" seafood ingredients, you may wish to add a "warming" chicken element by preparing top stock with chicken bone, chicken feet, and gizzards and combining it with water to total 2½ quarts of cooking liquid.

Sea cucumbers soften and melt away if they come into contact with oil for too long. Always cook sea cucumbers separately and add to the pot for only the last 30 minutes of cooking.

This elaborate soup makes an even more impressive presentation when it is served from a traditional ceramic soup pot. For banquets, serve it in a porcelain tureen with matching bowls and spoons.

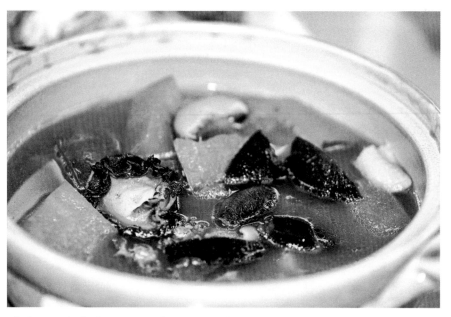

Abalone and Chicken Soup with Winter Melon and Black Mushroom (opposite page)

Abalone and Chicken Soup (Version 1) 鮑魚雞湯（一）

This recipe calls for fresh abalone. Bob Hong recommended using smaller, cultivated abalones as they are much more tender than the larger abalones, which require pounding. The abalone should be added into the soup whole and sliced before serving for better form and texture.

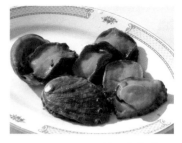

Pearl Abalone

6 small "Pearl" abalones, rinsed and cleaned
3 thin slices (about ⅛-inch thick) peeled fresh ginger
2 stalks green onions
1 whole chicken (approximately 2 pounds), skin and fat removed
1 pork loin (approximately 1 pound)
2 tablespoons cooking wine

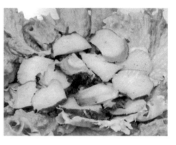

Sliced Pearl Abalone

Feiseui: Cook abalones along with the ginger and green onions in 1 quart of boiling water for 10 minutes. Clean out the guts with a sharp knife. Cook chicken in 2½ quarts of boiling water for 10 minutes, drain, and rinse with cold water. Cook pork loin in 1 quart of boiling water for 10 minutes, drain, and rinse with cold water.

In a large pot, combine abalone, chicken, pork, and cooking wine with 3 quarts of cold water. Bring to a boil over high heat and cook for an additional 30 minutes. Remove chicken and pork; place in the refrigerator to chill. Reduce heat to medium and cook for 2½ hours more, covered with the lid of the pot elevated by a pair of bamboo chopsticks set across the rim so that steam may escape.

Before serving the soup, chop the chicken and arrange it on a platter. Slice the pork. Remove the abalones from the soup, thinly slice them, and arrange on platters. Season the soup with salt to taste. Serve hot with the chicken, abalone, and pork as side dishes along with finely chopped ginger, green onions, and oyster sauce as condiments.

Serves 6.

Suggestions and Variations:

Bob Hong added chunks of winter melon and black mushroom to the abalone and chicken soup, creating a soup and cold side dishes.

Abalone and Chicken Soup (Version 2) 鮑魚雞湯(二)

Dried abalones are available year-round and worldwide. They are treasured for their unique flavor and texture. Reputedly, abalones nurture the yin and our essential energy.

> 4 small dried abalones
> 1 whole chicken (approximately 2 pounds), skin and fat removed, and cut into medium-sized pieces
> ¾ pound lean pork
> 4 dried scallops
> 6 jujube dates, rinsed
> 1 whole Mandarin orange peel
> 3 thin slices (about ⅙-inch thick) peeled fresh ginger
> 2 green onions

Place dried abalones in a pot of boiling water, cover, and soak overnight. Discard the whole pot of water and prepare another pot of hot water. Repeat this process, using fresh water each time, every 8 to 10 hours until the abalones yield to the touch. Clean the abalones and remove their intestines with a sharp knife. Put abalones in 1 quart of boiling water with ginger and green onions and cook for 30 minutes. Drain and rinse with cold water. Thinly slice.

Feiseui: Cook chicken in 2 quarts of boiling water for 10 minutes, drain, and rinse with cold water. Cook pork in 1 quart of boiling water for 5 minutes, drain, and rinse with cold water. Cut into ½-inch slices.

Soak dried scallops in warm water for 30 minutes. Reserve their soaking liquid.

Rinse and soak Mandarin orange peel in cold water for 30 minutes, drain, scrape off and discard the white pith on the inside of the peel. Chop coarsely into small pieces.

In a large pot, bring 3 quarts of water to a boil and add abalone, chicken, pork, scallops (and soaking liquid), jujube dates, and orange peel. Cook over high heat for 30 minutes. Reduce heat to medium and simmer, covered, for 2½ hours. Strain the soup and serve the broth hot with the solids on the side, offering soy sauce or oyster sauce as condiments.

Serves 6.

Most of the time, dried abalones do not get tender with just one soaking. Their reconstitution needs to be started two or three days in advance, repeating the soaking process several times. The bigger the abalone, the longer the process will take.

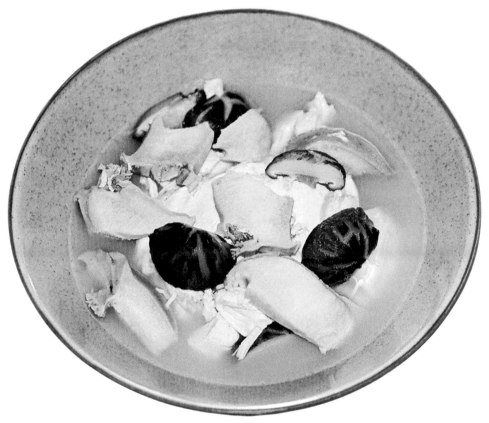

Abalone and Chicken Soup

Cordeceps and Chicken Soup (Version 1) 冬蟲草煲雞湯

The Miraculous Mushroom of the Himalayas

Prized for their rareness and medicinal value, cordeceps are found only on the Tibetan plateau. They are miniature mushrooms in the summer, while in the winter, they are parasites inside the larvae of a special kind of moth. Pairing chicken with pork for the cooling and moistening effect of pork, this soup tonifies the kidneys and lungs. It is said to be effective in treating back pain and asthma.

> 10 black dates
> 1 pound pork
> 1 whole chicken, cut into medium-sized pieces
> 8 pieces codonopsitis (each stick measuring 6–8 inches in length)
> 12 slices dried wild yam
> 2 tablespoons dried dragon-eye meat (about ½ ounce)
> 28 poria cocos in 2½-inch rolls, (2 ounces)
> ¼ cup foxnuts
> 24 cordeceps (each piece measuring approximately 2 inches long)
> ¼ cup wolfberries

Soak dates in cold water for 30 minutes, drain, and remove pits.

Feiseui: Cook pork in 2 quarts of boiling water for 5 to 10 minutes, drain, and rinse with cold water. Cook chicken in 2 quarts of boiling water for 5 to 10 minutes, drain, and rinse with cold water.

In a large pot, combine dates, pork, chicken, codonopsitis, wild yam, dragon-eye meat, poria cocos, foxnuts, and cordeceps with 5 quarts of cold water. Bring to a boil and cook over high for 30 minutes. Reduce heat to medium, cover with the lid elevated by a pair of bamboo chopsticks set across the rim of the pot, and continue to cook for 2 hours. Add wolfberries and simmer for an additional 45 minutes. Serve hot.

Serves 6–8.

Suggestions and Variations:

In China, ducks are as available as chickens. Traditionally cordecep soups are made with duck because duck meat is considered more yin-nourishing and less drying and hot than chicken. When you use a duck for the above recipe, you may omit the pork.

In general, ducks have a thick layer of subcutaneous fat. Be sure to remove the skin before parboiling the duck. Even so, there will be quite a lot of fat to skim off.

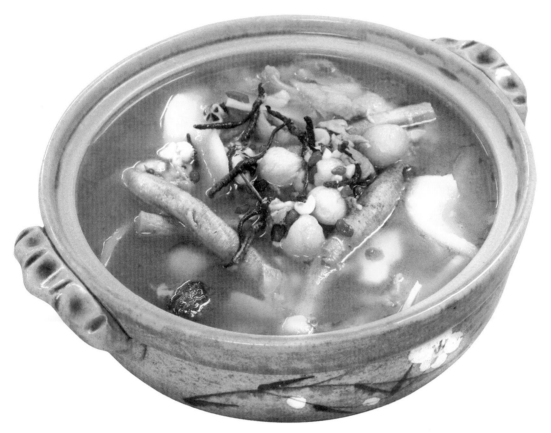

Cordeceps and Chicken Soup

Cordeceps and Chicken Soup (Version 2) 冬蟲草燉雞湯

This recipe demonstrates the dahn (steaming or double-boiling) method of making tonic soups.

> **1 bunch cordeceps (approximately 12 pieces), rinsed with cold water**
> **2 boneless, skinless chicken breasts, fat removed, cut into large chunks**
> **1 chunk peeled fresh ginger (the size of your thumb), crushed**
> **1 tablespoon cooking wine**

In a lidded dahnjung (double-boiling container), combine cordeceps, chicken, ginger, and wine with 4 cups of boiling water. Cover the dahnjung and place it inside a pot filled with enough hot water to come halfway up the side, cover, and steam for 30 minutes over high heat. Reduce heat to medium and continue to steam, covered, for 2 hours more. Season to taste with salt. Serve hot.

Serves 4.

SUGGESTIONS AND VARIATIONS:

Instead of chicken breast, you may use duck breast or any kind of small game bird such as partridge, squab, or quail for this recipe.

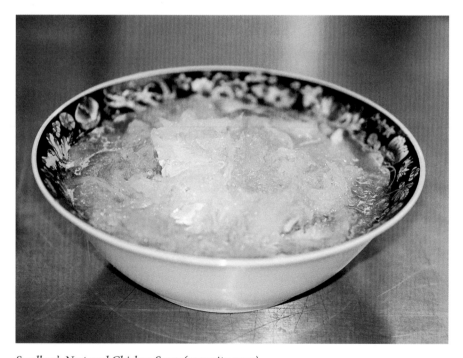

Swallow's Nest and Chicken Soup (opposite page)

Swallow's Nest and Chicken Soup 燕窩湯

Swallow's nest is rich in protein, calcium, and phosphorus. It helps to promote rejuvenation and maintain a healthy immune system. Swallow's nest can be served in sweet (meatless) or savory (with meat) preparations.

> **1 boneless, skinless chicken breast,**
> **¾ pound pork loin**
> **10 ounces swallow's nest**
> **1 chunk peeled fresh ginger (the size of a walnut), crushed**
> **½ teaspoon sea salt**

Soak swallow's nest in warm water for 4 hours or until softened. Drain and rinse.

Feiseui: Put chicken and pork in a pot of boiling water, cook for 10 minutes, drain, and rinse with cold water.

Put parboiled chicken, pork, ginger, swallow's nest, and salt in a dahnjung (double-boiling container) along with enough hot water to barely cover the ingredients. Cover the dahnjung and place it in a big steamer filled with enough hot water to come half way up the side of the *dahnjung*. Cover and steam on high heat for 30 minutes. Reduce heat to medium and continue to steam, covered, for additional 2 hours more. Serve hot.

Serves 4.

SUGGESTIONS AND VARIATIONS:

Swallow's nest can be cooked with coconut milk or regular milk and some rock crystal sugar (or a dash of stevia) for a delicious sweet soup.

Fritillary Bulb and Partridge Soup 川貝鷓鴣湯

To Stop Coughing

This soup is reputed to soothe a dry throat and smooth a hoarse voice. Partridge is said to be less warming than chicken. Do not make chicken soup when you have a heat condition.

> 1 partridge
> ½ pound lean pork
> ¼ cup large, Southern apricot kernels
> 1 tablespoon small, Northern apricot kernels
> ⅓ cup fritillary bulbs, rinsed
> 6 honey or brown dates

Feiseui: Cook partridge in 2 quarts of boiling water for 10 minutes, drain, and rinse with cold water. Cook pork in 2 quarts of boiling water for 10 minutes, drain, and rinse with cold water.

In a large pot, combine the partridge, pork, both types of apricot kernels, fritillary bulbs, and dates with 2½ quarts of water and bring to a boil. Cook over medium-high heat for 30 minutes. Reduce heat to medium, cover with lid elevated by a pair of bamboo chopsticks set across the rim of the pot, and simmer for 2 hours more. Strain and serve the broth hot.

Serves 4.

SUGGESTIONS AND VARIATIONS:

If you use a thermal cooker, after initial feiseui and boiling everything for 30 minutes on high, place the inner pot in the thermos for 6 to 8 hours.

You may peel and core one pear, cut it in large chunks, and add to the soup with other ingredients.

Sea Cucumber, Dried Scallop, and Selfheal Soup
海參干貝夏枯草湯

This soup is said to lower high blood pressure. Sea cucumbers and dried scallops are rich in protein, iodine, and calcium.

> 3 small sea cucumbers (about the size of your middle
>   finger)
> 4 dried scallops
> 1 ounce kelp
> 4 cups selfheal (1 ounce), rinsed well
> 1 chunk peeled fresh ginger (the size of a walnut), crushed
> 2 green onions, trimmed and cut into 3 pieces each
> 1 teaspoon cooking wine

Put sea cucumbers in a pot of boiling water, remove from heat, and let sit, covered, overnight. Drain and discard liquid. Soak the sea cucumbers in cold water for another 24 hours. Drain and discard liquid. Cook the sea cucumbers in 1 quart of boiling water with ginger, green onion, and wine for 15 minutes. Drain and clean the sea cucumbers, removing their intestines. Rinse with cold water and each into 3 pieces. Set aside.

Rinse and soak dried scallops in warm water for 1 hour. Reserve the liquid.

Rinse kelp and soak in a big bowl of cold water for 3 hours until softened. Drain and cut into 1-inch pieces.

In a 6-quart pot, bring 2 quarts of water to a boil and add sea cucumbers, scallops along with their soaking liquid, and kelp. Bring to a boil and cook for 15 minutes. Reduce heat to medium, cover with a lid elevated by a pair of bamboo chopsticks set across the rim of the pot, and cook for 30 minutes more.

In a small pot, combine selfheal with 3 cups of water and bring to a boil over high heat. Reduce heat to medium and simmer uncovered for 15 to 30 minutes. Strain, reserving liquid and discarding the selfheal. Add the reserved liquid to the sea cucumber and scallop soup and bring soup to a boil. Serve hot.

Serves 4.

Crabmeat, Yellow Chive and Dried Scallop Bisque
蟹肉韭黃瑤柱羹

Crabmeat, especially whole pieces of leg meat, is considered top-of-the-line among crustaceans, valued over shrimp and even lobster. Crabmeat is paired with delicate yellow chives in many expensive soups for banquets.

12 dried scallops
1 skinless, boneless chicken breast, cut into thin strips
¼ teaspoon salt
¼ teaspoon sugar
¼ teaspoon vegetable oil
1 teaspoon cornstarch
2 ounces bamboo pipe
2 thin slices (about ⅛-inch thick) peeled fresh ginger
1 green onion
6 dried black mushrooms
3 ounces bamboo shoots, julienned
6 ounces cooked crabmeat (leg meat only, if possible)
2 ounces yellow chives, cut into 1-inch pieces

THICKENING MIXTURE:

¼ teaspoon salt
¼ teaspoon sugar
1½ tablespoons cornstarch
¼ cup water

Rinse and soak dried scallops in warm water for 1 hour. Reserve the soaking liquid. Steam for 1 hour, reserve the steaming liquid, and shred the scallops by hand.

In a medium bowl, combine the chicken with the salt, sugar, vegetable oil, and cornstarch and marinate for 30 minutes.

Soak bamboo pipe in cold water for 1 hour until softened. Drain and cut off and discard the ends. Cook along with ginger and green onion in 1 quart of hot water for 3 minutes. Drain, rinse with cold water, and cut crosswise into ½-inch pieces.

Rinse and soak dried black mushrooms in hot water for 30 minutes, until soft. Drain, reserving the liquid. Cut off and discard the stems and cut mushrooms into thin strips.

In a large pot, combine scallops, chicken, bamboo pipe, mushrooms, and bamboo shoots with 1½ quarts of boiling water. Cook over high heat for 30 minutes. Reduce heat to medium, add crabmeat and chives, and cook for 5 minutes more.

In a small bowl, combine thickening mixture ingredients. Remove hot soup from heat and stir in thickening mixture. Serve hot.

Serves 4–6.

SUGGESTIONS AND VARIATIONS:

Similar ingredients are cooked with long-life noodles for birthday celebrations.

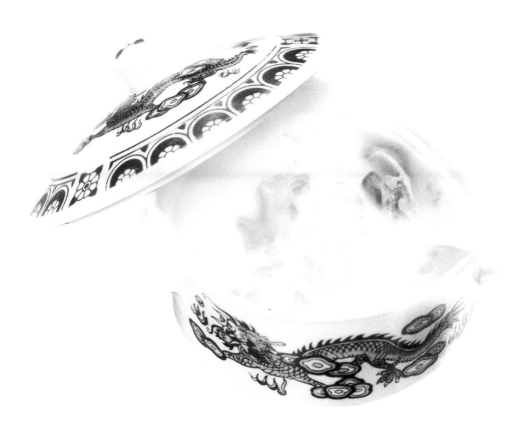

Hasmar Bisque with Sliced Abalone (next page)

Hasmar Soup or Bisque 雪蛤膏

This soup is essential for maintaining a wrinkle-free and youthful appearance. Ninety-nine-year-old Wai Tak Lau credits her smooth skin to her regular consumption of Hasmar Soup, not the use of cosmetics. Hasmar Soup is naturally thick and creamy.

4 ounces deer tendon
2 tablespoons dried hasmar
1 chicken breast bone with most of the meat carved off
1 pound pork neck bone
¼ pound chicken gizzards
½ pound chicken feet (claws cut off)

Soak deer tendon in a pot of hot water overnight. Drain, discarding the liquid. Put tendon in the inner pot of a thermal cooker and cover with fresh water. Bring to a boil, cook for 30 minutes, and place the inner pot inside the thermos to slow-cook overnight. Drain, discarding the liquid. If the tendon is not yet soft, boil again and keep it in the thermos for another 8 hours. Discard liquid and cut tendon into small pieces.

In a medium bowl soak dried hasmar in 2 quarts of water overnight. They will expand to fill the bowl and change from yellow to snowy white in color. Pick off any dark parts and retain the fatty white parts. Set aside.

Feiseui: In a large pot, combine the chicken and pork bones with 2½ quarts of boiling water and cook for 10 minutes until the scum rises to the top. Drain and rinse. In a large pot, boil chicken feet and chicken gizzards for 10 minutes. Drain, discarding liquid, and rinse.

In a large pot, combine chicken and pork bones, deer tendon, chicken feet, and gizzards with 3 quarts of cold water. Bring to a boil and cook, covered with a lid elevated by a pair of bamboo chopsticks set across the rim of the pot, over medium heat for 3 to 5 hours. The broth will become gelatinous and creamy. Add the hasmar and cook, stirring, over medium heat for 5 to 10 minutes more. Serve hot.

Serves 4.

SUGGESTIONS AND VARIATIONS:

As deer tendon takes a long time to reconstitute and to cook, this ingredient is a perfect candidate for the pressure-cooker.

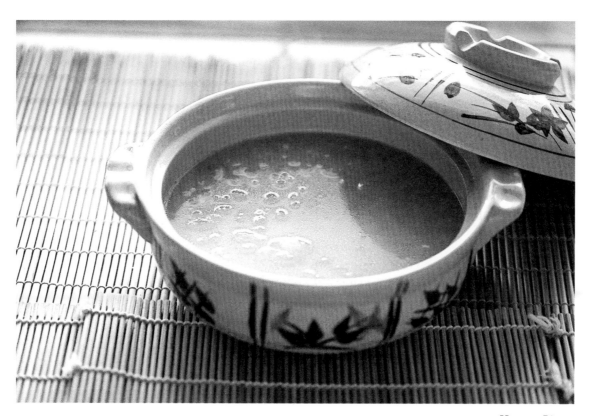

Hasmar Bisque

Winter Melon Bowl 冬瓜盅

To make this soup you have to overcome a few obstacles. First, you have to find a small winter melon, weighing 10 pounds or less and measuring fewer than 8 inches in diameter. You almost have to grow one yourself in your own backyard because you are not likely to find one that size in your neighborhood market since mature winter melons weigh upwards of 20 pounds and are sold cut up into wedges. Restaurants are able to get them at around 15 pounds and fewer than 12 inches in diameter because they have access to specialty growers.

Secondly, you have to have a steamer wide enough for the girth of the winter melon, and deep enough for its height with enough space for removal after the soup is cooked inside the melon tureen, steaming hot.

Thirdly, you have to have the tools and skills for carving a design on the hard rind of the winter melon. It is fun for a sculptor but daunting for a novice.

Ultimately, this is a job best left to the five-star restaurants. The following instructions have been derived from observing the chefs at work in the kitchen of Koi Gardens Restaurant in Dublin, California.

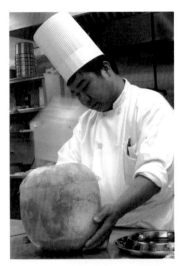

CARVING

The sous chef Fai Go 輝哥 uses a sharp-pointed pick to outline the Chinese character fu 福, meaning "blessings," and a pair of koi fish, freehand on the rind of the melon. The lines are thin and shallow dents like pencil marks, no more than 1/16 of an inch deep, barely scratching off the dark green surface of the rind. This is the first time I've seen this carving style. Compare with the bolder lines used by Martin Yan in his cookbook *The Chinese Chef,* copied by me using pumpkin carving tools.

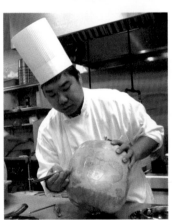

Fu 福 Design Carved by Fai Go

MAKING THE TUREEN

The top of the winter melon is then cut off about 5 inches from the calyx to form a lid with a zigzag pattern at the opening. If so desired, the lid may be put back on later.

After the seeds and pulp are removed, the inside is rinsed clean. The outside, with the carved design, is then covered in plastic wrap, placed in a heat-resistant bowl measuring 12 inches in diameter and 3 inches deep. The whole thing is put inside the steamer and steamed for 1 hour.

After 1 hour, the winter melon is taken out and the Chinese character *fu* 福 and the koi fish stand out like relief figures as a result of heat. The tureen, or steaming urn, for the soup is made.

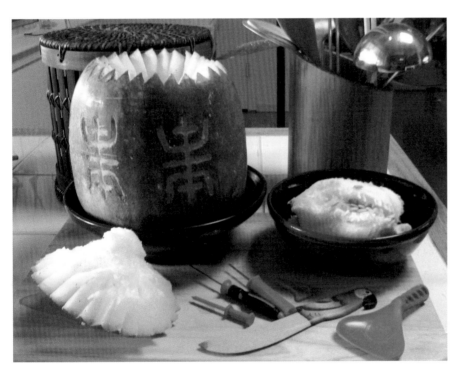

Longevity Design Carved by Teresa with Pumpkin-Carving Tools

The chef scoops out the clear liquid in the hollow and replaces it with top stock. Then he puts in the prepared ingredients—diced ham, roast pork, roast duck, shark's fin, etc., and returns the winter melon bowl to the steamer; there the soup and bowl continue to cook for 1½ hours.

MAKING THE SOUP

Koi Gardens uses richer ingredients than my Eight Jewel Diced Melon Soup. They include shark's fin, finely diced Smithfield ham, and finely diced roast duck, probably 3 ounces each, with crabmeat (leg pieces) as garnish. The soup inside the winter melon tureen does not require the inclusion of winter melon dice.

For a fancy vegetarian Winter Melon Bowl, vegetarian mock shrimp, mock crabmeat, mock ham, and mock shark's fin would achieve similar effects.

SERVING THE SOUP

When the winter melon bowl exits the steamer, the chef removes the plastic wrap on the design and places big leg pieces of cooked crabmeat and blanched green loofah diamonds on the rim of the bowl for garnish and flair.

The winter melon bowl is carted out to the dining room where the maître d' serves the first bowl of soup with an even amount of the ingredients, especially the fancy garnish for each diner.

The winter melon bowl is soft, translucent, and ready to eat, but the melon is not served. I suspect there is the risk of scraping a hole through the skin, then the soup may leak out, and the tureen may collapse.

Our party requested the melon off the wall of the tureen and the waiter obliged. He carefully scooped out the melon without causing damage to the winter melon bowl. To me, the melon itself is the most delicious part.

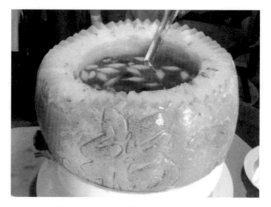

Steamed Winter Melon Bowl

Turtle Soup 水魚湯

Wai Kuen Szeto and her family used to celebrate Thanksgiving with a "Turtle Soup" until soft shell turtles ceased to be available in the U.S., since they are now on the brink of extinction and under protection by the Chinese government. Though I have a recipe, I am not going to publish it. Instead, I have included the following "Turtle Soup" by Lewis Carroll, the song sung by the Mock Turtle in *Alice's Adventures in Wonderland*.

> Beautiful Soup, so rich and green,
> Waiting in a hot tureen!
> Who for such dainties would not stoop?
> Soup of the evening, beautiful Soup!
> Soup of the evening, beautiful Soup!
>
> Beau—ootiful Soo—oop!
> Beau—ootiful Soo—oop!
> Soo—oop of the e—e—evening,
> Beautiful, beautiful Soup!
>
> Beautiful Soup! Who cares for fish,
> Game, or any other dish?
> Who would not give all else for two
> Pennyworth only of beautiful Soup?
> Pennyworth only of beautiful Soup?
>
> Beau—ootiful Soo—oop!
> Beau—ootiful Soo—oop!
> Soo—oop of the e—e—evening,
> Beautiful, beauti—FUL—SOUP!

16
Soupy Snacks and Light Meals

The staple of the Cantonese people is rice, mainly polished white rice. In peaceful and prosperous times, porridge (juk 粥), noodles (fan 粉 and min 麵), and dumplings are all treated like snacks. Under such a premise there evolved a colorful snack culture. In the morning, there is dim sum to go with tea. In the evening, there is siu ye 宵夜, nightime snacks which include porridge, noodles, and wontons, as well as sweet porridges (tong seui 糖水). There are also seasonal specialties like New Year cake, sweet round dumplings of the First Full Moon, rice dumplings wrapped in bamboo leaves on the fifth day of the fifth moon, moon cakes in Mid-Autumn, dumpling soup to herald in winter, and deep-fried sesame puffs for Chinese New Year's Eve. Some snacks such as potstickers and buns in a small bamboo steamer are not indigenous to Guangzhou, but they found their way to Hong Kong in the second half of the twentieth century, further enriching the culinary culture of the greater Pearl River Delta region.

At times of flood and famine, philanthropists were known to set up soup kitchens to feed the displaced population. It is amazing how far a bowl of rice soup could go to provide comfort and hope as well as nourishment to the body.

This chapter covers all soupy snacks including porridges, noodle soups, wonton soups, dumpling soups, and sweet soups.

Rice Soups 粥

Rice soup, by any other name—like congee, porridge, gruel, juk, or jook—is rice soup. After hours of cooking, the rice grains break down to a creamy constitution and yield a pleasingly sweet taste. During recovery from illness, rice soup provides a smooth transition from a liquid diet to solid food, gently gearing up the digestive mechanism. To plain rice soup, herb decoctions or powders may be added for distinct medicinal purposes. Later on, some solid ingredients may be added to enhance both the healing value and flavor.

In the *Book of Jook,* Bob Flaws has listed many rice soups made with single herbs, and with traditional herbal formulas. I will not duplicate those here, but have chosen instead to highlight recipes meant to illustrate various procedures for making medicinal rice soups. The Schisandra Rice Soup demonstrates a decoction, the Hoelen Rice Soup involves using medicinal herbs in powder form, while the Dispel Dampness Juk recipe guides you step-by-step through the preparation of a mixed bean soup. Once you have mastered the simple techniques of decoction, grinding, soaking, and straining of medicinal herbs, you can prepare any rice soup recommended by a traditional Chinese doctor or herbalist, tailored to your personal needs.

Graduating from a medicinal meal, the rice soup takes on a gourmet twist in the hands of Cantonese chefs. In a restaurant, a teahouse, or at home, a rice soup becomes a light meal or fancy snack, or may even be treated like a soup to complement fried noodle dishes.

RICE SOUP RECIPES

Plain Rice Soup	白粥
Leftover Rice Soup	冷飯粥
Rice Soup with Gingko Nuts and Bean Curd Skin	白果腐竹粥
Schisandra Rice Soup	五味子粥
Hoelen Rice Soup	茯苓粥
Dispel Dampness Juk	去濕粥
Thousand-Year Egg and Salted Pork Rice Soup	皮蛋鹹瘦肉粥
Roast Duck Carcass Rice Soup	掛爐鴨殼粥
Turkey Porridge	火雞粥
Frog Leg Congee	田雞粥
Beef Congee with Silky Egg	滑蛋牛肉粥
Dried Flatfish and Peanut Congee	柴魚花生粥
Lobster Trim Porridge	龍蝦頭尾粥
Cistanche and Lamb Rice Soup	肉蓯蓉羊肉粥
Sampan Congee	艇仔粥

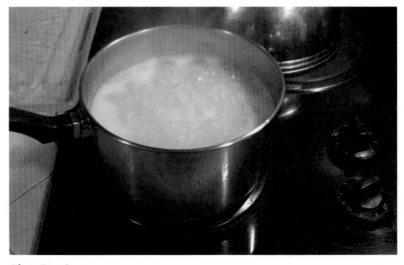

Plain Rice Soup

Plain Rice Soup 白粥

The foundation of all medicinal rice soups is plain rice soup. To make a good pot of plain rice soup requires some care. Here is the usual way to prepare it. Most Chinese people use long-grain white rice, though some prefer the short-grain.

Some people warn that one should never stir the rice soup while it is cooking, lest it will stick to the bottom and scorch the pot. Others, however, insist that it is the stirring that makes a rice soup smooth. Li-Min Wang, author of *Si-Ji Yang-Sheng-Zhou (Nurturing Rice Soups for the Four Seasons)* wrote that her mother told her, "There is no secret to making gruel; just stir it thirty-six times through and through." A movie 喬家大院 *Qiao Jia Da Yuan (The Big Courtyard of the Qiao Family)* also shows scenes of stirring the rice soup. I have tried it both ways and neither method scorched the pot. From my own experience, the only time the bottom got scorched is when I reheated a pot of rice soup that had cooled off. It is best to ladle it out and reheat in the microwave oven. Alternatively, you may boil 1 or 2 cups of water in a separate pot and then stir in the thickened rice soup on low heat.

1 cup short- or long-grain white rice

METHOD 1: USING AN OLD-FASHIONED CERAMIC POT

Rinse the rice.

Put 3 quarts of cold water in a ceramic pot and bring to a boil over high heat. Add the rice and return to a boil. Continue to cook over high heat for 30 minutes, stirring occasionally.

Reduce heat to medium-low and simmer uncovered for 2 hours, stirring occasionally. Do not add cold water during the course of cooking. If more liquid is needed, add hot water.

METHOD 2: USING A RICE COOKER

Many rice cookers include a porridge setting. This recipe requires a 5-quart rice cooker. If you do not have such a large rice cooker, simply halve the ingredients to make a smaller batch. Your pot should be no more than ⅔ full to start with to avoid boiling over.

Rinse the rice. Place the rice along with 2½ quarts of cold water into the rice cooker. Choose the porridge setting and set the cooking time for 2 to 3 hours and turn the rice cooker on. Before serving, if the rice soup is too thick, add hot water and stir well.

Leftover Rice Soup 冷飯粥

For myself, I rarely start making rice soup from scratch. I usually use leftover rice. It is easier and takes less time. This is also a plain rice soup.

Li-Min Wang, author of *Nurturing Rice Soups for the Four Seasons* (in Chinese), also prefers making the plain rice soup from leftover rice, her reason being that, according to Chinese doctors, a rice soup made from scratch with cold water is "cold" in nature and not agreeable for people with cold constitutions. For such people, it would upset the stomach and cause nausea.

Leftover Rice Soup is not smooth and pasty. You can still see the individual grains of rice in it. While it may not be up to restaurant standards, it is just as good tasting and easy to digest as the rice soup prepared from scratch.

2 cups leftover cooked rice

METHOD 1: USING A STAINLESS-STEEL STOCKPOT

Put 3 quarts of cold water in a stainless-steel stockpot and bring to a boil over high heat. Add the leftover rice and return to a boil.

Place a pair of bamboo chopsticks across the brim of the pot and put the lid of the pot on top of the chopsticks, leaving a gap for steam to escape.

Continue to cook over high heat for 30 minutes, stirring occasionally. Reduce heat to medium-low and simmer uncovered for 1 hour more, stirring occasionally.

METHOD 2: USING A RICE COOKER

Use a 5½-quart rice cooker or reduce the quantities by half with a smaller rice cooker.

Place the cooked rice and cold water in the rice cooker and choose the porridge setting. Set the cooking time for 1 hour and start the cooker. Usually the rice soup gets very thick. Mix in some hot water before serving.

Rice Soup with Gingko Nuts and Bean Curd Skin 白果腐竹粥

Quenching Thirst, Dousing Fire

Plain rice soup gets dressed up as a healing soup with the addition of gingko nuts and dried bean curd skin, a thin layer of film formed on the surface of boiled soy milk. Reconstituted bean curd skin is nutritious and the gingko nut is said to be anti-pyretic, soothing dry mouth and dry throat.

> 1 cup long- or short-grain white rice, rinsed
> 2 sheets dried bean curd skin
> ½ cup gingko nuts (about 2 ounces)

Shell the gingko nuts, blanch them in boiling water, remove the skin, and remove the green embryo in the seed using a tooth pick.

Rinse the dried bean curd skin and soak in hot water for 30 minutes. Drain, discarding the soaking liquid, and cut the reconstituted bean curd skin into small pieces.

In a ceramic pot, bring 4 quarts of cold water to a boil over high heat. Add the rice, bean curd skin, and gingko nuts and return to a boil. Continue cooking over high heat for 30 minutes, stirring occasionally. Reduce heat to medium-low and simmer uncovered for 2 hours. Do not add cold water during the course of cooking. If more liquid is needed, add hot water and stir well.

Serves 8.

Schisandra Rice Soup 五味子粥

Fresh as Springtime

The schisandra seed proffers all five tastes (sour, sweet, bitter, pungent, and salty), hence its Chinese name wu-wei-zi, "seed with five flavors." Nonetheless, as the sour taste dominates, a lot of sugar needs to be added. Its taste is refreshing like the pomegranate or raspberry and it is good for the liver, and for springtime.

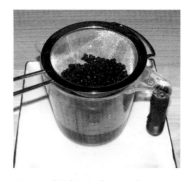
Strained Schisandra Seeds

> **2 ounces schisandra seeds**
> **1 cup rock crystal sugar (or ¼ teaspoon stevia)**
> **1 teaspoon pinenuts, whole or ground (optional)**
> **1 pink azalea blossom or dendrobium nobile orchid for garnish (optional)**
> **4 cups Plain Rice Soup (see recipe on page 297)**

Soak schisandra seeds in 2 cups of water for 8 to 12 hours. Strain the soaking liquid through cheesecloth or a fine strainer. Reserve the liquid and discard the seeds.

In a small stainless steel pot, dissolve the sugar (or stevia) in 1 cup of water. Mix in the schisandra liquid and bring to a boil. Strain the liquid into a clean bowl.

Pour the pinkish, sweetened schisandra liquid into the plain white rice soup. Add pine nuts or pine nut powder, if using, and stir well. Serve hot or at room temperature. Garnish with a few azalea petals or a whole blossom, if available, to accentuate the color and the season.

Serves 4.

SUGGESTIONS AND VARIATIONS:

Instead of mixing it into porridge, the schisandra liquid is very pretty in a noodle soup with broad, clear mung bean noodles.

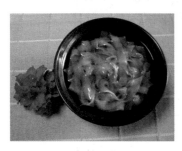
Broad Mung Bean Noodles in Schisandra Broth

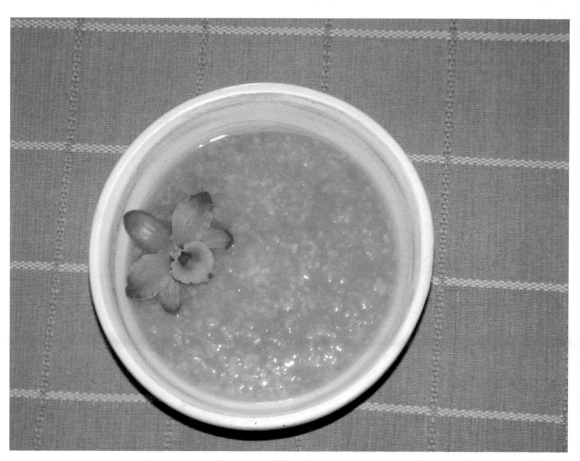

Schisandra Rice Soup Garnished with a Dendrobium Orchid

Hoelen Rice Soup 茯苓粥

A Rice Soup for Sleeplessness

Hoelen is also known as poria cocos or tuckahoe. It is a fungus growing at the root of pine trees. Its function is to soothe the mind and calm the spirit. In the old days, a hoelin cake would be given to a young child suffering from uneasy sleep. This rice soup fortifies heart and spleen and helps people with insomnia.

> **1¾ ounces poria cocos**
> **4 cups Plain Rice Soup (see recipe on page 297)**

Grind the poria into powder.

In a large pot, combine the ground poria powder, 2 cups of hot water, and the rice soup. Cook, stirring, over medium heat until hot. Season to taste with salt or sugar if desired.

Serves 4.

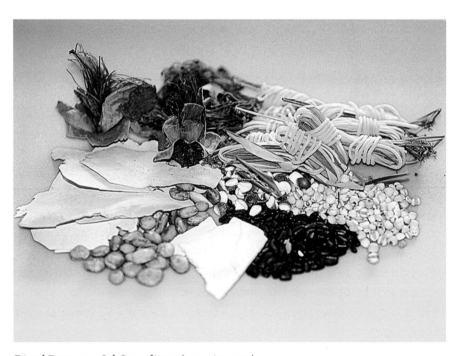

Dispel Dampness Juk Ingredients (opposite page)

Dispel Dampness Juk 去濕粥

A Summer Soup to Counter Bloating

This is an established formula for treating edema, the accumulation of fluid in the face, abdomen, and/or lower extremities. Dispel Dampness Juk combats summer heat which leads to inhibited urination, stomach stagnation, and discomfort due to bloating. In spite of its name, this is a juk that does not use rice. Beans and other grains are used instead for their diuretic properties. Some of the ingredients of Dispel Dampness Soup are not items you would normally stock in your pantry, but you can easily have them assembled in a Chinese herb store for about $2.

Bordering between medicine and food, this soup does not taste bad, but it does not taste great, either. It is bland. To make it more palatable, you might want to add salt or sugar, provided that it is not the cause of the water-retaining condition.

> **1 package of Dispel Dampness Juk ingredients, including aduki beans, pearl barley, foxnuts, poria cocos, dried hyacinth beans, dried kapok flowers, and rush pith**
> **2 pounds winter melon**

Soak all the beans overnight. Discard soaking liquid.

Rinse and soak foxnuts and pearl barley in cold water for 30 minutes. Set aside.

Scrub the skin, remove pulp and seeds from the winter melon, and cut it into 2-inch chunks, leaving the rind on.

Rinse remainder of the packaged herbs and place the herbs in a mesh cloth bag.

In a 5-quart inner pot of a thermal cooker, cook aduki beans, hyacinth beans, foxnuts, pearl barley, and the bag of herbs in 3 quarts of boiling water for 30 minutes. Add winter melon and return to a boil. Cook an additional 15 minutes. Place the inner pot into the thermal cooker and let the soup slow-cook for 6 to 8 hours. Before serving, remove the inner pot from the thermos and bring the soup to a boil again on the stove, anywhere from 15 to 30 minutes. Remove the mesh bag of herbs and serve soup hot or at room temperature.

Serves 6.

Thousand-Year Egg and Salted Pork Rice Soup 皮蛋鹹瘦肉粥

Gather the Heat and Beat It

This soup uses the thousand-year egg and pork to gather heat and beat excesses in the system. It is a treat I enjoyed as a child whenever I had a sore throat.

> **1 pound pork loin, cut into 2-inch cubes**
> **2 sheets dried bean curd skin**
> **2 cups cooked white rice**
> **2 "thousand-year" eggs, shelled and diced**
> **1 teaspoon salt**
> **1 cup cilantro, chopped (optional)**
> **1 green onion, chopped (optional)**

Sprinkle pork with salt and refrigerate for 6 hours or overnight. Rinse.

Rinse the dried bean curd skin and soak in hot water for 30 minutes. Drain and discard the soaking liquid. Cut bean curd skin into small pieces.

In a large pot, combine pork, bean curd skin, cooked rice, and diced "thousand-year" eggs with 3 quarts of boiling water and return to a boil, stirring occasionally. Reduce heat to medium-low and simmer uncovered for 1½ hours, stirring occasionally. Add hot water as needed. Serve hot, garnished with chopped cilantro and green onions, if using.

Serves 6–8.

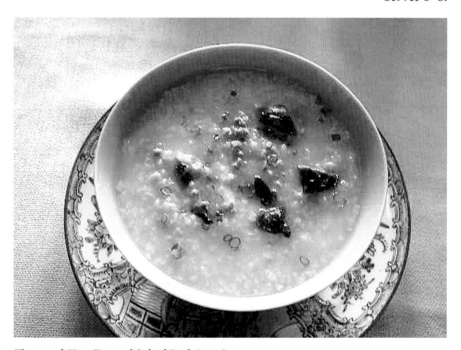

Thousand-Year Egg and Salted Pork Rice Soup

Roast Duck Carcass Rice Soup 掛爐鴨殼粥

This is my father's favorite. Of course, Ah-Bu made it best. I remember vividly my own happy anticipation of this delicious rice soup even when the family was still at dinner enjoying the roast duck the day before. As the roast duck is marinated with spices and stuffed with cilantro, its rich flavor is passed on to the soup in the next round of cooking.

- 1 roast duck carcass
- 2 sheets dried bean curd skin (optional)
- 1½ cups long-grain white rice, rinsed
- 2 bamboo shoots, sliced
- 2 "thousand-year" eggs, shelled and smashed into a paste (optional)
- 1 cup cilantro sprigs, cut into 1-inch pieces
- ½ head iceberg lettuce, shredded

In a ceramic pot, combine the roast duck carcass with 3 quarts of water and boil over high heat for 30 minutes. Skim off any scum and fat that rise to the top.

If using dried bean curd skin, rinse it and soak in hot water for 30 minutes. Drain and discard the soaking liquid. Cut bean curd skin into 1 inch wide strips, then into 2-inch lengths. Naturally there are broken and irregular pieces.

Add bean curd skin (if using), rice, bamboo shoots, and "thousand-year" eggs (if using) to the soup pot with the duck carcass along with 2 more quarts of hot water. Bring to a boil again over high heat. Reduce heat to medium-low and simmer for 2 hours.

Carefully remove all of the duck bones and skim off any additional scum and fat. Stir in the cilantro and serve hot, with shredded lettuce on the side.

Serves 6–8.

Turkey Porridge 火雞粥

Served the day after Thanksgiving, this is a distinctly Chinese-American adaptation of the Cantonese Roast Duck Carcass Rice Soup. After the family feasted on roast turkey, the housewife would carve out the left-over meat to go into sandwiches and pot pies. As for the carcass, it is too big to go into the soup pot all at once. I would recommend using only one half and freeze the other half for later. Serve with *yauh-ja-gwai* (Chinese long doughnut), if available.

> 1½ cups long- or short-grain white rice, rinsed
> ½ roast turkey carcass
> 1 cup bamboo shoots, sliced (approximately 8 ounces)
> 1 canned abalone, sliced (approximately 6 ounces)
> 1 cup cilantro sprigs, chopped

Place the turkey carcass in 3 quarts of water in a stainless steel pot and bring to a boil over high heat. Cook for 30 minutes and skim off any scum and fat that rise to the surface.

Transfer the turkey carcass to a ceramic pot and add the rice and bamboo shoots, along with 4 quarts of cold water. Bring to a boil over high heat and cook for 30 minutes. Reduce heat to medium-low and simmer for 2 hours, stirring occasionally. Remove any bones and skim fat. Leave the morsels that have fallen from the carcass. Add abalone, if using, and half of the cilantro and simmer for an additional 15 minutes. Stir in the rest of the cilantro and serve hot.

Serves 8.

Frog Leg Congee 田雞粥

Frogs are called tìhn gāi 田雞 in Cantonese, literally "chicken of the rice paddies." Though frozen frog legs are more readily available, Cantonese cooks prefer fresh ones, claiming that their flavor is superior. In the latter case, the frog is cut up like a chicken into bite-size pieces.

4 dried scallops
12 frog legs
½ teaspoon salt
½ teaspoon sugar (optional)
¼ teaspoon ground white pepper
1½ tablespoon soy sauce
2 tablespoons cornstarch
1 tablespoon cooking wine
1 teaspoon vegetable oil
1½ cup long- or short-grain white rice, rinsed
5 cups soup stock, chicken or homemade top stock (optional)
¼ cup finely shredded green onion
¼ cup finely shredded ginger

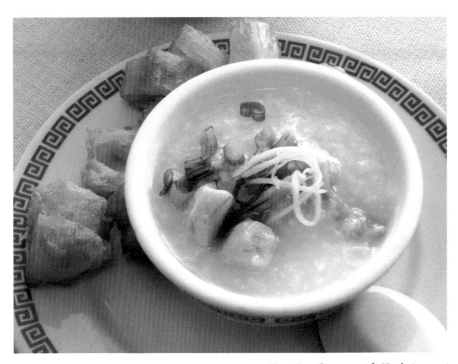

Frog Leg Congee with Yauh-ja-gwai

Rinse and soak dried scallops in warm water for 1 hour. Reserve the soaking liquid and shred the scallops by hand.

Cut frog legs into halves. In a medium bowl, combine frog legs with salt, sugar (if using), soup stock (if using; if not, replace with same amount of water), white pepper, soy sauce, cornstarch, and wine to marinate for 30 minutes.

In a large pot, combine rice, scallops along with their soaking liquid, and soup stock with 2½ quarts of water. Bring to a boil, cook over high heat for 30 minutes, reduce heat to medium-low, and simmer uncovered for 2 hours. Add hot water if more liquid is needed. Stir. Add frog legs, increase heat to high, and return to a boil. Cook for 5 to 10 minutes, stirring occasionally. Serve hot, garnished with green onion and ginger shreds.

Serve with yauh-ja-gwai (long doughnut), if available.

Serves 6.

Beef Congee with Silky Egg 滑蛋牛肉粥

A High Protein Rice Soup

This recipe cuts out the egg yolk for those who worry about their cholesterol level. If cholesterol is not your concern, you may use the whole egg. Again, nothing should be wasted unless it is bad for your health.

> **4 dried scallops**
> **12 ounces flank steak, sliced**
> **1½ tablespoons soy sauce**
> **½ teaspoon sugar (optional)**
> **1 tablespoon rice wine**
> **2 tablespoons cornstarch**
> **½ teaspoon salt**
> **1½ cups rice**
> **1 tablespoon vegetable oil**
> **5 cups soup stock, beef or homemade top stock**
> **4 egg whites**
> **3 tablespoons finely chopped green onion**
> **3 tablespoons finely chopped ginger**

Rinse and soak dried scallops in warm water for 1 hour. Reserve the soaking liquid and shred the scallops by hand.

In a medium bowl, combine beef with soy sauce, sugar (if using), salt, rice wine, cornstarch, and oil and marinate for at least 30 minutes. For better results, keep marinated beef in the refrigerator for 1 hour.

In a medium-size bowl, lightly beat egg whites by hand (with a fork or a pair of chopsticks) until it has an even consistency but without being frothy.

In a large pot, combine rice, scallops, and the scallop soaking liquid with the soup stock and 2½ quarts of water. Bring to a boil, cook over high heat for 30 minutes, reduce heat to medium-low, and cook for 2 hours. Add hot water if more liquid is needed. Stir. Add beef and continue to cook for 10 minutes until beef turns brown, stirring occasionally. Remove from heat and stir in the beaten egg white. Serve hot, garnished with green onion and ginger.

Serves 6.

Dried Flatfish and Peanut Congee 柴魚花生粥

This is a folk recipe. Dried and salted fish are Cantonese soul food and one has to acquire a taste for it if one does not grow up in the culture.

Highly nutritious, this simple rice soup is comforting and warming on stormy days when fishermen cannot go out to sea and fresh catch is not available.

> ½ cup raw peanuts, shelled and blanched
> 2 tablespoons vegetable oil
> 4 pieces dried flatfish (about ½ ounce)
> 1½ cup rice
> 5 tablespoons finely chopped green onion
> 5 tablespoons finely chopped fresh ginger
> 5 cups soup stock, chicken or homemade top stock (optional)

Rinse the flatfish and pat dry.

Soak peanuts in warm water for 30 minutes, drain, and discard soaking water.

In a frying pan, heat vegetable oil and add the dried fish pieces. Cook on medium until golden brown on both sides. Drain oil and chop finely.

In a large pot, combine fish, peanuts, and rice with soup stock (if using; if not, replace with same amount of water) plus 2½ quarts of water. Bring to a boil and cook uncovered over high heat for 30 minutes. Reduce heat to medium-low and cook uncovered for 2 hours, stirring occasionally. Add hot water if it appears to be too thick, and stir. Serve hot, garnished with chopped green onion and ginger.

Serves 6.

SUGGESTIONS AND VARIATIONS:

The dried fish fillets may be simply shredded and put directly without frying in the soup pot with the raw peanuts. Pan-frying the fish gives it a stronger aroma and taste.

Lobster Trim Porridge 龍蝦頭尾粥

The Chinese are frugal people. After feasting on lobster, stir-fried or baked, they'll save the leftover head, the tail-end, and the claws to make a rice soup. The flavor sealed in during baking or stir-frying will be released into the soup upon boiling. Lobster rice soup is a delicacy.

2 cups cooked white rice
lobster trim from 2 lobsters
3–5 thin slices of fresh ginger, finely shredded
2 green onions, finely shredded
½ cup chopped cilantro

In a large pot, combine lobster trim, rice, and ginger with 3 quarts of water, bring to a boil, and cook over high heat for 30 minutes. Reduce heat to medium-low and simmer for 1 hour. Serve hot, garnished with cilantro and green onion.

Serves 6.

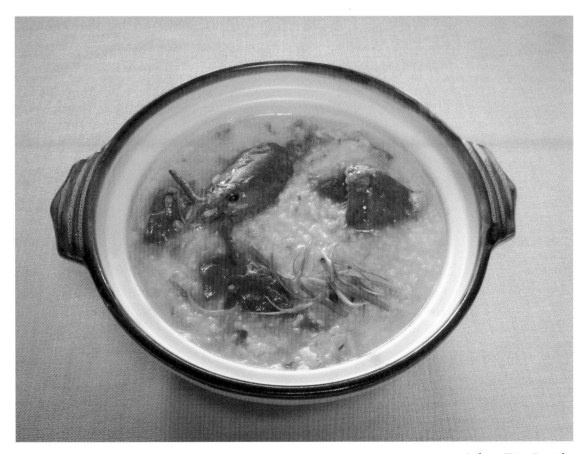

Lobster Trim Porridge

Cistanche and Lamb Rice Soup 肉蓯蓉羊肉粥

This soup improves libido in both men and women. Both major ingredients warm the system. Cistanche is also used to treat infertility.

¼ pound ground or minced lamb
½ teaspoon salt
½ teaspoon sugar
½ teaspoon soy sauce
1 teaspoon cornstarch
1 teaspoon vegetable oil
¼ ounce cistanche, rinsed
½ cup cooked rice
1 teaspoon chopped ginger
1 teaspoon chopped green onion

In a medium bowl, mix lamb with salt, sugar, soy sauce, and cornstarch. Add oil to seal in the flavor. Marinate for at least 30 minutes.

In a medium-size pot, combine cistanche and rice with 1½ quarts of boiling water. Cook over high heat uncovered for 30 minutes, stirring occasionally. Reduce heat to medium and continue to cook for another 30 minutes, uncovered. Return to high heat, stir in minced lamb, bring to a boil, lower heat, and simmer uncovered for 15 minutes. Serve hot, garnished with ginger and green onion.

Serves 2.

SUGGESTIONS AND VARIATIONS:

If ground lamb is not available in the butcher's, buy some shank meat or lamb chop and mince by hand. It is much easier than you may think.

Sampan Congee 艇仔粥

Along the riverbank of Pearl River's waterways and hugging the coastline of the South China Sea beyond Pearl River's estuary live the Daan People 蛋家, one of China's many ethnic minorities, on wooden boat houses. Some reside on bigger boats with sails called junks while others stay in smaller boats called sampans. The smaller sampans are also their means of transportation. This Sampan Congee and the Dried Flatfish and Peanut Rice Soup might very well be the culinary creation of the Daan People.

¼ pound dried squid
1½ pound pork neck bone
½ pound fresh squid
½ pound fresh scallops
¾ pound prawns, shelled and deveined
½ ounce fresh ginger, finely chopped
½ jellyfish, shredded (pre-packaged)
1 cup deep-fried peanuts with skin (like Spanish peanuts)
12 deep-fried egg roll skins, crumbled into small pieces
1½ cup rice, long- or short-grain white rice, rinsed
¼ cup finely chopped cilantro
¼ cup finely chopped green onion
2 yau ja gwai (Chinese long doughnut), cut into bite-size pieces

Rinse and soak jellyfish in hot water for 30 minutes. Drain.

Rinse and soak dried squid in hot water (removed from heat) overnight, covered and removed from heat. Repeat if the squid is still hard. Rinse and score lengthwise and crosswise, and cut into bite-sized pieces.

Clean fresh squid, score lengthwise and crosswise, and cut into bite-sized pieces.

Feiseui: Cook pork neck bone in 2 quarts of boiling water for 10 minutes, drain, and rinse with cold water.

In a large pot, combine pork neck bone and rice with 5 quarts of boiling water. Cook over high heat for 30 minutes. Reduce heat to medium and cook for 1 hour more. Discard pork neck bone. Add dried and fresh squid, scallops, prawns, and ginger. When prawns begin to turn pink and squid begin to curl (about 5 to 10 minutes), remove from heat. Serve hot, garnished with jellyfish, peanuts, crumbled egg roll skin, green onions, cilantro, and yau ja gwai on the side.

Serves 6–8.

SUGGESTIONS AND VARIATIONS:

It is difficult to rehydrate dried squid to the same pliability as fresh squid. Some people suggested soaking it with some baking soda; some even suggested the use of boric acid. As I am wary of these chemicals, I tried using papaya powder, a meat tenderizer, instead.

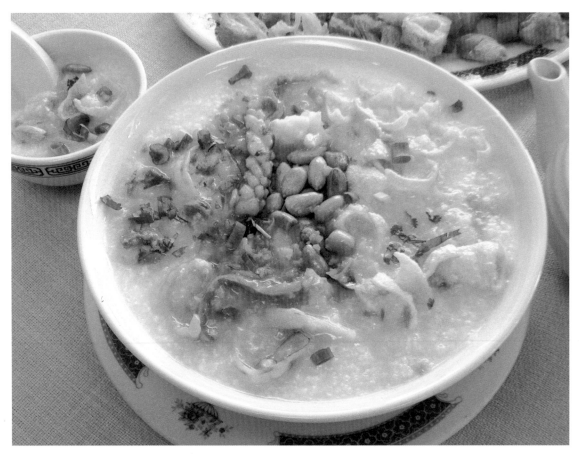

Sampan Rice Soup

Noodle, Wonton, and Dumpling Soups 粉 麵 雲 吞 湯 圓

Rice has always been the main staple for southerners living south of the Yangtze River. The Cantonese have always treated noodles as snacks or light meals. Cantonese housewives never bothered to make noodles from scratch. Noodles are always bought from stores.

Rice noodles do not keep well under refrigeration. I always try to get them from the store on the same day they are delivered.

NOODLE, WONTON, AND DUMPLING SOUP RECIPES

Seafood Noodle Soup	三鮮湯麵
Shrimp and Black Mushroom Noodle Soup	冬菇蝦仁湯麵
The Grand Mix Noodle Soup	什錦湯麵
Spicy Shredded Pork Noodle Soup	榨菜肉絲湯麵
Roast Pork and Broad Rice Noodle Soup	叉燒湯粉
Shrimp and Pork Wonton Soup	鮮蝦雲吞
Winter Solstice Savory Dumpling Soup	鹹湯圓
(see recipe under Festive Soups)	
Plain Dumplings (see recipe under Festive Soups)	無餡湯圓
Crabmeat, Yellow Chives, and Long Life	蟹肉韭黃伊麵
Noodle Soup (see recipe under Festive Soups)	

Seafood Noodle Soup 三鮮湯麵

Noodle Soups are usually the combination of stir-fried or sautéed food and cooked noodles made into a soup. With meat and vegetables, pasta and broth, it is a meal unto itself.

   1 rehydrated sea cucumber, cut into bite-sized pieces
   3 slices fresh ginger, 1/16-inch thick
   ⅔ pound shrimp, shelled and deveined
   ½ teaspoon salt, for marinating shrimp
   1 pound tender Chinese greens, trimmed and cut into 3-inch
      pieces
   1½ pounds precooked round noodles
   4 tablespoons vegetable oil
   6 green onions, cut into 1-inch sections
   1 pound fresh squid, scored lengthwise and crosswise, and cut into
      bite-sized pieces
   2 tablespoons rice wine
   1 tablespoon soy sauce
   4 cups top stock

In a medium pot, combine sea cucumbers and ginger with 3 cups of water and boil for 30 minutes to get rid of any chalky smell. Drain, discarding liquid, and rinse.

In a bowl, combine shrimp and salt and set aside for 15 minutes. Rinse and drain.

In a pot of hot water, add noodles. Heat for 3 minutes, separating noodles with chopsticks. Drain and rinse noodles with cold water.

Cook greens in boiling water for 5 minutes uncovered, drain, and set aside.

In a frying pan, heat the vegetable oil and stir-fry green onions on high heat for about 10 seconds or until it slightly wilts. Do not brown or burn it. Add sea cucumbers, squid, and shrimp. Stir-fry quickly (for 2 to 3 minutes). Add wine and soy sauce, stir-fry until the liquid evaporates. Drain the oil. Bring 4 cups of top stock and 4 cups of water to a boil, add noodles and greens, and cook for another 3 minutes. Place noodles in a bowl, top with seafood, garnish with greens, and pour soup on top. Serve immediately.

Serves 6.

Chinese tender greens include choi sam (heart of baby bok choy), yau choi (rape), gaai laan (Chinese broccoli), snow pea tendrils, and even peapods. Romaine lettuce is also acceptable.

As noodles absorb liquid and become soggy, do not let them sit in the soup for too long before serving.

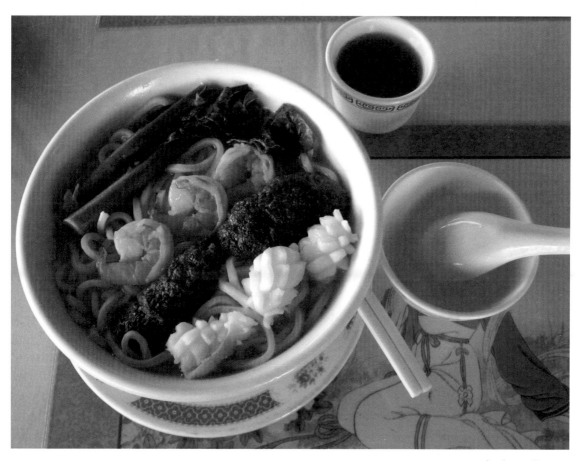

Seafood Noodle Soup

Shrimp and Black Mushroom Noodle Soup 冬菰蝦仁湯麵

This is also a combination of a savory dish and cooked noodles. The making of the dish involves several cooking techniques including stir-fry, sautée, and blanching.

1 pound shrimp, cleaned and deveined
1 package round noodles (1 pound)
12 dried black mushrooms
1 teaspoon soy sauce
1 teaspoon sugar
1 tablespoon plus 3 teaspoons cornstarch, divided
2 cloves garlic, crushed
1 tablespoon oyster sauce
2 teaspoons salt, divided
pinch of ground white pepper
5 tablespoons vegetable oil, divided
1 egg white, beaten
1 pound *yauh choi* (tender Chinese greens), trimmed
1½ pounds pork neck bone
1 tablespoon of cooking wine

Feiseui: Cook pork neck bone in 2 quarts of boiling water for 10 minutes, drain, and rinse with cold water. Put pork neck bone into another pot with 2½ quarts of water. Cook over high heat for 10 minutes. Reduce heat to medium-low and simmer for 30 minutes. Discard the bones and save the liquid.

Rinse and soak dried black mushrooms in hot water for 30 minutes, until soft. Reserve soaking liquid and cut off and discard mushroom stems. In a small bowl, combine the mushrooms with soy sauce, sugar, and 1 teaspoon of the cornstarch and marinate for 30 minutes.

In a small bowl, combine shrimp with ½ teaspoon of salt and let sit for 15 minutes. Rinse with cold water, pat dry, then combine with white pepper and ½ teaspoon salt and 1 teaspoon cornstarch. Mix shrimp with egg white. Set aside.

In a frying pan, heat 1 tablespoon of the vegetable oil on high heat. Add garlic and cook, stirring, until browned. Add mushrooms and continue to cook for 5 minutes more. Pour in the mushroom soaking liquid and an additional cup of water and simmer covered for 1 hour.

In a small bowl, combine 1 tablespoon of the cornstarch and the oyster sauce with 2 tablespoons of water and stir into frying pan with mushrooms and garlic. Remove pan from heat.

Cook noodles in 3 quarts of boiling water for 5 minutes. Drain. Rinse with cold water.

Cook yauh choi in 1 quart of boiling water with the 1 tablespoon of the vegetable oil and 1 teaspoon of salt for 2 minutes. Drain.

In a hot frying pan, swirl in the remaining 3 tablespoons of vegetable oil and add shrimp. Stir-fry until they begin to turn pink, then add cooking wine. Drain the oil.

Place cooked noodles in a bowl. Top with shrimp, mushrooms, and yauh choi. Pour in soup and serve immediately.

Serves 4.

SUGGESTIONS AND VARIATIONS:

If yellow chives are available, substitute 2-inch pieces of the delicate chive (6–8 ounces) for the yauh choi. I also like to use snow pea tendrils.

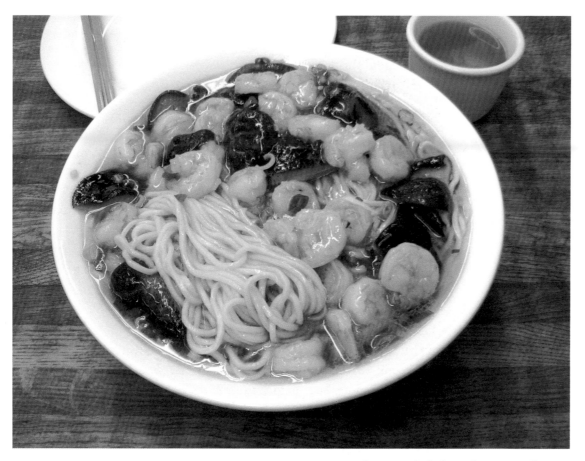

Shrimp and Black Mushroom Noodle Soup

The Grand Mix Noodle Soup 什錦湯麵

"The Grand Mix" refers to a required combination of liver and gizzards. Chicken giblets are preferred. Other ingredients include bamboo shoots, black mushrooms, green peas, shrimp, chicken and/or meat in the stir-fry mix that tops a noodle soup.

⅔ cup tiger lily buds
6 dried black mushrooms
4 ounces chicken breast, cut into bite-sized pieces
3 ounces pork liver, cut into bite-sized pieces
3 duck or chicken gizzards, scored lengthwise and crosswise and
     cut into halves

MARINATE:

1 teaspoon rice wine
¼ teaspoon salt
¼ teaspoon sugar
¼ teaspoon ground black pepper
¼ pound shrimp, peeled and deveined
½ teaspoon salt for marinating shrimp
½ cup diced or sliced carrots
½ cup green peas
1 bamboo shoot, sliced
1 pound *choi sam* (heart of baby bok choy), trimmed and halved
2 tablespoons vegetable oil
1 cup of water
1½ pounds precooked round noodles
1¼ teaspoons salt
2 tablespoons soy sauce
1 teaspoon sugar
1 cup of water

Soak tiger lily buds in warm water for 20 minutes, drain, remove hard ends, and tie into knots.

Rinse and soak dried black mushrooms in hot water for 30 minutes, until soft. Remove the stems and halve or quarter the mushroom caps.

In a medium bowl, combine chicken, liver, and gizzards with rice wine, ¼ teaspoon salt, soy sauce, sugar, black pepper, cornstarch, and oil. Marinate for 30 minutes.

In a separate bowl, mix shrimp with 1 teaspoon of salt. Let sit for 15 minutes, rinse, drain, and pat dry.

In a skillet, heat 2 tablespoons of oil on high heat, add chicken, liver, and gizzards, cook for 5 minutes on high heat, add 1 cup of water, cover, and cook for an additional 5 minutes on medium-high heat. Reduce heat, cover, and let simmer for 10 more minutes on medium-low heat.

In a large pot, bring 2½ quarts of water to a boil. Add mushrooms, carrots, peas, bamboo shoots, lily buds, and choi sam. Boil uncovered for 10 minutes. Add shrimp and continue to boil uncovered for 5 minutes. Add chicken, liver, and gizzards to the soup. Turn off the heat.

In a separate pot, add noodles to hot water and cook for 3 minutes, separating with chopsticks.

Place noodles in a bowl, top with meat and vegetables, pour soup over the top, and serve immediately.

Serves 6.

Spicy Shredded Pork Noodle Soup 榨菜肉絲湯麵

This is more of a Northern or Sichuan-style noodle soup, but very popular among Cantonese these days. The noodles are made to order fresh from kneaded dough in the kitchen of New Yen Ching Restaurant. Fresh noodles are also available prepackaged in the grocery stores.

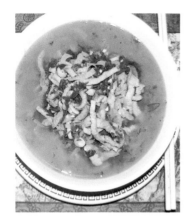

Spicy Shredded Pork Noodle Soup

1 pound pork loin, shredded
¼ teaspoon sugar
¼ teaspoon cornstarch
1½ tablespoons soy sauce, divided
2 ¾ teaspoons vegetable oil, divided
6 ounces Szechuan preserved turnip (*ja choi* 榨菜), rinsed, thinly
    sliced, and shredded
5 green onions, cut into 1-inch lengths (optional)
3 slices ginger root, about ⅟₁₆-inch thick, shredded
1½ teaspoons rice wine
1½ pound fresh noodles
6 cups top stock (optional)

In a medium bowl, combine pork with sugar, cornstarch, and ¼ teaspoon each of the soy sauce and vegetable oil.

In a heated wok or frying pan, swirl in 1½ teaspoons of the vegetable oil and add the turnip and pork. Stir-fry for 3 to 5 minutes. Remove from heat and set aside.

In another frying pan, heat 1 teaspoon of the vegetable oil and add green onion and ginger. Stir-fry for 1 minute, add rice wine, and combine with pork and preserved turnip.

Bring 6 cups of top stock or water to a boil. Stir in the remaining soy sauce.

Put fresh noodles in a pot of boiling water and return to a boil. Add 1 cup of cold water and bring to a boil once more. Rinse with cold water and drain.

Place noodles in a bowl. Top with pork and preserved turnip stir fry. Pour hot soup over it and serve immediately.

Serves 6.

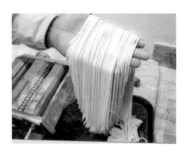

Freshly Made Noodles

Suggestions and Variations:

Preserved potherb mustard green stir-fried with shredded pork is another favorite topping for noodle soup.

Roast Pork and Broad Rice Noodle Soup 叉燒湯粉

Southern Chinese people make pasta and pastry out of white rice powder. Broad rice noodles from the Sa Ho 沙河 district near Canton are so popular that Sa Ho Fan 沙河粉 (or ho fan 河粉) has become the common term for Cantonese rice noodles. They are light, smooth and silky in a soup.

Chinese roast pork (*cha siu* 叉燒) can be bought in the deli department of Asian grocery stores, made fresh daily.

> **1 pound tender Chinese green, cut into 3-inch pieces**
> **12 ounces fresh broad rice noodles (sa ho fan)**
> **9 ounces roast pork, sliced**
> **1 tablespoon finely chopped green onion (optional)**
> **1½ cups soup stock, chicken or top stock**

Cook greens in boiling water for 2 minutes. Drain.

Combine soup stock with 1½ cups of water and bring to a boil. Add rice noodles and cook for 3 minutes, separating with chopsticks as needed.

Put noodles into a bowl and top with roast pork, greens, and green onions. Ladle broth over the top and serve immediately.

Serves 4.

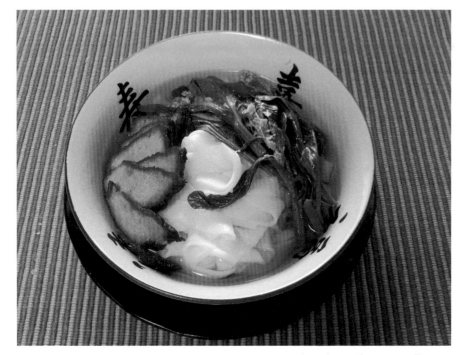

Roast Pork and Broad Rice Noodle Soup

Besides roast pork, braised beef brisket is a favorite with broad rice noodle soup. Usually the vegetable to go with braised beef brisket is baby bok choy or romaine lettuce.

The Chinese deli also offers roast duck. Chopped pieces (with bone attached) make delicious topping for noodle soups of any kind.

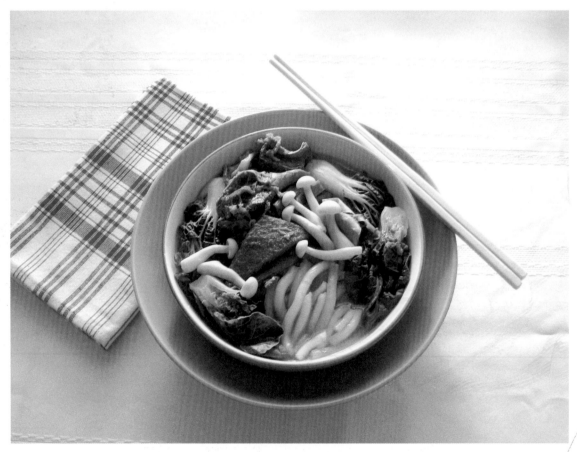

Braised Beef Brisket and Round Rice Noodle Soup with Baby Bok Choy and Mushroom

Shrimp and Pork Wonton Soup. 鮮蝦雲吞

There are two kinds of wonton wrapping or wonton skin. The common ones are square ones. The Cantonese created another kind, round in shape, with a little bit of baking soda added to the dough to give a different mouthfeel. Both kinds are available in Asian grocery stores.

Wontons

½ pound shelled shrimp, deveined and coarsely chopped
⅓ pound pork, minced
½ teaspoon rice wine
¾ teaspoon salt
⅛ teaspoon black pepper
1 tablespoon cornstarch
¼ cup bamboo shoots, finely chopped
1 teaspoon minced fresh ginger
1 package of wonton skin (about 60)

Soup

3 cups soup stock, chicken or top stock
3 cups water
1 dash ground white or black pepper
2 tablespoons soy sauce
½ cup purple laver or nori
1 cup chopped cilantro
1 cup chopped celery
2 tablespoons chopped green onion
1 teaspoon vegetable oil
1 teaspoon sesame oil
1 egg beaten evenly but not frothy

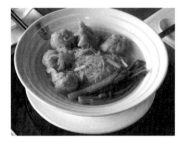

*Wonton Noodle Soup,
Hong Kong Style*

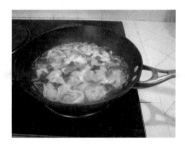

Wonton Cooking

TO MAKE WONTONS:

In a medium bowl, combine shrimp, pork, rice wine, salt, pepper, cornstarch, bamboo shoots, and ginger.

Lay a wonton wrapper on your work surface and add a teaspoon of filling to the center. Fold as shown below. Repeat with remaining wrappers until all of the filling has been used up. Set aside. The wontons may be frozen for later use.

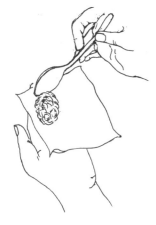

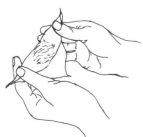

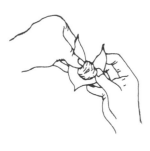

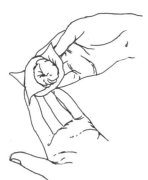

Steps in Making Wonton

TO MAKE GARNISH:

Heat a wide, flat nonstick skillet, spray on some vegetable oil, turn down the heat, pour in the beaten egg, spread the egg evenly over the surface of the skillet by tilting, and let it form a very light, paper-thin layer. Remove from heat as soon as it is formed. Keep the color light yellow instead of dark yellow or brown. When the egg cools, shred it into fine strips. Set aside.

TO MAKE SOUP:

In a large pot, bring 6 cups of water to a boil and add wontons. Cook until wontons float to the surface (about 10 minutes). Add a cup of cold water and bring the soup to a boil and the wontons to the surface again (about 5 more minutes).

In a medium pot, bring soup stock and water (3 cups each) to a boil. Combine soy sauce, purple laver, celery, and green onion, bring to a boil, cook for 5 minutes uncovered, and turn off heat.

Ladle wontons and hot soup into six individual medium-size bowls. Garnish with cilantro and shreds of paper-thin egg, and sprinkle with ground pepper and sesame oil. Serve immediately.

Serves 6.

SUGGESTIONS AND VARIATIONS:

By adding minced bamboo shoot, black mushroom, and dried scallop to the ingredients above, Cantonese chefs created yet another kind of dumplings called séui gáau 水餃, available at teahouses but not as popular as wontons.

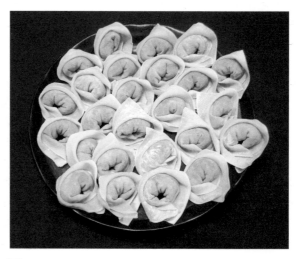

Wontons

Sweet Soups 糖水

In the Pearl River Delta region, a sweet soup is called tong-seui 糖水, meaning "sweetened water." A sweet soup is mostly starchy, with ingredients like grains (such as glutinous rice, wheat berry, and pearl barley), dried legumes (such as red beans, aduki beans, mung beans, and broad beans), taro, yam and sweet potato.

Due to its thick and smooth texture like that of a rice soup, a sweetened bean soup is also called a *juk*. I have tried cooking lotus seeds, beans, rice, and other grains in a thermal cooker. Granted, this cooking method saves energy, yet, without the roll-boiling process on the stovetop, the ingredients do not burst open to release the starch and the soup stays relatively thin and clear. To *juk* devotees, this is simply not acceptable.

Traditionally, rock crystal sugar is used instead of refined sugar. Considering the fact that rock crystal is obtained from a supersaturated sugar solution, strictly speaking, it is still a refined sugar. For diabetics with a sweet tooth, it is best to substitute with stevia. Since stevia is 300 times as sweet as sugar, it takes only 0.16 teaspoon of stevia to get the sweetness of 1 cup (48 teaspoons) of sugar. Since it is hard to measure out 0.16 teaspoon accurately, just use a dash. It won't hurt to use ¼ teaspoon of stevia for ease of measurement in these soup recipes that call for 1 cup of sugar. I have tried it and it tastes fine.

A sweet soup with red beans is an all-time favorite, though the cooler green mung beans are preferred in summer.

Sweet Soup Recipes

Red Bean Sweet Soup	紅豆粥
The Wedding Tea = Red Jujube, Lotus Seed, and Egg Tea (see recipe under Festive Soups)	新抱茶
Lotus Seed, Lily Bulb, and White Woodear Sweet Soup	蓮子百合雪耳糖水
Mung Bean, Kelp, and Rue Sweet Soup	海帶綠豆臭草粥
Black Sesame Seed Gruel	芝麻糊
Walnut Gruel	核桃糊
Sweet Almond Tea	杏仁茶
A Congee of Seven Jewels	七寶粥、臘八粥
Ground Sesame Seed Paste Dumplings	芝麻餡湯圓
Taro Sweet Soup With Osmanthus Flowers	桂花芋頭糖水
Sweet Swallow's Nest Treat	冰糖燕窩
Purple Rice and Dumpling Soup	紫米圓肉湯圓

Red Bean Sweet Soup 紅豆粥

A Warming Dessert

The Chinese red beans (hóngdòu 紅豆) are different from what the Japanese call aduki beans, which are chìxiǎodòu 赤小豆 in Mandarin Chinese. Red beans are round while the aduki beans are flatter and elongated.

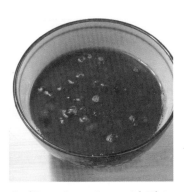

Red Bean Sweet Soup with Plain Dumplings

¾ cup red beans
½ piece dried Mandarin orange peel, soak and scrape off inside, and finely shred
1 cup rock crystal sugar or 0.16 teaspoon stevia powder

Soak red beans overnight. Drain and discard soaking liquid.

Put the red beans and Mandarin orange peel in 2 quarts of hot water and bring to a boil. Reduce heat to medium and continue to cook at a rolling boil for 1 to 2 hours, covered with a lid set atop a pair of chopsticks laid across the rim of the pot to allow steam to escape, until the beans expand and burst open. Add sugar or stevia powder, stir, and boil for another 5 to 10 minutes until the sugar is dissolved. Serve hot or at room temperature.

Serves 4.

SUGGESTIONS AND VARIATIONS:

Bean soups are ideal candidates for thermal cooking. The beans get softened without falling apart. Slow-cooking in the thermos avoids boiling over and scorching. Boil again on stove top if you like it mushy.

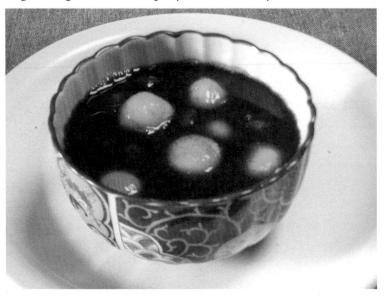

Red Bean and Plain Dumpling Soup

Lotus Seed, Lily Bulb, and White Woodear Sweet Soup
蓮子百合雪耳糖水

Comforting and Delightful

A sweet soup with lotus seeds, lily bulbs, and white woodears is an all-time favorite. White woodear lubricates the system and soothes the spirit, promoting good sleep and good complexion.

> 4 ounces lotus seeds
> 1 ounce dried lily bulbs
> 12 jujube dates, pitted
> 1 white woodears
> 1 cup rock crystal sugar or 0.16 teaspoon stevia powder
> 6 quail eggs, hard-boiled and shelled

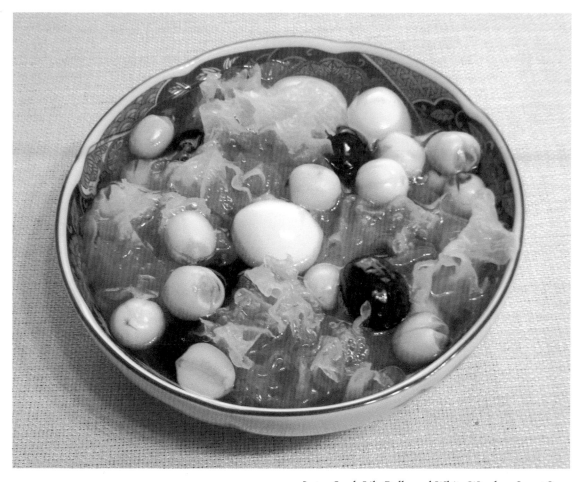

Lotus Seed, Lily Bulb, and White Woodear Sweet Soup

Soak white woodears in cold water for 1½ hours. Drain, cut off hard end, and break into small florets.

Soak lotus seeds for at least 3 hours in cold water. Drain and remove any green embryo in the center. Rub off the brown membrane on the outside of the seed.

Rinse lily bulb scales and jujube dates separately, in cold water.

In a large pot, put lotus seeds and dates in 2 quarts of hot water and bring to a boil. Reduce heat to medium and continue to boil for about 1½ hours, until the lotus seeds soften. Add additional hot water to the soup as needed. Add white woodears and lily bulb scales and continue to cook 30 minutes more. Add rock crystal sugar (or stevia powder, if using) and boil for about 10 minutes until sugar is well dissolved.

Serve hot or at room temperature, garnishing each bowl with a hard-boiled quail egg.

Serves 6.

SUGGESTIONS AND VARIATIONS:

It is not easy to remove the brown skin of the dried lotus seed, but they can be purchased already blanched. As it takes a long time for lotus seeds to soften, you may substitute canned lotus seeds in order to save time. Simply add them toward the end of cooking, just before you add the sugar.

For a fruity variation, add bite-size ripe papaya cubes into the soup toward the end of cooking. This makes a vibrant dessert for festive occasions.

Mung Bean, Kelp, and Rue Sweet Soup 海帶綠豆臭草粥

Grandma's Recipe for Zits

One of teenagers' worst growing pains is acne. Zits are not only annoying and unsightly, they are unhealthy. The skin condition reflects an overheated internal system, aggravated by fatty and spicy food. Kelp and mung beans are anti-pyretic. Mung bean is a known antidote for poison.

Rue, with its pale foliage and prolific yellow blooms, makes an attractive complement in the garden. It is a favorite because its strong odor naturally wards off pests. Bruised rue in beer has been used as a folk remedy both in America and Europe for snake bite because of its ability to expel poison from the system.

The soup does not taste bad at all, but for teenagers growing up in the Western culture, it may take some getting used to.

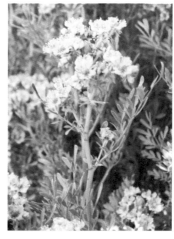

Rue Plant

> 1½ cups mung beans (approximately 12 ounces)
> 6 strips kelp (approximately 3 ounces)
> 3–4 sprigs rue
> 1 piece Mandarin orange peel (approximately ¼ ounce)
> 1 cup rock crystal sugar or 0.16 teaspoon stevia powder

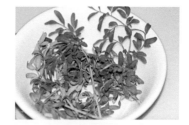

Rue Prigs

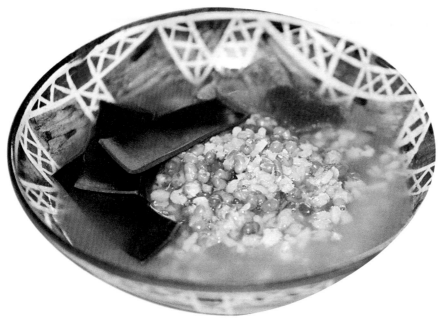

Mung Bean, Kelp, and Rue Sweet Soup

Soak mung beans overnight. Drain and discard soaking liquid.

Soak kelp in cold water for 1 hour. Drain and cut into 1 inch wide strips.

Soak Mandarin orange peel in cold water for 30 minutes. Drain and scrape off and discard the white pith on the inside of the peel. Cut into fine shreds or small pieces.

In a large pot, combine mung beans, kelp pieces, and orange peel with 2 quarts of hot water. Bring to a boil, reduce heat to medium, and continue to cook at a rolling boil for 1 hour. Add hot water if needed. Stir in rue and sugar (or stevia) and continue to boil over medium heat for 30 minutes. Remove rue sprigs. Serve hot or at room temperature.

Serves 6.

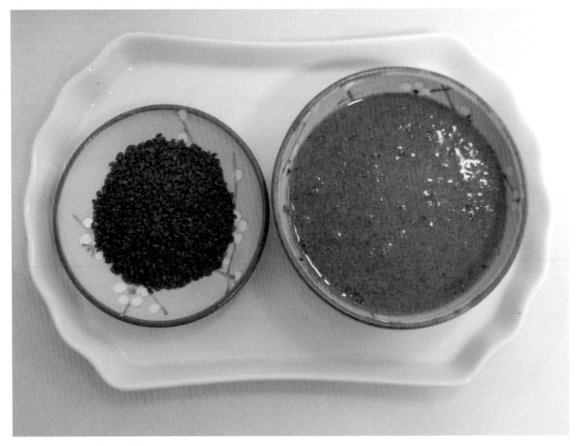

Sesame Seeds and Gruel (opposite page)

Black Sesame Seed Gruel 芝麻糊

To Smooth and Lubricate the Skin

There are black, white, and yellow sesame seeds. Black sesame seeds are the type that are used the most for medicinal purposes. They are approximately five percent fat and are rich in calcium, as well as phosphate and iron. Black sesame seeds lubricate both the skin outside and the intestines inside, help with constipation, and improve one's complexion and hair.

> **4 ounces black sesame seeds (approximately ¾ cup), rinsed, drained, and dried**
> **¾ cup rock crystal sugar or 0.16 teaspoon stevia powder**
> **3 tablespoons cornstarch**

Heat a small frying pan over low heat and stir-fry sesame seeds without oil until they become aromatic.

Place sesame seeds in a blender with 1 cup of water and blend at high speed for 2 to 3 minutes.

In a saucepan, dissolve the rock crystal sugar (or a dash of stevia powder) in 5 cups of hot water. Stir in sesame seed mixture over low heat.

In a small bowl, mix cornstarch with 3 tablespoons of water and stir into the sesame seed mixture.

Serve hot or at room temperature.

Serves 6.

SUGGESTIONS AND VARIATIONS:

Black sesame seed gruel mix is available in powder form in cans, making for an instant snack. As the mix is already sweetened, there is no need to add sugar.

Instead of cornstarch you may use rice powder. Some people may grind 3 tablespoons of raw white rice with the sesame seeds.

Walnut Gruel 核桃糊

More Brain Power to You

The Chinese believe that, because walnut kernels are shaped like the hemispheres of the brain, walnuts are beneficial to the brain. So did the Greeks and Romans. Besides the power of suggestion, walnuts provide fair amounts of omega-3 fatty acids, essential to brain health, which is associated with a vast array of physical and mental functions including anti-inflammation, immune enhancement, ability to concentrate, and fine and gross motor skills.

In TCM, walnut is used to treat symptoms related to kidney deficiency such as asthma, seminal emission, or constipation. This recipe is good for preventing constipation in the elderly.

> **4 ounces shelled walnuts, in halves (approximately 1⅓ cups)**
> **¾ cup rock crystal sugar or ⅕ teaspoon stevia powder**
> **3 tablespoons cornstarch**

Soak walnuts overnight. Drain, remove skin, and rinse.

Put walnuts in a blender with 1 cup of water and blend at high speed for 2 to 3 minutes.

In a saucepan, dissolve rock crystal sugar (or stevia powder) in 5 cups of hot water. Stir in the walnut mixture over low heat.

In a small bowl, combine cornstarch with 3 tablespoons of water and stir into the walnut mixture to thicken it as well as making it smooth.

Serve hot or at room temperature.

Serves 6.

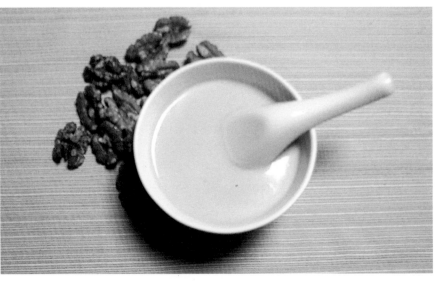

Walnut Gruel

Sweet Almond Tea 杏仁茶

A Cosmetic Drink that also Soothes Your Throat

Chinese almonds are not almonds. They are apricot kernels. There are two kinds of apricot kernels: the Southern and the Northern. The Northern kind is bitter and used primarily for medicine, whereas the Southern kind tastes sweet and is used both for food and medicine. The ratio of Southern apricot kernels to Northern apricot kernels is 4:1.

Apricot kernels can soothe a sore throat and reduce coughing and hoarseness. The drink helps improve skin complexion, clear voice, and get rid of bad breath. This sweet soup is called a tea because it has a thin consistency even lighter than milk.

> **4 ounces sweet almond or large, Southern apricot kernels**
> **(approximately 1 cup)**
> **¼ cup bitter, Northern apricot kernels (1 ounce)**
> **1 cup white rice**
> **1 cup rock crystal sugar or ¼ teaspoon stevia powder**
> **6 red jujube dates, pitted (optional)**

Soak apricot kernels in cold water for 2 hours, drain, and remove the skin. If you are able to buy blanched almonds, you may skip these steps as these will be pre-soaked and with skins already removed.

Soak rice for 1 hour. Drain.

In a mortar, crush and grind apricot kernels and rice with a pestle for 10 minutes. It should be of the consistency of cornmeal, with some grainy pieces. With repeated grinding and straining, it should get finer until it is like a paste. Add 1 cup of water and strain, reserving the liquid.

Grind the kernels and rice mixture again, add 1 cup of water, and strain again. Repeat several times until the mixture is ground to a paste.

In a large pot, combine water with the liquid from straining, to total 2½ quarts (10 cups) of liquid. Add rock crystal sugar or stevia powder. Cook on medium heat for 5 minutes while stirring constantly. If using jujube dates, soak for 10 minutes in hot water, then sliver the jujube dates, add them to the milky liquid, and continue to boil for 2 minutes on medium heat until jujube date slivers float to the top. Serve hot or at room temperature.

Serves 6.

Instead of using mortar and pestle, you may use a blender to reduce grinding time. You still need to run water through several times to extract the essence from the paste.

If Chinese apricot kernels are not available, almonds may be substituted. Incidentally, the name for apricot kernels and almonds is the same in Chinese, *hahng yàhn* in Cantonese or *xìng-rén* in Mandarin.

Almond tea mixture is available in powder form, canned, already sweetened.

Sweet apricot kernels or blanched almonds may be boiled whole with honey dates, or with fresh loquats when in season to make a sweet tea. It helps to stop coughing, soothe the lungs, and dissolve phlegm.

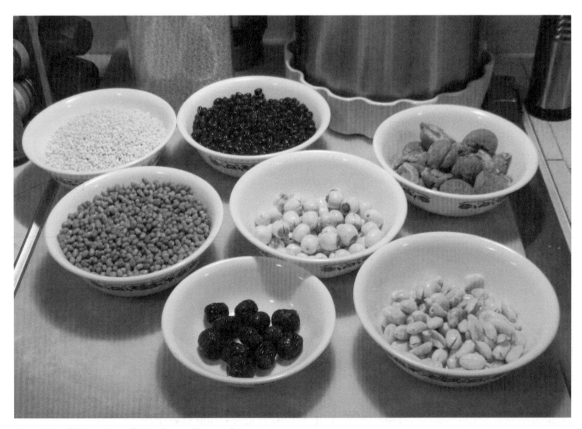

Seven Jewel Soup Ingredients (opposite page)

A Congee of Seven Jewels 七寶粥、臘八粥

Wintry Soul Food

This congee consists of grains, legumes, and nuts. Traditionally, only seven ingredients, including rice, are used, but more and more ingredients, even meat, have been added to the basic requirement of seven. Obviously, the original meaning has been lost.

The Congee of Seven Jewels is steeped in Buddhist culture. Ever since Buddhism became popular in China around the 5th century AD, people have made pilgrimages to mountain temples to commemorate the date of Buddha's nirvana on the eighth day of the twelfth moon by the lunar calendar. The monks would prepare cauldrons of congee to feed the faithful. Hence, the congee is also called Buddha's congee or *Laahp-baat-juk* 臘八粥, meaning the "Twelfth-Moon and Eighth-Day Congee," with *laahp* referring to the last month of the year and *baat* meaning "eight." The congee nourishes the soul as well as the body.

The congee always starts with rice, either plain or sweet white rice. Other grains like pearl barley, corn, oats, and sorghum may be added. The most popular legumes to use are red beans and mung beans. Other choices include yellow soybeans, hyacinth beans, and aduki beans. Among seeds and nuts, the Chinese favor lotus seeds, peanuts, and chestnuts, to be augmented by gingko nuts, sweet apricot kernels or almonds, and pine nuts. Dried longan and red jujube dates are added to sweeten the pot. There are many options.

From year to year, the eighth day of the twelfth moon of the lunar year falls on different days on the solar (or Western) calendar, mostly during the month of January. One must consult a lunar calendar to determine which day it is.

> 1 cup sweet glutinous rice, rinsed
> ½ cup red beans
> ½ cup mung beans
> ½ cup raw peanuts, shelled
> ½ cup lotus seeds
> ½ cup chestnuts, shelled
> 12 red jujube dates
> 1 cup rock crystal sugar or ¼ teaspoon stevia powder

Soak red and mung beans, jujube dates, lotus seeds, peanuts, and chestnuts separately overnight or for at least 6 hours. Drain and discard the liquid.

Remove the brown skin from the chestnuts, but you may keep the skin of the peanuts. Remove the skin and green embryo from the lotus seeds, if any.

In the inner pot of the thermal cooker, combine beans, lotus seeds, peanuts, chestnuts, and rice with 4 quarts of water and bring to a boil over high heat. Add the sugar (or stevia powder) and jujube dates, reduce heat to medium, and continue to boil for 30 minutes.

Place the inner pot, covered, into the thermal cooker. Cover the outside lid and let cook overnight. The congee should be ready by the next morning. Serve hot.

Heat the congee in the inner pot on the stove if you desire a more mushy texture. Stir constantly and add hot water if needed. Serve hot.

Serves 6–8.

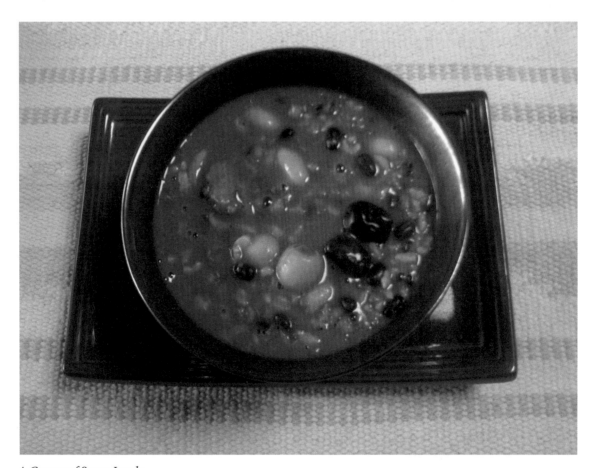

A Congee of Seven Jewels

Ground Sesame Seed Paste Dumplings 芝麻餡湯圓

For Family Gatherings at Full Moon

The round dumplings symbolize the full moon as well as reunion. The dumpling soup may be served as a dessert soup any time of the year, but is a must on the first full moon and the eighth (mid-autumn) full moon.

FILLING:

¼ cup black sesame seeds
1 ounce lard or pork fat, finely minced (optional)
½ cup confectioners sugar or ⅛ teaspoon stevia powder

WRAPPING:

1 cup glutinous rice powder
¼ cup boiling water
2 tablespoons cold water

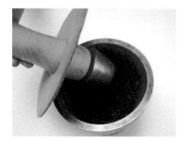

Pounding Sesame Seeds in a Mortar

FOR THE FILLING:

In a dry frying pan, stir-fry sesame seeds over low heat (for about 30 seconds) until they yield their aroma. Grind into a fine powder, either in a spice grinder or with a mortar and pestle.

In a small bowl, combine pork fat, if using, with sugar and sesame seed powder. Refrigerate for about 30 minutes, until the mixture becomes firm.

Divide sugar mixture into 20 parts and roll each into a ball. (If no fat is added, the filling may be runny. Use a spoon to handle it.)

FOR THE WRAPPING:

In a medium bowl, combine glutinous rice powder with boiling water and cold water. Knead into a smooth dough. Shape the dough into a roll about 2 inches in diameter. Cut into 20 pieces. Roll each piece of dough into a ball, then flatten it into a round patty, about 3 inches in diameter.

MAKING THE DUMPLINGS:

Lay one piece of the wrapping on your work surface and place one portion of filling in the center. Gather the edges of the wrapper around the filling and pinch to seal. Roll gently into a ball. Repeat until all filling and wrappers are used up. Yields 20 dumplings.

In a medium pot, bring 1½ quarts of water to a boil; add dumplings and let cook for 5 to 10 minutes over medium heat until they rise to the surface. Add 1 cup of cold water and let cook until the dumplings rise again.

Ladle dumplings and soup into serving bowls and serve hot or at room temperature.

Serves 4–6.

SUGGESTIONS AND VARIATIONS:

One may use red bean paste as filling for the dumplings (see recipe under Festive Soups on pages 201–202).

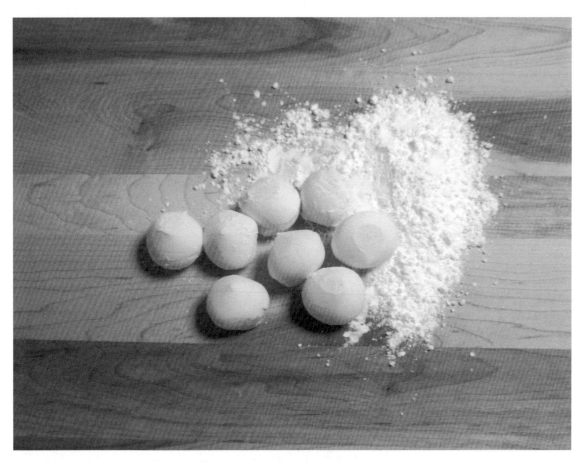

Dumplings with Sesame Seed Paste Filling

Taro Sweet Soup with Osmanthus Flowers 桂花芋頭糖水

A Sweet-Scented Soup for Autumn

Taro or *yù tóu* 芋頭 (*wuh táu* in Cantonese), is the root out of which Hawaiian poi is made. Poi is made by mashing or pounding taro into a mush. The small taro, however, can be eaten whole, boiled, as in this recipe. A larger variety called banlong-wu in Cantonese may also be used for this soup, cut in ½-inch or 1-inch dice.

As raw taro may cause skin irritation for some people, do not peel it prior to cooking. Never eat raw or half-cooked taro either, because it may cause itching in the throat.

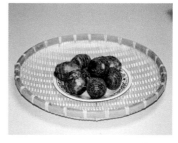

Small Taro

    1½ pounds small taro roots
    1 cup rock crystal sugar or 0.16 teaspoon stevia powder
    2 tablespoons candied or dried sweet-scented osmanthus flowers

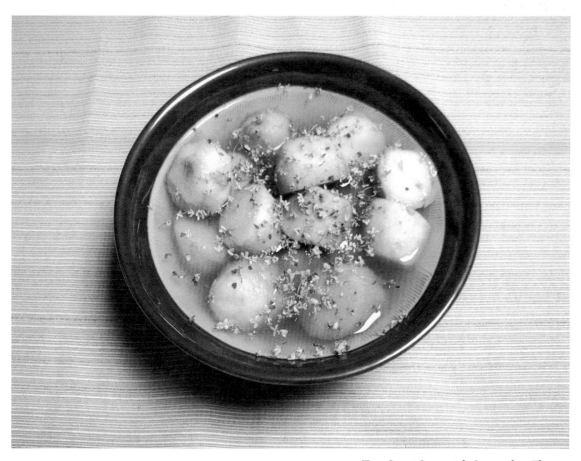

Taro Sweet Soup with Osmanthus Flowers

Place the whole scrubbed taro in a large pot. Add enough water to cover half of the taro and bring to a boil over high heat. Reduce heat to simmer for 2 hours. Drain taro and cool by running cold tap water over it. Remove outer skin which comes off easily after boiling. For small taro, leave whole or cut in half.

Place the cooked taro in 2 quarts of water and bring to a boil over high heat. Reduce heat to medium, continue to boil for 10 minutes. Add sugar or a dash of stevia powder, and stir until dissolved. Sprinkle osmanthus flowers into the soup for additional aroma and flavor. Serve hot.

Serves 6.

Suggestions and Variations:

You may use the larger banlong-wu (diced or cubed) or sweet potatoes for this soup.

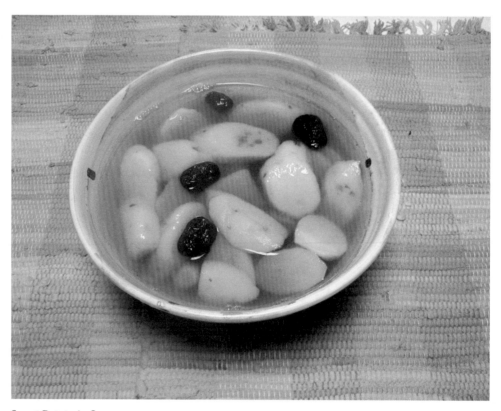

Sweet Potato in Soup

Sweet Swallow's Nest Treat 冰糖燕窩

Ageless Beauty

The swallow's nest is prized for its collagen that reputedly preserves youthful complexion and smooth skin. It is pricey because of its rarity. Cleaned and ready-to-use nests from Indonesia go for $800 to $1,200 per ½-pound box in 2008. Swallow's nest is commonly referred to in English as "bird's nest."

2 ounces swallow's nest (6–8 pieces)
1 cup rock crystal sugar or ¼ teaspoon of stevia powder
6 cherries (fresh or from a jar)

Rinse swallow's nest in 6 cups of boiling water. Soak for 1 hour and drain. Repeat soaking and draining process until nest is 2 or 3 times bigger than its original size. If there are feathers remaining in the nest, add a few drops of oil and then rinse it off.

In a medium pot, bring 6 cups of water to a boil, add sugar (or stevia powder), and cook until dissolved. Add reconstituted nests and cook for 5 minutes. Serve hot or cold, garnishing each bowl with a cherry.

Serves 6.

SUGGESTIONS AND VARIATIONS:

Substitute the expensive swallow's nest with the more affordable white wood-ears. This makes an even more attractive dessert because, unlike the gel from the swallow's nest, the snowy white fungi retain their showy floret form after cooking.

Any kind of fresh cherries will do for garnish. I do not pit them but you may choose to do so. If cherries are not in season, use the bright red ones preserved in heavy syrup.

Purple Rice Soup with Plain Dumplings 紫米圓肉湯圓

To Tonify Blood

Black glutinous rice mixed with white rice turns purple upon cooking. With red jujube dates and dragon-eye fruit, it makes a delicious dessert soup. If this soup is shared with younger children, remove the date pits ahead of time.

> **6 jujube dates, rinsed**
> **12 dragon-eye fruit, rinsed**
> **2 tablespoons each black glutinous rice and white glutinous rice**
> **2 tablespoons honey**
> **30 plain dumplings (see recipe on page 205)**

Soak rice in water for 30 minutes.

In a large pot, bring 1½ quarts of water to a boil. Add rice, dates, and longan meat. Bring to a boil again and roll-boil, uncovered, for 30 minutes. Reduce heat to medium and simmer for another 30 minutes. Stir in honey,

Put dumplings in a pot of hot water and bring to boil. When the dumplings float to the surface, add 1 cup of cold water and bring to a boil again. Scoop dumplings into cold water to cool.

Add dumplings to soup. Serve hot or at room temperature.

Serves 6.

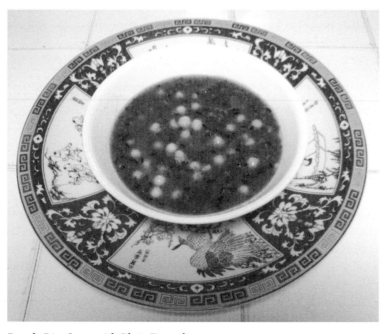

Purple Rice Soup with Plain Dumplings

Selected Bibliography and Further Reading

Albala, Ken. *Beans: A History.* Oxford and New York, New York: Berg, 2007.

Alley, Lynn. *The Gourmet Slow Cooker.* Berkeley, California: Ten Speed Press, 2003.

Ansel, David. *The Soup Peddler's Slow & Difficult Soups: Recipes & Reveries.* Berkeley, California: Ten Speed Press, 2005.

Bensky, Dan and Andrew Gamble. *Materia Medica.* Revised edition. Seattle, Washington: Eastland Press, 1993.

Bensky, Dan and Randall Barolet. *Formulas & Strategies.* Seattle, Washington: Eastland Press, 1990.

Blonder, Ellen and Annabel Low. *Every Grain of Rice.* New York, New York: Clarkson N. Potter, 1998.

Brown, Simon G. *Modern-Day Macrobiotics.* Berkeley, California: North Atlantic Books, 2005.

Burros, Marian. *Cooking for Comfort.* New York, New York: Simon and Schuster, 2003.

Canfield, Jack, Mark Victor Hansen, Maida Rogerson, Martin Rutte, and Tim Clauss. *Chicken Soup for the Soul at Work.* Deerfield Beach, Florida: Health Communications, Inc., 1996.

Chang, Chung-Ching. *Chin Kuei Yao Lueh: Prescriptions from the Golden Chamber.* Translated into English by Wang Su-yen and Hong-yen Hsu. Oriental Healing Arts Institute of the United States, 1983.

Chang, Dr. Stephen T. *The Great Tao.* San Francisco, California: Tao Publishing, 1985.

Chang, K.C., ed. *Food in Chinese Culture.* New Haven, Connecticut: Yale University Press, 1977.

Chen, Helen. *Helen Chen's Chinese Home Cooking.* New York, New York: William Morrow, 1994.

Chopra, Deepak, MD *Grow Younger, Live Longer.* New York, New York: Three Rivers Press, 2001.

Cohen, Misha Ruth, OMD, L. Ac. with Kalia Doner. *The Chinese Way to Healing: Many Paths to Wholeness.* New York, New York: The Berkley Publishing Group, 1996.

Davidson, Alan, ed. with Helen Saberi. *The Wild Shores of Gastronomy: twenty years of the best food writing from the journal Petits Propos Culinaires.* Berkeley, California: Ten Speed Press, 2002.

Flaws, Bob. *The Book of Jook.* Boulder, Colorado: Blue Poppy Press, 1995.

Flaws, Bob. *The Tao of Healthy Eating.* Boulder, Colorado: Blue Poppy Press, 1998.

Finnegan, John. *The Facts About Fats: A Consumer's Guide to Good Oils.* Berkeley, California: Celestial Arts, 1993.

Gardner, Erle Stanley. *Gypsy Days on the Delta,* New York, New York: William Morrow, 1967.

Gillenkirk, Jeff, and James Motlow. *Bitter Melon.* Seattle, Washington: University of Washington Press, 1986.

Goettemoeller, Jeffrey. *Stevia Sweet Recipes: Sugar-Free Naturally!* Bloomingdale, Illinois: Vital Health Publishing, 1998.

Grossinger, Richard, *Planet Medicine: Origins.* Revised Edition, Berkeley, California: North Atlantic Books, 2005.

Gifford, K. Dun and Sara Baer-Sinnott. *The Oldways Table: Essays and Recipes from the Culinary Think Tank.* Berkeley, California: Ten Speed Press, 2007.

Huang, Parker Po-fei. *Cantonese Dictionary.* New Haven, Connecticut: Yale University Press, 1970.

Hsiung, Deh-Ta. *Chinese Regional Cooking.* New York, New York: Mayflower Books, 1997. Originally Published in U. K. by Macdonald Educational Limited. London. 1979.

Kaptchuk, Ted J., OMD. *The Web That Has No Weaver.* New York, New York: Congdon and Weed, 1983.

Kingston, Maxine Hong. *The Woman Warrior.* New York, New York: Vintage Books, 2000.

Kingston, Maxine Hong. *China Men.* International edition. New York, New York: Vintage Books, 1989.

Kushi, Michio. *The Book of Macro-biotics: The Universal Way of Health, Happiness, and Peace.* Tokyo: Japan Publications, Inc., 1987.

Lai, Him Mark, Joe Huang, and Don Wong. *The Chinese of America 1785–1980.* San Francisco, California: Chinese Cultural Foundation, 1980.

Leung, Doreen. *Kwan Tong Pou (Delicious and Healthy Soup Recipes From Celebrities).* In Chinese. Hong Kong: Hong Kong China Gas Company, Ltd., 1987.

Li, Dong-Yuan. *Li Dong-Yuan's Treatise on the Spleen & Stomach: A Translation of the Pi Wei Lun.* Translated from Chinese by Yang, Shou-Zhong & Li Jian-Yong. Boulder, Colorado: Blue Poppy Press, 1993. Newly translated and annotated by Bob Flaws. Boulder, Colorado: Blue Poppy Press, 2004.

Lin, Yu Tang. *The Importance of Living.* New York, New York: The John Day Company, 1937.

Liu, Jilin, and Gordon Peck, editors. *Chinese Dietary Therapy.* Hong Kong: Churchill Livingstone, 1995.

Minnick, Sylvia Sun. *Samfow: The San Joaquin Chinese Legacy.* Fresno, California: Panorama West Publishing, 1988.

Molony, David. *The American Association of Oriental Medicine's Complete Guide to Chinese Herbal Medicine.* New York, New York: Berkley Books, 1998.

Moskowitz, Reed C., MD *Your Healing Mind.* New York, New York: William Morrow and Company, 1992.

Ni, Maoshing, and Cathy McNease. *The Tao of Nutrition.* Santa Monica, California: SevenStar Communications, 1993.

Ni, Maoshing, *The Yellow Emperor's Classic of Medicine.* A new translation of the *Neijing Suwen* with commentary. Boston, Massachusetts and London: Shambhala, 1995.

Oliver, Mary. *White Pine.* Orlando, Florida: Harcourt, Inc., 1991

Peterson, James. *Splendid Soups.* New York, New York: John Wiley & Sons, 2001

Pitchford, Paul, ed. *Healing with Whole Foods*. Berkeley, California: North Atlantic Books, 1993.

Pfaelzer, Jean. *Driven Out: The Forgotten War Against Chinese Americans*. New York, New York: Random House, 2007.

Pollan, Michael. *The Omnivore's Dilemma: A Natural History of Four Meals*. New York, New York and London: The Penguin Books, 2006.

Pollan, Michael. *In Defense of Food: An Eater's Manifesto*. New York, New York: The Penguin Press, 2008.

Reid, Daniel P. *Chinese Herbal Medicine*. Boston, Massachusetts: Shambhala Press, 1992.

Reid, Daniel P. *Traditional Chinese Medicine*. Boston and London: Shambhala Press, 1996.

Rachel Naomi Remen, MD *Kitchen Table Wisdom*. New York: Riverhead Books, 1996.

Reuben, Carolyn. *Antioxidants: Your Complete Guide*. Rocklin, CA: Prima Publishing, 1995.

Reuben, Carolyn. *Cleansing the Body, Mind and Spirit*. New York: Berkley Books, 1998.

Robbins, John. *Diet for a New America*. Tiburon, California: H. J. Kramer Book in a joint venture with New World Library, 1987.

Salter, Tina with Steve Siegelman. *Nuts: Sweet and Savory Recipes from Diamond of California*. Berkeley, California: Ten Speed Press, 2002.

Schell, Hal. *Cruising California's Delta*. Stockton, California: Schell Books, 1995.

Schlosser, Eric. *Fast Food Nation*. New York, New York: Perennial, 2002. Originally published by Houghton Mifflin, 2001.

Swahn, J. O. *The Lore of Spices*. New York/Avenel: Crescent Books, 1991.

Swanson, Heidi. *Super Natural Cooking*. Berkeley/Toronto: Celestial Arts, 2007

The French Culinary Institute. *Salute to Healthy Cooking: From America's Foremost French Chefs*. Emmaus, Pennsylvania: Rodale Press, 1998.

Tierra, Michael. *Planetary Herbology*. Twin Lakes, Wisconsin: Lotus Press, 1992.

Tierra, Michael. *The Way of Chinese Herbs*. New York/London/Toronto: Pocket Books, 1998.

Tsukiyama, Gail. *Women of the Silk*. New York, New York: St. Martin's Press, 1991.

Tsukiyama, Gail. *The Language of Threads*. New York, New York: St. Martin's Griffin, 2000.

Waghorn, Annita. *Historic Archaeological Investigations of the City Center Cinemas Block Bounded by Miner Avenue and Hunter, El Dorado, and Channel Streets, Stockton, California*, A report prepared for The Redevelopment Agency of the City of Stockton. Rohnert Park, California: Anthropological Studies Center, Sonoma State University, 2004.

Wang, Li-Min. *Si-Ji Yang-Sheng-Zhou. (Nurturing Rice Soups for the Four Seasons)* In Chinese. Taipei: Lian He Wen Xue, 2000.

Weil, Andrew, MD. *Eating Well for Optimum Health: The Essential Guide to Bringing Health and Pleasure Back to Eating*. New York, New York: Alfred A. Knopf, 2000.

Weil, Andrew, MD. *Spontaneous Healing*. New York, New York: Fawcett Columbine, 1995

Weil, Andrew, MD. *8 Weeks to Optimum Health*. New York, New York: Alfred A. Knopf, 1997

Weil, Andrew, MD. and Rosie Daley. *The Healthy Kitchen*. New York: Alfred A. Knopf, 2003.

Yan, Martin. *Chinese Cooking for Dummies*. New York, New York: Wiley Publishing, Inc., 2000.

Yan, Martin. *Martin Yan's Chinatown Cooking: 200 Traditional Recipes from 11 Chinatowns around the World*. New York, New York: William Morrow, 2002.

Yan, Martin. *Martin Yan's China*. San Francisco, California: Chronicle Books, 2008.

Young, Grace. *The Wisdom of the Chinese Kitchen: Classic Family Recipes for Celebration and Healing*. New York, New York: Simon and Schuster, 1999

Young, Grace and Alan Richardson. *The Breath of a Wok: Unlocking the Spirit of Chinese Wok Cooking through Recipes and Lore*. New York, New York: Simon and Schuster, 2004.

Yung, Judy, Gordon H. Chang, and Him Mark Lai. *Chinese American Voices from the Gold Rush to the Present*. Berkeley, California: University of California Press, 2006.

Xie, Zhufan and Jiazhen Liao. *Traditional Chinese Internal Medicine*. Beijing: Foreign Language Press, 1993.

Zhao, Zhuo and George Ellis. *The Healing Cuisine of China*. Rochester, Vermont: Healing Arts Press, 1998.

Appendix A:
Pronunciation Guide for
Mandarin and Cantonese

The most convenient way to describe a Chinese syllable is by its initial, final, and tone. An initial may be a consonant or a semi-vowel. A final may be a simple vowel or a diphthong, with or without a nasal or stop ending, and in the case of Mandarin Chinese, a retroflex vowel.

Mandarin

Pinyin has symbols for 20 initials, 2 semi-vowels, 6 vowels, 1 retroflex vowel, 9 diphthongs, 4 triphthongs, 16 nasal finals, and 4 tones.

Initials

b (*bā* "father") as in s<u>p</u>a
p (*pù* "shop") as in <u>p</u>ull
m (*mǐ* "rice") as in <u>m</u>e
f (*fū* "husband") as in <u>f</u>ood
d (*dì* "younger brother") as in s<u>t</u>eed
t (*tā* "he/she/it") as in <u>t</u>ar
l (*lā* "pull") as in <u>l</u>ast
n (*nǐ* "you") as in <u>n</u>iece
g (*gē* "song") as in s<u>k</u>i
k (*kū* "cry") as in <u>c</u>ool
h (*hú* "lake") as in <u>h</u>ouse
zh (*zhī* "know")
ch (*chī* "eat") as in ar<u>ch</u>er
sh (*shí* "ten") as in wa<u>sh</u>er
z (*zǐ* "seed")
c (*cì* "thorn") as in zi<u>ts</u>
s (*sī* "silk") as in <u>s</u>ilk
j (*jī* "chicken") as in <u>J</u>ill
q (*qī* "seven") as in <u>ch</u>eat
x (*xì* "drama") as in o<u>c</u>ean or con<u>sci</u>ence

Semi-Vowels

y (*yi* "one") as in <u>y</u>am
w (*wǔ* "five") as in <u>w</u>ater

Vowels

i (*yī* "one") as in t<u>ea</u>
  (*si* "silk") as in s<u>i</u>n
u (*gǔ* "bone") as in f<u>oo</u>d
ü (*lü* "green") as in sh<u>e</u>
a (*mǎ* "horse") as in <u>a</u>rt
o (*pò* "broken") as in f<u>a</u>ll or f<u>ou</u>r
e (*gē* "song") as in bigg<u>e</u>r

Retroflex Vowel

er (*ér* "son") as in h<u>er</u>

Diphthongs and Triphthongs

ia (*jiā* "home") as in <u>ya</u>
ie (*xiě* "write") as in <u>ye</u>s
ua (*huā* "flower") as in g<u>ua</u>va
uo (*guǒ* "fruit") as in <u>wa</u>ter
üe (*yùe* "moon")
ai (*mǎi* "buy") as in b<u>uy</u>
ei (*gěi* "give") as in s<u>ay</u>
ao (*gāo* "tall") as in h<u>ow</u>
ou (*gǒu* "dog") as in <u>low</u> or g<u>oa</u>t
iao (*xiào* "laugh")
iou/iu (*lìu* "six") as in ch<u>ew</u> or <u>you</u>
uai (*kuài* "fast") as in w<u>ide</u>
uei/ui (*gùi* "expensive") as in <u>weigh</u>

Nasal Finals

There are 16 compound sounds that are spelled with nasal consonants after vowels.

an (*mǎn* "full") as in tw<u>ine</u>
en (*gēn* "root") as in h<u>unt</u>
ang (*fāng* "square")
eng (*péng* "friend") as in st<u>ung</u>
ong (*dōng* "east") as in <u>only</u>
ian (*qián* "front")
in (*jìn* "near") as in g<u>in</u>

iang (*liàng* "bright") as in y<u>oung</u>

ing (*bīng* "ice") as in s<u>ing</u>

iong (*xióng* "bear")

uan (*duăn* "short") as in <u>wan</u>d

uen/un (*dùn* "slow-cook") as in t<u>une</u> or <u>wound</u>

uang (*guāng* "light")

ueng/weng (*fēng* "bee")

ü*an/yuan* (*yuăn* "far")

ü*n/yun* (*yún* "cloud")

The four tones are marked by pitch graphs:

1. level: ā (*mā* "mother")
2. rising: á (*má* "hemp")
3. dipping: ă (*mă* "horse")
4. falling: à (*mà* "scold")

Cantonese

Cantonese has 17 initials, 2 semi-vowels, 6 vowels, 10 diphthongs, 17 nasal finals, and 17 corresponding stop finals. Cantonese has 8 (or 9) tones, divided into the yin (higher pitch) and yang (lower pitch) sets. The yang set is signified by the symbol *h* after the vowel.

Notations inside square brackets [ ] are International Phonetic Alphabet (IPA) symbols, slightly modified according to the Yale dictionary.

Initials

The 17 consonantal initials are:

b [p] (*bīn* "edge") as in s<u>p</u>in

p [p'] (*pa* "fear") as in <u>p</u>ick

m [m] (*mò* "slow") as in <u>m</u>ore

f [f] (*fo* "lesson") as in <u>f</u>ast

d [t] (*dìn* "crazy") as in s<u>t</u>unt

t [t'] (*tìn* "sky") as in <u>t</u>oad

n [n] (*nìhn* "year") as in <u>n</u>eat

l [l] (*léi* "pear") as in <u>l</u>oose

s [ɕ] (*sàan* "mountain") as in <u>s</u>and

ch [tɕ'] (*chìn* "thousand") as in <u>ch</u>in

j [tɕ] (*jíe* "older sister") as in <u>j</u>am

g [k] (*gàm* "gold") as in s<u>k</u>in

k [k'] (*kàhn* "diligent") as in <u>k</u>ick
gw [kw] (*gwok* "nation") as in s<u>qu</u>ab
kw [k'w] (*kwàih* "palm tree") as in <u>qu</u>ick
ng [ŋ] (*ngóh* "I") as in si<u>ng</u>er
h [h] (*hóu* "good") as in <u>h</u>ot

Semi-Vowels

y [y] (*yeh* "night") as in <u>y</u>es
w [w] (*wàhn* "cloud") as in <u>w</u>and

Syllabic m and ng

Cantonese uses two nasal sounds as syllables and as words:

m [m] (*m̀h* "not") as in English <u>mmm</u>, an expression for approval
ng [ŋ] (*ńgh* "five") as in English si<u>ng</u>

Finals

There are 6 vowels, 10 diphthongs, 17 nasal finals, and 17 corresponding stop endings in Cantonese. Here are some pronunciation guides:

Vowels

aa/a [aː] (*gàa* or *gà* "home") as in gar<u>a</u>ge
e [ɛː] (*jē* "umbrella") as in s<u>e</u>veral
eu [oeː] (*hèu* "boots") as in h<u>er</u>
i [iː] (*si* "silk") as in s<u>ee</u>
o [ɔː] (*sō* "a comb") as in s<u>ou</u>rce
u [uː] (*gū* "auntie") as in g<u>oo</u>d

Diphthongs

aai [aːi] (*gāai* "street") as in h<u>i</u>gh
aau [aːu] (*bāau* "bun") as in h<u>ow</u>
ai [ai] (*gāi* "chicken") as in k<u>i</u>te
au [au] (*lāu* "coat") as in s<u>ou</u>th
ei [ei] (*géi* "how many") as in h<u>ay</u>
eui [ψü] (*heui* "go")
iu [iːu] (*síu* "few, not many") as in f<u>ew</u>
oi [ɔːi] (*hòi* "open") as in t<u>oy</u>
ou [ou] (*gòu* "tall") as in g<u>o</u>
ui [uːi] (*bui* "back") as in bet<u>wee</u>n

Nasal Finals

aam [aːm] (*sàam* "three") as in al<u>arm</u>
aan [aːn] (*chāan* "meal") as in bl<u>ind</u>
aang [aːŋ] (*chāang* "pot")
am [am] (*gām* "gold") as in <u>gum</u>
an [an] (*jàn* "true") as in <u>gun</u>
ang [a ŋ] (*gāng* "bisque") as in s<u>ung</u>
eng [ɛːŋ] (*sèng* "fishy smell") as in s<u>ang</u>
eun [en] (*chèun* "spring")
eung [oeːŋ] (*hèung* "fragrant")
im [iːm] (*yìhm* "salt") as in s<u>eem</u>
in [iːn] (*chìn* "thousand") as in s<u>een</u>
ing [eːŋ] (*sing* "holy") as in s<u>ing</u>
on [ɔːn] (*gòn* "dry") as in bey<u>ond</u>
ong [ɔːŋ] (*góng* "harbor") as in g<u>ong</u>
un [uːn] (*bun* "half") as in lag<u>oon</u>
ung [oŋ] (*dùng* "winter")
yün/yun [yüːn] (*syùn* "sour")

Stop Finals

The final p, t, k sounds in Cantonese are unreleased or arrested stops:

aap [aːp] (*ngaap* "duck") as in h<u>arp</u> (without the <u>r</u>)
aat [aːt] (*maat* "wipe") as in sm<u>art</u> (without the <u>r</u>)
aak [aːk] (*gaak* "separate") as in b<u>ark</u> (without the <u>r</u>)
ap [aːp] (*gap* "pigeon") as in s<u>upp</u>er
at [aːt] (*gwāt* "bone") as in b<u>utt</u>er
ak [aːk] (*bāk* "north") as in b<u>uck</u>
ek [ɛːk] (*sehk* "stone") as in s<u>ack</u>
eut [ɥt] (*chēut* "go out")
euk [oeːk] (*geuk* "feet")
ip [iːp] (*dihp* "plate") as in d<u>eep</u>
it [iːt] (*dit* "fall") as in str<u>eet</u>
ik [ɪk] (*yihk* "wing") as in s<u>ick</u>
ot [ɔːt] (*hot* "thirsty") as in h<u>ot</u>
ok [ɔːk] (*gok* "horn") as in h<u>ock</u>
ut [uːt] (*fut* "wide") as in f<u>oot</u>
uk [ok] (*luhk* "six") as in l<u>ook</u>
yüt/yut [yüːt] (*syut* "snow")

The tones are marked according to their pitch contours:

1. high-level: ā (*gām* "gold")
2. high-rising: á (*gám* "brocade")
3. mid-level: a (*gam* "forbid")
   (unmarked)
4. extra-high falling: à (*gàt* "tangerine")
   (with stop final)
5. high-falling: à (*sàn* "new")
6. low-falling: àh (*sàhn* "spirit")
7. mid-rising: áh (*sáhn* "crazy")
8. low-level: ah (*sahn* "careful")
   (unmarked)

APPENDIX B:
Contributors to the Cookbook

Interviewers

Diane Barth

Diane Barth first interviewed the elderly at Jene Wah Senior Citizens Center as a reporter for the local newspaper. Diane worked as a newspaper reporter in Sacramento, covering politics, and in Stockton, covering urban affairs and immigration issues. She studied at the University of California, Berkeley, where she received her BA in Journalism. She has put in countless hours in her own kitchen, where her simmering soups are stock for her husband and thirteen-year-old son.

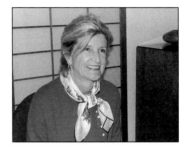

Diane Barth

Elizabeth (Beth) D. Luna

Beth turned ninety when this cookbook project started in 2003 and she is still going strong. Beth has been active with the Sierra Club and the Peace and Justice Network, writing for *Connections,* selling ads, and distributing the newspaper.

Beth has two children, eight grandchildren, seventeen great-grandchildren, and one great-great-grandchild. Beth attributes her alertness of mind and agility of body to the gift of good genes from her parents and to a simple way of life that includes a sensible vegetarian diet, rest, and exercise. She averages seven hours of sleep per night and a rest break after lunch.

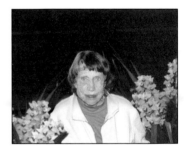

Beth Luna

Eileen Phillips

Eileen Phillips, a graduate of the University of the Pacific, was raised in California and Pennsylvania. She recently retired after a thirty-five-year career with the San Joaquin County Human Service Agency, where, in her capacity as a Program Analyst with the Department of Aging, she worked with Jene Wah, Inc. for more than a decade and came to know the Chinese seniors very well. Upon her retirement in February of 2007, Eileen joined Jene Wah's board of directors.

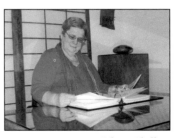

Eileen Phillips

It was Eileen who suggested that profiles of the senior chefs be included in this cookbook. She was also the first to volunteer to do interviews.

Photographers

Fritz Chin

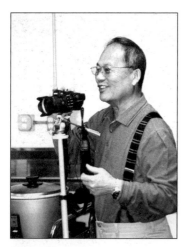

Fritz Chin

Fritz Chin and his wife Lisa started Fritz Chin Photography in 1973 on the Miracle Mile of Stockton. Together they have built a thriving business and a legacy. Their success is evidenced by the fact that family portraits by Fritz Chin are proudly displayed in people's homes while all high school graduates treasure their senior pictures taken by Fritz Chin. Weddings and special events fill their appointment book.

Fritz and Lisa finally found time to travel when their son Arnold took over the family business in 2003. Fritz also joined the board of directors of Jene Wah, Inc. at that time.

Calixtro Romias

Calixtro Romias

Calixtro Romias has been a professional photographer for more than thirty years, working for *The Stockton Record* newspaper. He has been published in *USA Today, Washington Post, Esquire* magazine, *Asian Weekly,* and other newspapers.

Calixtro resides in Stockton with his wife Donna S. Yee, who is a graphic artist by trade and an excellent photographer. They met while attending San Joaquin Delta College photography classes; they have been married for nearly thirty years. Calixtro's current long-term project is examining the issues of homelessness among veterans.

Calixtro became involved with this cookbook project because of close ties to the Asian culture and his love of food and travel. He and Donna have traveled numerous times to China to explore the country, food, and culture. His hobbies include running to keep fit, tai chi to relax, and traveling for adventure.

Photo Credits

Ben Clark (page 72, Sea Turtle, Hawaii)

Kathy Crump (page 17, Blue Heron)

Barbara Flaherty (page 16, Scene of San Joaquin Delta)

Janet Fong (page 72, Sea Turtle, Panama)

Julie Low (page 48, Bronze Hot Pot)

Robert Hong (page 255, Vegetarian Hot Pot)

Charles Hwang (page 19, Mausoleum and Memorial of 72 Martyrs)

Mary Wei (page 48, Tibetan Hot Pot)

Tony Wong (page 55, Pantry)

Yi-Po Anthony Wu (page 24, Jene Wah's Ribbon Cutting Ceremony)

Profiles of Soup Contributors

Lai King Chan

Lai King Chan and her husband tried for years to have a child. They were frequently separated due to immigration law and his decision, during World War II, to join the United States Army. After the war, he returned to China for a time and they had a baby girl who died at only eight months. Devastated, he was nonetheless forced to return to the U.S. to find work. When the amnesty law took effect, she followed. She was forty-three, her child-bearing years past, and her nest empty. Her husband broached the subject one day: "I want a son," he said.

The Chans adopted a five-year-old from an agency in Hong Kong. At first the child didn't behave, but he grew into a loving child who wanted to emulate his father. When he finished high school, he joined the army and took active part in the first Persian Gulf War. Now a police officer, he remains a devoted son and frequently picks his mother up from Jene Wah for lunch at the Chinese restaurant across the street from the police station and for dim sum on the weekends.

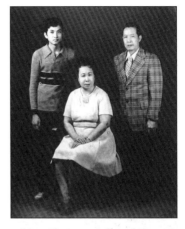

Mrs. Chan, seated, with her son and husband

Wai Ying Lee Tam

Wai Ying Lee was born in a small farm village set among lychee orchards and tiers of rice paddies that flooded with water from the mountains. As a child, she climbed fruit trees, swam in ponds, and cultivated silkworms. She learned to pound fishcake from fresh carp she had caught herself only hours before, gathered black mushrooms in the woods, and minced chicken or pork for homemade sausage.

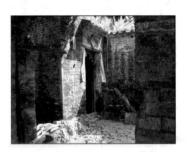

Lai King Chan's Old Village in Xinhui

When she and her sisters were kept from attending school, even though their brothers got to attend, she began sneaking out to attend evening classes. "My mother knew, but she couldn't stop me," she says. "At least I can write my own letters."

But this agrarian life changed with the turbulent times that beset China in her teens. Her father died, and even though they were not landowners, the Communists began to harass her mother. The family fled to Hong Kong, where an uncle introduced her to her husband, who ran a large hotel in the city. Eventually her children moved to the U.S., obtained residency, and sponsored their parents.

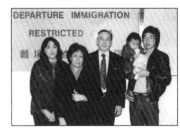

Mrs. Tam at Hong Kong Airport, departing for U.S.

Wai Ying and her husband now share a one-bedroom apartment in downtown Stockton. She regularly sees her children and grandchildren, all

Americanized by now. "There was no future for our children there," she explains. "We had to let them come to America, and then we followed."

Wai Kuen Szeto

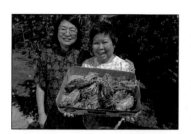

Wai Kuen Szeto showing off her homemade dried cabbage to Teresa Chen

Like many Chinese peasants, Wai Kuen Szeto's family did not own very much land. Their humble plot of less than an acre was considered acceptable, and she did not find the conversion to communal life under Communist rule at all painful. "I don't mind working, I'm good at that," she says.

In fact, Szeto was considered a model comrade. She was judged a Class One worker for producing the biggest turnips in the brigade and also served as one of the chefs for the commune, preparing meals for more than 400 people when rations were imposed during a famine. Her husband was a cow herder before liberation and a cow herder after liberation; he died a cow herder.

Today, her lush backyard garden reveals some of her skills and a continued capacity for hard work. Long bean vines weave along the lattice of a vertical trellis, casting mottled shadows on the bok choy and chard below. On a raised bed of heavy planks, yellow squash blossoms bump against a carpet of green leaves; hidden underneath are baby winter melons that will eventually weigh more than 30 pounds.

But while she still does the gardening, these days it's her daughter and daughter-in-law who make the soup. In old China, it was considered great fortune to have four generations under one roof. A visit to Wai Kuen Szeto's home in Stockton, full of bustling great-grandchildren, reveals that this now rare tradition is still intact.

Shu Shing Tan

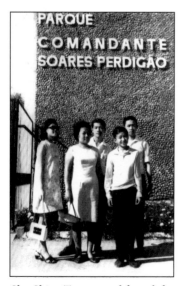

Shu Shing Tan, second from left, with her children in Brazil

At the age of twenty, Shu Shing Tan moved from Toishan to Mozambique. "I was different from other Toishan village girls because my parents sent me to Hong Kong for a high school education," she says. "I was considered more adventurous."

Her new husband owned a cocktail bar and an auto repair shop, and she was a valuable business partner, expanding their ventures with a collection of rental properties. Together, they would have one daughter and three sons. When Mozambique's Marxist-Leninist rebels declared independence from Portugal in 1976, Shu Shing Tan's family property was confiscated and their bank accounts were frozen. Luckily, she was a Portuguese citizen and had some relatives in Brazil. The couple moved again—to yet another country where they knew neither the language nor the customs. Beginning anew in Sao Paolo, they opened a deli.

Eventually their daughter left for Vancouver to study, married a Chinese American, and petitioned for her mother to immigrate to the United States. By then, Shu Shing Tan's husband had passed away, and her sons were scattered across the world. She herself had lived on three continents. She added a fourth by moving to San Francisco in 1983 and kept busy by shuttling between the West Coast and the East Coast to visit her grandchildren. When her youngest son moved to Stockton, she finally decided to settle down—but not slow down. With her new free time, she plans to learn a classical Chinese instrument.

Yuk Hung Hong

It wasn't until immigration law was relaxed to allow children to sponsor their parents that Yuk Hung Hong came to the United States. Her husband had been living in San Francisco and had sponsored both sons but not her. He had been reluctant after his sons were exhaustingly interrogated upon their arrival—Bob for months on Angel Island and Bevin in an Oakland County Jail.

To make good with his wife, Yuk Hung Hong's husband retired and moved out of his room in the Hong Residential Hall in San Francisco. They moved to Stockton, into the home of their son Bevin.

Initially, Mr. Hong was awkward in his newfound role as husband, father, father-in-law and grandfather. But Yuk Hung Hong took naturally to family life, adapting to her role as the wife of a man who took off thirty years ago and never returned to China.

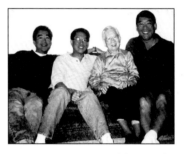

Mrs. Hong, second from right, with her grandsons

Outgoing and spunky, Yuk Hung Hong went to work when she decided she needed extra money to spoil her grandchildren. She also learned how to build up her social security benefits. With smart money-management skills, she was able to buy the expensive ingredients she needed for her favorite soups.

When she passed away in 2005, her grandchildren reminisced about her cooking. Bevin Jr. drew a laugh at the memorial service with this recollection: "Grandma had a soup for everything," he said. "A soup to fatten you up, a soup to help you lose weight, and a soup to get rid of zits."

Yuen Chin Lee

Yuen Chin was fifteen years old when she married a widower twenty-six years her senior. Her husband, Mr. Lee, was a potato farmer in the San Joaquin Valley. He traveled back and forth to China, and Yuen Chin had two children: a girl and a boy.

In 1950, her husband told her to go to Hong Kong to await immigration. She brought her son but had to leave her daughter behind because her husband

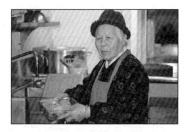

Yuen Chin Lee in Jene Wah's kitchen

did not bother to put the girl on the application. After twelve years of waiting, she and her son were finally allowed to come to the U.S.

Shortly after their arrival, Mr. Lee, then seventy years old, was hit by a car. As he could no longer farm, Yuen Chin found a job at the Tri-Valley Cannery, where she worked for the next twenty-five years, supporting her family. She now lives with her son, Robert, a graduate of the University of the Pacific. Before going to work he drops her off at Jene Wah, where every morning she makes the coffee for everybody. To this day, Yuen Chin's only regret is that she has never had the opportunity to see her daughter, still living in China and now with five children of her own, again.

Lin Chan

Lin Chan was born in Shuntak, a county known for its culinary innovations. On the eve of Japanese occupation, Lin and her husband went to work for his elder brother in his restaurant in Hong Kong. Later, they opened their own restaurant, which she kept going even after her husband died from liver cirrhosis due to excessive drinking. However, Hong Kong was growing rapidly—its population tripled in ten years—and her restaurant was razed by the urban development commission to build high-rise apartment buildings.

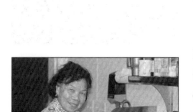

Lin Chan in Jene Wah's kitchen

A widow with four children to support, she went to work in a store that specialized in expensive dried seafood and valuable medicinal herbs, handling rare delicacies like shark's fin, eucommia bark, and sea cucumbers that others might only enjoy once or twice in a lifetime. She became an accomplished chef, learning to work deftly with sophisticated ingredients that require special handling.

Under the impression that her daughter would enjoy a better life in the United States, Lin married her off to a man in Golden Mountain, but was heartbroken when she discovered how hard life could be for immigrants in the United States. A devoted mother, Lin moved here to help her daughter with babysitting—and the preparation of nutritious gourmet meals.

Yin Kan Lau

The daughter of an elementary school principal in a bustling seaside port, Yin Kan Lau attended school from an early age. She married into a comparatively wealthy family—her husband's father was a butcher in the United States who regularly sent money home to his only son.

Yin Kau Lau and her husband had four children, three born in Toishan and a fourth born in Hong Kong, the city she grew to love after moving there in

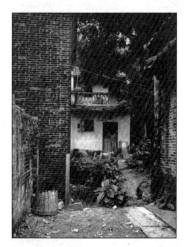

Mrs. Lau's old family home in Taishan, China

1950. "My village was overrun by bandits…. Everyone was leaving and there was such turmoil in the country," she says.

The couple lived in Hong Kong for fourteen years. When their immigration papers arrived, Yin Kan Lau's family moved to Stockton, where her father-in-law owned a grocery store in the heart of Chinatown. He bought the family a two-story house and Yin Kan Lau's husband went into the grocery business himself. Her younger children finished middle school and high school in Stockton, and her eldest son, Francis, who had already finished high school in Hong Kong, went to San Joaquin Delta College. He would later become a civil engineer and two-term president of Jene Wah's Board of Directors.

Still, despite her family's success in the United States, Yin Kan Lau misses chatting with her old friends in teahouses for hours on end. "After moving to Hong Kong, I never missed China very much," she says. "But here, I miss Hong Kong."

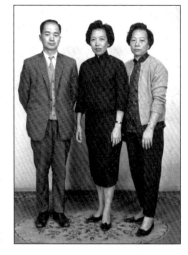

Mrs. Lau (right) with her sister and brother-in-law in Hong Kong

Sun Ma

When Sun Yuet was born, there were already two girls in the family. Her father, a U.S. citizen who commuted between San Francisco and Toishan, registered her as a son and gave her a boy's name, intending to sell her papers, which could fetch as much as $2,000, a hefty sum in the 1930s.

Despite the Communist takeover, Sun's father-in-law was classified as a Canadian laborer, not a capitalist, and her mother-in-law deposited all their money in the cooperative and voluntarily turned in her husband's handgun. Later, they would have no trouble leaving China.

While Sun was living in Hong Kong, her brother and nephew petitioned for her status to be changed from male to female on her records. With the problem rectified, she and her husband immigrated to the U.S. in 1972 and went straight to work, never stopping until retirement thirty years later.

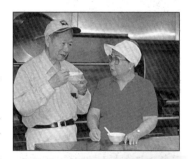

Mr. and Mrs. Ma after test cooking a soup

Sun Kwong

Sun Kwong was born in 1930 in Toishan, China to a farming family with six children. When she was about eleven, the Japanese Army came into her village. Sun remembers hiding under the bed with her sisters and disguising their faces so the soldiers would not find them attractive.

At the age of seventeen, Sun Kwong entered into an arranged marriage. The wedding and marriage were both very happy as both Sun and her husband "fell in love at first sight." They had four children.

Sun Kwong's husband was a successful businessman in Canton who left for Hong Kong to avoid the Communists, leaving Sun and the children behind.

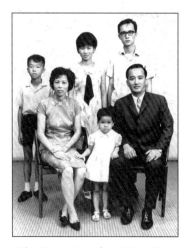

The Kwong Family in Hong Kong

She was not allowed to join him so she made up a story, claiming that he was taking a second wife and she had to go to Hong Kong to stop him. She swayed the authorities, and the reunited family operated their own clothing factory in Hong Kong. One of their daughters eventually immigrated to the United States, and sponsored her mother in 1976. After retirement, Sun's husband followed in 1982. Today, Sun Kwong is an American citizen.

Kim and Henry Yip

In 1951, Henry Yip was twenty-four, out of a job, and had two young daughters to feed. He made up his mind to go to the United States, where his cousin owned a restaurant. At the time, U.S. law only permitted 100 Chinese immigrants per year. Henry's father lived in Stockton, but didn't have citizenship. To circumvent the law, Henry's father contacted a man who had concocted a list of "sons" and was offering their papers for sale. Mr. Yip purchased a paper for Henry, who was then able to come the U.S. under an assumed name.

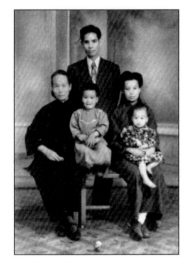

Henry Yip, standing, and Kim Yip, right, before his immigration to the United States

In the 1960s, in an attempt to stamp out the practice of fraudulent documentation, the U.S. State Department promised amnesty to those who confessed and surrendered their passports. Wanting to do the right thing, Henry went to confess and was promptly stripped of his citizenship and ability to leave the country. Not only could he no longer visit his family, but now there was no chance that he could send for his wife, Kim, or his children.

In the meantime, Kim and the girls had moved to Hong Kong. A resourceful single mother, Kim was reading the newspaper one day and found a list of countries that would allow anyone born in that country to apply for U.S. immigration under their quotas. Kim had been born in Malaysia, but moved to China at the age of five. She wrote to the Malaysian government. "I'm so lucky she is so smart," Henry says. "She did what I could not do."

Kim and her children were finally approved for immigration to the U.S. and boarded a plane for California. The family's reunion at the San Francisco Airport marked the end of a thirteen-year separation. Today, Kim and Henry, who eventually took over the restaurant, own their own home in Stockton and recently celebrated their sixtieth wedding anniversary and Henry's eightieth birthday.

Wai Tak Lau

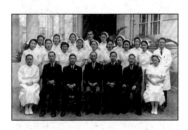

Wai Tak Lau (2nd row, 2nd from left) at nursing school graduation

While growing up, Esther Chan remembered her mother rarely smiling. Wai Tak Lau lived a hard life, beginning with her rejection by her own parents because she was a blue baby—deprived of oxygen during a strenuous labor.

Raised by her aunt and uncle, Esther's mother would eavesdrop on the tutoring sessions provided for her male cousins and eventually became a nurse and a midwife, moving to the countryside after the Japanese invasion to work as a nurse at a school affiliated with the Baptist Church. The school was forced to retreat further and further inland as the Japanese advanced. En route, she met Mr. Yip, a teacher for the boy's school, and they married in 1944. Esther was born prematurely a year later, just before the end of the war.

When the Communists took over after the war, Wai Tak Lau's husband was thrown in a Mongolian prison camp as a counter-revolutionary like many other educated individuals. To escape similar persecution, Wai Tak Lau escaped to Hong Kong with the help of a family friend. A year later, the same friend helped Esther, then only nine years old, escape as well.

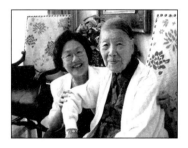

Esther Chan and her mother, Wai Tak Lau

After eight years in jail, Wai Tak Lau's husband was released. Esther remembers going back with her mother for a visit. But her father desperately yearned to reunite with his family on a more permanent basis. He contracted with a smuggler to take him across the border. The smuggler was apprehended, and Wai Tak Lau's husband was sent to a labor camp where he died, never to see his wife or daughter again.

Esther, the much-loved director of Jene Wah, got her first teaching job in 1965, coinciding with her mother's retirement from nursing. After her retirement, Wai Tak Lau, who joined the Chinese Baptist Church in 1958, earnestly took up cooking, perfecting her slow-cooking soup recipes. She moved to Stockton in 1991, and then, at age ninety-six, Wai Tak Lau lost her only daughter, Esther. She surprised and impressed everyone with her strength.

A great-grandson, Isaac Doi, was born in November, 2007. The little fellow is so happy and lovable that he filled Wai Tak Lau's life with many, many smiles.

Robert Hong

When Bob Hong was twelve, his father brought him to the United States. Together they crossed the Pacific Ocean, bound for San Francisco. But when they arrived, only his father was allowed to enter the country. Bob, who could hardly speak any English, was detained and interrogated on Angel Island.

Several months later, Bob was finally allowed ashore. But he was not reunited with his father, then living alone in bachelor quarters in San Francisco. Instead, his father sent him to live with another family from the same clan. The Hongs in Stockton are all from Gujeng Village in Sunwui, cousins tracing back many generations to when their ancestors migrated to the Pearl River Delta. Bob moved to Stockton, eventually graduating from St. Mary's High School.

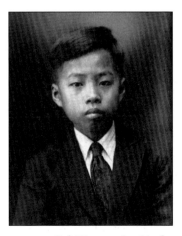

Bob Hong at Age Twelve

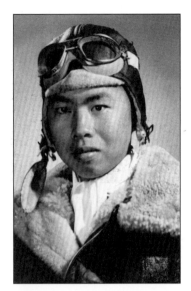

Bob Hong in his Air Force uniform

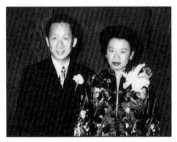

Mr. and Mrs. Yim on their wedding day

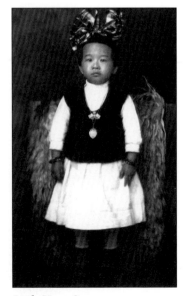

Little Hang Seung

After serving in WWII, Bob went to the University of California at Berkeley on the GI Bill. He met and married Meeyoke, a native of Stockton. When he graduated, they moved to Oakland, where Bob got a job with the Internal Revenue Service. In 1983, Bob took an early retirement from the IRS, and he and Meeyoke moved back to Stockton to be near their elderly parents. Bob also began a busy life of public service.

In the last decade, Bob has been an important member of Stockton civic life. He served on the Planning Commission of the City of Stockton, on the board of directors for United Way of San Joaquin and the Sister City Association, and as two-term president of Jene Wah. In addition, he is an ardent martial arts practitioner. Both Bob and Meeyoke practice Yang-style taichi chuan, shibashi qigong, and liutong chuan. An avid traveler, Bob has also trekked the Himalayas several times.

Thelma Yim

Thelma was born Leung Hang Seung in San Francisco. She attended both Chinese and American schools, but her social life in Chinatown, which was highly segregated according to which region in China your parents came from, was restricted to other youths from Heungshan. In her teens, she joined the Chik Char Music Club to play the butterfly harp and sing Cantonese songs. There she met Vincent Yim, her future husband.

Thelma's mother was widowed at age twenty-nine with five children. All the kids chipped in and helped her. Thelma's brothers were drafted during WWII. It was not until the war was over that Thelma and Vincent met again and started to date. They were married in 1948. By then, Vincent already owned his Temple Bell store in Stockton, an art curio store stocking beautiful things from China that he would run for forty-three years. A natural leader, Vincent was also active in the Chinese community. Because their first child, Thelmvina, needed special care, Thelma was a full-time housewife for many years before she took a job to work in the public library.

Eventually, Vincent developed a prolonged illness, but Thelma never complained. Instead she complimented Vincent for never complaining and looked forward to seeing him every morning in the nursing home. But now that Vincent has passed away, and her son, Johnny, has his own family, Thelma says she does not feel like cooking her special dishes anymore.

Lai Kuen Lee

Lai Kuen Wong married Po Pui Lee in the countryside of Toishan. Shortly after their first son was born, Po Pui Lee went to Toishan City to sell Western cigarettes smuggled into China via Macao, a Portuguese colony. When the border was closed in 1956, he left for Hong Kong to find work. When he saved enough money, he sent for his family. Only their four-year-old daughter was allowed to emigrate with Lai Kuen Lee. The two older boys had to stay behind.

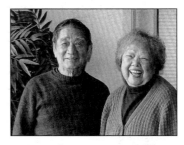

Mr. and Mrs. Lee at Jene Wah

With the money he saved, Mr. Lee bought his own van for transporting construction materials under government contract. But after a riot in 1966, the Hong Kong government stopped issuing new orders. So he took out a new license and became a taxi driver.

It wasn't until 1982 that their second son was allowed to leave China. He settled in Hong Kong. Their daughter Connie married a man from Stockton in 1986 and, after she became a U.S. citizen herself, sponsored her parents and the family of her eldest brother to immigrate to the United States. Half a century later and half a world away, the family is finally together again.

About the Author

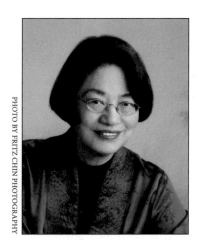

Teresa M. Chen, PhD, and her husband, Yi-Po Anthony Wu, MD, founded Pacific Complementary Medicine Center (PCMC) in Stockton, California, in 1993. Dr. Chen oversees community outreach and health education, organizes seminars, conferences and workshops, leads breathing and Liu Tong exercise classes, lectures to college extension and community groups, and contributes articles about food, nutrition, exercise, and complementary medicine to publications such as *APA (Asian Pacific American) News and Review* and *Connections,* an alternative newspaper published by the Peace and Justice Network. She also edits and writes for PCMC's newsletter and website at www.wuway.com. Their professional ethics can be summed up in the motto *jing ye le qun* 敬業樂群 meaning "Revere your work and endow the community with joy."

Named the Chinese Cultural Society of Stockton's 2007 Citizen of the Year, Dr. Chen has also served on the board of the United Way of San Joaquin and of Jene Wah, Inc., a Chinese multi-service and senior citizen center. She has developed and secured funding from San Joaquin County for an Asian Nutrition Lunch program and an acupuncture-based chemical-dependency treatment program. Raised in Hong Kong, Dr. Chen graduated from Radcliffe College and received her PhD in Linguistics from the University of Hawaii. Before settling in Stockton, she was a researcher at the University of California at Berkeley and taught at San Francisco State University.

Index

~~~